Gynecologic Oncology

Controversies in Cancer Treatment

Harvey A. Gilbert, M.D.

Series Editor

Gynecologic Oncology

Controversies in Cancer Treatment

Edited by
Samuel C. Ballon,
M.D., C.M.

Associate Professor of Gynecology and Obstetrics
Director, Section of Gynecologic Oncology
Stanford University School of Medicine
Stanford, California

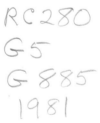

G. K. Hall Medical Publishers
Boston, Massachusetts

G. K. Hall Medical Publishers
70 Lincoln Street
Boston, Massachusetts 02111

81 82 83 84 / 4 3 2 1

Gynecologic oncology.

(Controversies in cancer treatment)

Bibliography.
Includes index.
1. Generative organs, Female–Cancer. I. Ballon,
Samuel C. II. Series. [DNLM: 1. Genital neoplasms,
Female–Therapy. WP 145 G9966]
RC280.G5G885   616.99′465   81-2005
ISBN 0-8161-2156-7   AACR2

CONTRIBUTORS

Michael L. Berman, M.D.
Associate Professor of Obstetrics and Gynecology
Director, Division of Gynecologic Oncology
University of California
Irvine, California

Richard C. Boronow, M.D.
Clinical Professor of Gynecology and Obstetrics
University of Mississippi Medical Center
Jackson, Mississippi

Stephen K. Carter, M.D.
Director, Northern California Cancer Program
Consulting Professor of Medicine
Stanford University School of Medicine
Clinical Professor of Medicine
University of California
San Francisco, California,

Thomas W. Castaldo, M.D.
Assistant Professor of Obstetrics and Gynecology
Division of Gynecologic Oncology
Cornell University Medical College
New York, New York

Donald G. C. Clark, M.D.
Attending Surgeon
Memorial Hospital for Cancer and Allied Disease
Memorial Sloan Kettering Cancer Centers
New York, New York

Carmel J. Cohen, M.D.
Professor of Obstetrics and Gynecology
Director, Division of Gynecologic Oncology
The Mount Sinai School of Medicine of the City University of New York
New York, New York

William T. Creasman, M.D.
Professor of Obstetrics and Gynecology
Director, Division of Gynecologic Oncology
Duke University Medical Center
Durham, North Carolina

Stephen L. Curry, M.D.
Assistant Professor of Obstetrics and Gynecology
Division of Gynecologic Oncology
The Milton S. Hershey Medical Center of the Pennsylvania State University
Hershey, Pennsylvania

Philip J. DiSaia, M.D.
Professor and Chairman
Department of Obstetrics and Gynecology
University of California
Irvine, California

Dorothy C. Donahue, R.N.
Head Nurse
Gynecology Service
Memorial Hospital for Cancer and Allied Diseases
Memorial Sloan-Kettering Cancer Center
New York, New York

Sarah S. Donaldson, M.D.
Associate Professor of Radiology
Division of Radiation Therapy
Stanford University School of Medicine
Stanford, California

Alex Ferenczy, M.D.
Associate Professor of Pathology and Obstetrics and Gynecology
McGill University and the Sir Mortimer B. Davis Jewish General Hospital
Montreal, Canada

Arlan F. Fuller, Jr., M.D.
Assistant Professor of Obstetrics and Gynecology
Division of Gynecologic Oncology
Harvard University School of Medicine
Boston, Massachusetts

Howard D. Homesley, M.D.
Associate Professor of Obstetrics and Gynecology
Director, Division of Gynecologic Oncology
Bowman Gray School of Medicine of Wake Forest University
Winston-Salem, North Carolina

Gary H. Johnson, M.D.
Associate Professor of Obstetrics and Gynecology
Director, Division of Gynecologic Oncology
University of Utah Medical Center
Salt Lake City, Utah

Howard W. Jones III, M.D.
Assistant Professor of Obstetrics and Gynecology
Division of Gynecologic Oncology

Vanderbilt University Medical School
Nashville, Tennessee

Walter B. Jones, M.D.
Associate Attending Surgeon
Memorial Hospital for Cancer and Allied Diseases
Memorial Sloan-Kettering Cancer Center
New York, New York

A. Robert Kagan, M.D.
Chairman, Department of Radiotherapy
Southern California Permanente Medical Group
Los Angeles, California

Garry V. Krepart, M.D.
Associate Professor of Obstetrics and Gynecology
University of Manitoba
Winnipeg, Canada

Emmet J. Lamb, M.D.
Professor of Gynecology and Obstetrics
Stanford University School of Medicine
Stanford, California

John L. Lewis, Jr., M.D.
Chief, Gynecology Service
Memorial Hospital for Cancer and Allied Diseases
Memorial Sloan-Kettering Cancer Center
Professor of Obstetrics and Gynecology
Cornell University Medical College
New York, New York

Alvaro Martinez, M.D.
Assistant Professor of Radiology
Division of Radiation Therapy
Stanford University School of Medicine
Stanford, California

George W. Morley, M.D.
Professor of Obstetrics and Gynecology
Director, Gynecologic Oncology Service
University of Michigan Medical Center
Ann Arbor, Michigan

C. Paul Morrow, M.D.
Professor of Obstetrics and Gynecology
Director, Division of Gynecologic Oncology
University of Southern California School of Medicine
Los Angeles, California

William A. Nahhas, M.D.
Assistant Professor of Obstetrics and Gynecology
Division of Gynecologic Oncology
The Milton S. Hershey Medical Center of the Pennsylvania State
    University
Hershey, Pennsylvania

Staffan R. B. Nordqvist, M.D., Ph.D.
Professor of Obstetrics and Gynecology and Oncology
University of Miami School of Medicine
Miami, Florida

Timothy J. O'Brien, Ph.D.
Assistant Professor of Obstetrics and Gynecology
Director, Gynecologic Oncology Research Laboratory
University of Southern California School of Medicine
Los Angeles, California

June A. O'Hea, R.N., B.S.N., F.N.P.
Assistant Director, Nursing Service
Memorial Hospital for Cancer and Allied Diseases
Memorial Sloan-Kettering Cancer Center
New York, New York

Roland A. Pattillo, M.D.
Professor of Obstetrics and Gynecology
Medical College of Wisconsin
Milwaukee, Wisconsin

Edmund S. Petrilli, M.D.
Assistant Professor of Obstetrics and Gynecology
Division of Gynecologic Oncology
Georgetown University School of Medicine
Washington, D.C.

David R. Popkin, M.D., C.M.
Associate Professor of Obstetrics and Gynecology
Director, Division of Gynecology and Gynecologic Oncology
McGill University
Royal Victoria Hospital
Montreal, Canada

William M. Rich, M.D.
Assistant Professor of Obstetrics and Gynecology
Division of Gynecologic Oncology
University of California
Irvine, California

Eugene C. Sandberg, M.D.
Associate Professor of Gynecology and Obstetrics
Stanford University School of Medicine
Stanford, California

John B. Schlaerth, M.D.
Assistant Professor of Obstetrics and Gynecology
Division of Gynecologic Oncology
University of Southern California School of Medicine
Los Angeles, California

Peter E. Schwartz, M.D.
Assistant Professor of Obstetrics and Gynecology

Yale University School of Medicine
New Haven, Connecticut

W. Gary Smith, M.D.
Assistant Professor of Obstetrics and Gynecology
Division of Gynecologic Oncology
University of Utah Medical Center
Salt Lake City, Utah

Hisham K. Tamimi, M.D.
Assistant Professor of Obstetrics and Gynecology
Division of Gynecologic Oncology
University of Washington School of Medicine
Seattle, Washington

Tate Thigpen, M.D.
Director, Division of Medical Oncology
The University of Mississippi Medical Center
Jackson, Mississippi

John C. Weed, Jr., M.D.
Assistant Professor of Obstetrics and Gynecology
Division of Gynecologic Oncology
Duke University Medical Center
Durham, North Carolina

To David, Marie, and John

CONTENTS

FOREWORD

Dr. Samuel C. Ballon, one of the current leaders in the field of gynecologic oncology, has assembled a talented and knowledgeable group of physicians who possess excellent credentials and expertise for the subjects they are presenting. He has introduced each subject in a succinct format that challenges the physician to continue reading every section and has highlighted those areas in which there is a difference of opinion.

Some of the arguments and counter-arguments in this book may result in disagreements of lengthy duration that will be debated in oncology meetings for a long time to come. This type of stimulation and controversy challenges physicians to think and to contribute to the literature, resulting in better patient care.

It is appropriate that Dr. Ballon selected Dr. John L. Lewis, Jr. as the first author in this book. The establishment of the role of the gynecologic oncologist was a controversial issue in gynecology during the early 1970s. Serving as a division director for the American Board of Obstetrics and Gynecology, Dr. Lewis was able to assemble and structure a committee to establish the Division of Gynecologic Oncology. The early controversies, often vitriolic, have vanished with an appreciation of what has been achieved. This committee, chaired by Dr. Lewis, has established a standard of practice and quality of care in gynecologic oncology that has led to the delivery of the best health care that has ever been achieved for women afflicted with tumors of the reproductive organs.

It is also appropriate that Dr. Richard C. Boronow, one of the founders and the tenth president of the Society of Gynecologic Oncologists, was asked to present another perspective on the role of the gynecologic oncologist. Drs. Lewis and Boronow have placed the field of gynecologic oncology into perspective, providing an understanding of how the contemporary gynecologic oncologist is a unique phenomenon in clinical medicine.

The two perspectives on DES (chapter 4) are unique to this book. Dr. Eugene Sandberg has adapted the scholastic method based on Greek logic, which was concerned with deduction, systematization, and formal logic, to present both sides of the DES controversy. This discussion and Dr. Staffan Nordqvist's perspective are well structured and filled with valuable material.

The most frustrating problem in gynecology—carcinoma of the ovary—is well covered. Five chapters deal with ovarian cancer, and they reflect an increasing frustration on the part of those involved in the management of patients with these diseases, as little impact on survival has been achieved in the past three decades. The authors have mastered the conglomeration of facts currently known about ovarian cancer and present them in a very direct and informative manner.

Limitations of space prohibit discussion of each section here, although each subject deserves special attention. Many of the other contributors to this comprehensive book not only helped structure present-day gynecologic oncology but have also trained many of the gynecologic oncologists who are now leaders in the field.

The authors' keen appreciation and understanding of patient care contribute to this book, which will have particular appeal to the practitioner. It is complete in that it also devotes a section to the specialized training of nurses in the care of gynecologic cancer patients. Although the role of nursing care for the gynecologic oncology patient is vital, only recently have these professionals become organized as a subspecialty of nursing.

A general feature of the book is the excellence of the citations in the literature by the many authors. All contributors have selected the most relevant and up-to-date items with respect to both original work and review articles.

This is a book that can be profitably read by every gynecologist who wishes to keep abreast of current trends in gynecologic malignancies.

Hugh R. K. Barber, M.D.
Professor and Chairman
Department of Obstetrics and
Gynecology
New York Medical College
Director, Department of Obstetrics
and Gynecology
Lenox Hill Hospital
New York, New York

SERIES PREFACE

The impetus for this series came from the intellectually and emotionally difficult experiences my colleagues and I have encountered when attempting to make decisions about the best treatments for patients who have cancer. The patient's and physician's anxiety about the disease and the toxic treatments necessary for its eradication hamper reasoned discussions and charge the atmosphere with hidden messages. The physician's own fears of death and failure to cure enhance the intensity of this interchange. Unfortunately the resultant decision in each patient's case often only partly rests on scientific doctrine. Science deals predominantly with measurable quantities such as survival, but the quality of life as it is perceived in each situation is equally important. Therefore discussion of controversy in cancer is not and should not be only a cataloging of scientific facts but must also contain intuitive and affective measurements of human value.

Each of the books in this series is unique. Some editors chose to explore a vast range of topics, others chose to narrow down the number of issues and explore them in greater depth. Not all sides of each issue are presented, for the editor felt in some cases that only one or two points of view should be elaborated. For some, only one point of view was thought necessary, in which instances the contributor included a discussion of the standard, accepted opinion in addition to setting forth his or her position. The series was conceived of as a whole; as a result some issues are discussed in only one book because of space constraints, but would have been appropriate for other books in the series as well. On the other hand, other controversies are included in more than one book and are addressed by a different group of discussants in each; these controversies were repeated because of their universal appeal and current interest.

The editors for these books were selected because they possessed the following attributes:

a high level of expertise in their fields;

respect of their colleagues as fine clinicians;

continual questioning of the standard dogmas, and spending their professional lives attempting to improve the standard of medical practice; and

they are kind, caring individuals who value the patient-physician relationship.

Controversy is inherent in oncology; I am hopeful that the reader will gain significant insights toward making better decisions in managing patients.

I would like to acknowledge Dolores Groseclose for editorial assistance and Deanne, Jason, and Jill Gilbert for their support.

Harvey A. Gilbert
Series Editor

INTRODUCTION

It is appropriate to consider the significance of this volume within the historical context of gynecologic surgery and the evolution of a group of professionals, within the specialty of gynecology and obstetrics, dedicated to improving techniques of diagnosis and treatment of malignant tumors of the female reproductive system. Early in the modern era of gynecologic surgery, physicians as well as patients developed a defeatist attitude about cancer, which is still being overcome by those seeking to acquire the knowledge and skills necessary for cancer treatment and prevention.

Abdominal hysterectomy as performed by Freund in 1878, Schroeder in 1879, and Wells in 1880 resulted in 75% mortality. In 1893, Schuchardt devised the technique of extended vaginal hysterectomy for cancer of the cervix and reported a 14% five-year survival. Schauta increased survival by this approach to 38.2%, excluding operative deaths. In 1898, Wertheim first performed his radical abdominal hysterectomy. From 1900 to 1910, he published numerous papers dealing with various problems associated with the operative treatment of cancer of the uterus. In 1911, he produced his important monograph based on 500 such operations (Ballon 1976).

The discovery of radium by the Curies also occurred in 1898. In 1906, Wickham and DeGras first applied it to cancer of the uterine cervix. Perhaps the earliest controversy in gynecologic oncology arose at this time, as both gynecologists and radiologists tried to establish and defend the superiority of their techniques. As late as 1954 Meigs declared, "with ultraradical surgery . . . operability (of patients with carcinoma of the cervix) could reach nearly 95%." In 1970, Parsons wrote, "in all too many instances, however, radiation therapy is given by radiologists who are primarily interested in diagnosis and give therapy in an indifferent way simply because they have the equipment and are presented with a certain number of patients to treat. Cobalt units are scattered like television sets all over the country. It is amazing to find that so few radiologists have had any more than a smattering of training to use them properly." Parsons argued that only 275 radiation therapists had the necessary experience with the problems of radiation therapy to acquire board certification in 1970. At that time, however, although a few institutions offered advanced training in radical pelvic surgery, the American Board of Obstetrics and Gynecology had not yet created a Division of Gynecologic Oncology to certify training programs as to their ability to produce individuals skilled in all modalities of gynecologic cancer detection and treatment.

At present, over 20 programs have been approved for the training of advanced clinical fellows in gynecologic oncology, and over 150 individuals have been certified by the American Board of Obstetrics and Gynecology. Five North American societies of gynecologic oncologists now exist, and an international journal serves as an organ of these societies to disseminate the rapidly expanding pool of new information. The gynecologic oncologist and radiation therapist have, for the most part, identified each other as a resource and have made strides toward the development of a team approach to women with reproductive tract tumors. A combination of radiation and operation no longer implies the radical use of each modality in sequence. Rather, it suggests that the therapist and gynecologist, informed by an understanding of the natural history and biologic behavior of the disease in question, tailor their approaches to patients so that treatment results can be improved without a corresponding increase in complications.

In spite of these advances, many disputes remain unsolved. In many medical centers, surgeons continue to defend their areas of responsibility on the basis of a defined set of operative techniques. The orientation of gynecologic oncologists toward the comprehensive care of women with pelvic cancer is disturbing to those who remain more concerned with technique rather than disease. Similarly, some medical oncologists, who may lack expertise in the treatment of solid tumors, continue to view chemotherapy of reproductive tract tumors with skepticism. The role of the gynecologic oncologist as the focal point for women with pelvic cancer or its complications continues to require emphasis. This role has been firmly established, and the precise definition of the breadth and scope of its influence needs further refinement.

As one volume in a series dealing with controversies in cancer medicine, this book covers some of the aspects of gynecologic oncology that continue to be debated both informally and in the scientific literature. This text reflects the progress that has been made in gynecologic oncology by the many individuals who have contributed to this volume and who are dedicated to the care of women with malignant tumors of the reproductive system.

The discussion of a controversial issue should attempt to define its basis as well as to describe the divergent views of the authors. No conscious attempt has been made, therefore, to present diametrically opposed viewpoints; rather, each issue has been approached from a slightly different perspective to define the problem and chronicle the continuing efforts toward its solution. Several chapters have only one contributor, since virtually all investigators recognize the issues in question and await further information for their resolution. For example, the improper design and interpretation of clinical trials require continuing education of the clinical investigator in statistics (Chapter 10). Recognition of this is seen in the requirement by the Division of Gynecologic Oncology that fellows in approved training programs complete a course in statistics.

The benefits and risks of exogenous estrogen administration to postmenopausal women have also been defined (Chapter 8). Interpretation of existing data suggests that both require further examination. With this awareness, appropriate techniques of hormone replacement should be developed for women who have undergone spontaneous or induced menopause.

The concluding chapter of this text deals with the specialized training of nurses in the care of women with reproductive cancers. That this is a topic worthy of discussion is evidenced by the increasing dependence of gynecologic oncologists and radiation therapists on nurses who are skilled in the practice of gynecologic oncology nursing.

The constraints of time and space as well as individual perceptions of various controversial issues have determined the topics covered in this text. Although the answers to many of these controversies will be found, new questions will most certainly arise. Clearly, there are sufficient problems to warrant a companion work.

References

Ballon, S. C. The Wertheim hysterectomy. *Surg. Gynecol. Obstet.* 142:920–924, 1976.

Meigs, J. V. *Surgical treatment of cancer of the cervix.* New York: Grune and Stratton, 1954.

Parsons, L. Damocles and the oncologist. In *Gynecological oncology,* eds. H. R. K. Barber, and E. A. Graber. Baltimore: Williams and Wilkins, 1970.

Chapter 1

*The Role of
the Gynecologic
Oncologist*

PERSPECTIVE:

John L. Lewis, Jr.

Gynecologic oncologists can be defined as clinicians who are trained in obstetrics and gynecology and, in addition, have special training, experience, and skills that qualify them to use all of the effective modalities of therapy in the treatment of patients with gynecologic malignancies; that is, radical pelvic surgery, radiation therapy, and chemotherapy. This area of subspecialization was identified as one of at least three areas within the discipline of obstetrics and gynecology in which the knowledge, skills, and techniques required to give the best clinical care available were beyond the scope of core residency training programs and the regular experience of practicing obstetricians and gynecologists. It is clear that there are still many areas of debate and controversy concerning this recent development and the role such individuals will play in the care of patients with gynecologic malignancies. The purpose of this presentation is to trace briefly the historical developments and the evolutionary process that led to the identification of this area of subspecialization, to outline the current standards for training and certification of such individuals, and to define the roles played by gynecologic oncologists in relation to patient care, teaching, and research in this field. Recognizing that the role such specialists will play is somewhat dependent upon the setting in which they work, variations in the function of a gynecologic oncologist will be discussed according to whether work is carried out in a university hospital, a core residency training program in obstetrics and gynecology, a specialized cancer institute, or in a community setting. Finally, some of the remaining debate concerning these individuals and how they function will be discussed. Obviously, these views are personal and therefore represent the biases I have in relation to the area of subspecialization. Many of these ideas are the result of a long period of cooperation and collaboration with others with whom I worked on the Division of Gynecologic Oncology of the American Board of Obstetrics and Gynecology when it was first established in 1970. I would not like to have them feel responsible, however, if some of these ideas are individual to me and not ones with which they would agree.

The underlying concept of the development of gynecologic oncology as an area of specialization is that one individual should have skills not only in radical pelvic surgery but experience and knowledge in the other areas of effective treatment of gynecologic malignancies. Such an individual is the ideal person to work in multimodality trials in which more than one form of therapy may be employed. It is not surprising that obstetrics and gynecology was the first area in which such a development was recognized and formalized, since this field of medicine has long been involved in studying and applying more forms of therapy than surgery alone. An example is the effort of gynecologists responsible for the care of women with cervical cancer to carry out tests of radiation sensitivity with trial doses of radiation to determine whether radiation therapy or surgery is the modality to be used definitively. In other words, the emphasis was on determining the best therapy for an individual patient's malignancy without having to take into account whether she first saw a gynecologic surgeon or a radiation therapist. Gynecologists were also early in developing and accepting on an international basis uniform classification and staging schemes. Finally, chemotherapy was adapted to special needs of patients with gynecologic malignancies long before recognition of this field as a subspecialty was considered.

In 1970, the Division of Gynecologic Oncology was established as one of the three areas of subspecialization within obstetrics and gynecology. The others were Fetal and Maternal Medicine and Reproductive Endocrinology. The division was charged with defining the knowledge and skills to be obtained by the gynecologic oncologist during a formalized period of training, outlining the standards of an approved training program, and examining for purposes of certification by the board those people who completed approved training programs and met certain other requirements. It was obvious that there were training programs in existence before 1970 that met the same goals as those later to be approved by the division. There were other programs, however, that because of the institution's lack of emphasis on all effective modalities of therapy or deficiencies in training personnel or clinical experience available to the trainee, did not provide the basic experience needed for subsequent competent functioning as a gynecologic oncologist. Other training programs emphasized only one form of therapy, such as radical pelvic surgery, or one investigative program, such as cervical cytologic screening activities, without any effort to train someone in surgery, radiation therapy, and chemotherapy. Therefore it was not surprising that one of the first means by which one could determine what a training program needed was to define what gynecologic oncologists should be able to do after they were trained. The program outlined below has been accepted in the United

States and may set a pattern for development and acceptance of this area of subspecialization in other parts of the world. At this time, however, it is not recognized or proposed that the program must have any effect outside the United States, although it is hoped that the strength of the ideas on which the program is based will result in such a development.

Training and Certification

In determining the contents of a training program in gynecologic oncology, it was first necessary to define the skills and knowledge one should have at the end of the training period. The process of gaining skills, learning techniques, and increasing one's factual knowledge is a continuing one, so there is no indication here that the process is completed at the end of the two-year training period. At the same time, it was necessary to outline the contents of the training program and the actual experience of the trainees so that they would be able to function independently at the end of the training period. The areas to be defined relate to surgery, radiation therapy, chemotherapy, gynecologic pathology, and all of the general medical and surgical knowledge and skills necessary for one to care for any patient. In relation to surgery, the trainee must be taught to carry out the standard radical surgical procedures as well as those procedures necessary to care for complications brought on either by the growth of the gynecologic malignancy or complications of the therapy, whether due to surgery, radiation, chemotherapy, or combinations of these. Training in radiation therapy must give the trainee information concerning basic principles of radiobiology and radiation therapy as well as practical skills in the planning of combinations of external and local radiation treatment and technical skills in the use of radiation applicators. Particular emphasis is placed on the complications of radiation therapy and the problems in evaluation of pelvic findings in patients following radiation therapy. Trainees are to learn the practical pharmacology of the currently available chemotherapeutic agents as well as experience in their administration and control of toxicity. Training in surgical pathology related to gynecologic malignancies has recently been reemphasized. In fact, interpretation of histologic material is now a portion of the oral examination of the Division of Gynecologic Oncology, which leads to certification as to special competence. Finally, an approved course in biostatistics has been added as one of the requirements for a training program. This emphasizes that the trainee must learn the principles of biostatistics which allow one to determine the significance of results of clinical trials as well as plan these trials appropriately.

To allow one to achieve these goals in a period of only two years, a training program must be carefully planned and meet certain guidelines if such a prodigious feat is to be accomplished. Evidence that it is possible comes from the performance of trainees who have finished such programs and have functioned very well in establishing gynecologic oncology service units in major university and residency programs over the last 10 years. The duration of the program must be a minimum of two years, and there is some evidence that certain trainees could benefit from an even longer program. More importantly, it must be carried out in an institutional setting in which there are not only appropriate physical facilities but personnel and clinical experience available to the trainee. The commitment of an institution to the development of a training program requires that it have not only the personnel necessary to carry out the clinical care for which it is responsible, but also that it has adequate teaching staff. This is true in teaching not only surgical techniques but the other clinical skills as well. In the past it has been required that such a training program be carried out in an institution that also has a clinical training program in radiation therapy, the justification for this being the need for didactic teaching in the principles of radiobiology and techniques of radiation therapy. One of the main needs is not only an adequate number of patients being cared for in the institution but a commitment of the institution to utilize these patients for the training of fellows. One of the most difficult judgments a training program director has to make is how to balance the need for excellent patient care with the need of the fellow to gain experience. For most of us, this consists of a large amount of supervision of trainees throughout most of their fellowship program, although it is obvious that, by the end of the program, they need to have the ability to carry out the procedures independently.

Certification as to special competence in gynecologic oncology by the American Board of Obstetrics and Gynecology has required that individuals meet the following requirements: completion of a core residency in obstetrics and gynecology; completion of an approved fellowship program in gynecologic oncology; passage of parts I and II of the American Board of Obstetrics and Gynecology basic exams; passage of a written examination in gynecologic oncology at the end of fellowship training; two years of practice as a gynecologic oncologist in an appropriate setting in which all effective forms of gynecologic cancer care are available; submission of an 18-month case list documenting this practice; submission of a thesis based on clinical or laboratory research related to gynecologic oncology; and passage of an oral examination that includes evaluation and interpretation of histopathologic slides (*Bulletin of the Division of Gynecologic Oncology* 1979). For those who were trained in gynecologic oncology before the approval of training programs in 1972, or who functioned as gynecologic oncologists on the basis of at least five years of clinical experience without formal training (the so-called grandfathers), certification was available if they met all of the same qualifications with the exception of having completed a two-year approved training program. Although this was a controversial decision at the time the division was established, all who now have the certificate have shared a common body of knowledge.

Role of the Gynecologic Oncologist

It is evident from the preceding discussion that gynecologic oncologists must work in an institutional setting in which all of the effective forms of gynecologic cancer therapy are available. It certainly does not require that they work in a setting that meets the rigid standards of a training program, since there are a limited number of such institutions in the country. We will discuss particular roles in relation to patient care, research, and teaching, but it should be emphasized that there are certain consequences of the kind of care gynecologic oncologists give that separate their work from that of others in the field of obstetrics and gynecology or other medical specialties. One of these is that by becoming involved in all of the therapeutic aspects of a malignancy, the gynecologic oncologist establishes a basic continuity of care that avoids many of the fragmenting aspects of the standard care of patients with malignancy. For example, it is not unusual for a patient to be seen in a family practitioner's office and then be sent to a surgeon for a diagnosis and primary therapy. Additive radiation therapy may be given by a different physician in a different setting, and if these two treatments do not result in a cure, the patient is sent to another physician, a medical oncologist, for subsequent chemotherapy. Many patients have recorded the increasing sense of doom that each subsequent referral gives them. Members of the gynecologic oncology service are involved with patients at all stages of these developments, whether they care for them alone or organize the service in such a way that gynecologists, radiation therapists, and medical oncologists all see the same patients in the same clinical area simultaneously.

Patient Care

In my opinion, a good gynecologic oncology service works closely and continuously with representatives of the other important areas pertaining to gynecologic cancer care. It is important that there be agreement about joint therapy protocols as well as investigative protocols within an institution for each stage of each gynecologic malignancy. These protocols may be those adapted from collaborative clinical trial groups or worked out independently in an institution on the basis of its own faculty's interest and experience. It is important, however, that all adhere to the same protocol so that what happens to the patient is not determined by the type of physician she sees first (that is, gynecologic oncologist, chemotherapist, or radiation therapist), but rather by what is appropriate treatment for her malignancy with consideration given to the staging, grading, and other prognostic factors as well as her own specific health status. It is apparent, then, that it is necessary for the representatives of the various specialties to have respect for each other and to cooperate in achieving this goal. It is here that the knowledge and skill gained in areas other than radical surgery and the willingness to utilize other modes of therapy separate the gynecologic oncologist from the gynecologist trained to operate on cancer patients.

Surgery

The surgery the gynecologic oncologist should be ready to perform includes the standard radical pelvic procedures (radical hysterectomy with node dissection, radical vulvectomy with node dissection, exenterative procedures) and reparative plastic procedures such as creation of a neovagina when indicated. In addition, the gynecologic oncologist must be able to take care of problems that arise involving the gastrointestinal tract and genitourinary system when they are directly involved with gynecologic cancer growth or damaged as a result of treatment, whether it be by surgery or radiation therapy. It is in these latter two areas that gynecologic oncology differs most from the standard gynecologic training programs in the past, for these were felt to be off limits to gynecologists. Achieving this knowledge and skill has resulted in less fragmentation of care of the gynecologic cancer patient. In the past this has been best represented by exenterative procedures in which the gynecologist removed the tumor, the general surgeon isolated the intestinal segment necessary for a conduit and prepared the stoma, and the urologist did the anastomosis between ureters and intestinal segment.

When exercising surgical judgment, there are two areas requiring particular comment. There is no other disease that demands so much in the way of competence and experience from a gynecologic oncologist as ovarian cancer. At the time of initial surgery a maximal effort to remove as much tumor as possible must be made so that subsequent chemotherapy will bring the most benefit to the patient. This involves not only the skillful removal of large amounts of tumor in the pelvis without damaging vital structures but also requires some bowel resection and reestablishment of continuity when such a procedure will make a significant difference in the amount of tumor left. One of the most interesting and demanding operations currently being done in gynecologic cancer cases is the so-called second-look procedure in ovarian cancer patients following effective initial treatment with chemotherapy. This requires not only evaluation of the undersurface of the diaphragm and retroperitoneal spaces but also careful evaluation of all of the peritoneal surfaces and abdominal contents.

Another type of surgery in which the gynecologic oncologist has unusual experience is that of operating in an irradiated field. Although past experience has shown the problems caused by trying to perform radical surgery in conjunction with full radiation therapy, there is no question that there are times when such a procedure represents the only opportunity a patient has to be cured. A candidate must learn the different types of dissection necessary in radiated organs and the problems of healing. No better example of this can be given than trying to determine how extensive biopsies should be to rule out recurrent disease after full radiation for cervical cancer. An aggressive biopsy may provide reassurance that cancer is not there and that the induration is only due to radiation therapy, but if it is followed by fistulization, a whole new set of problems begins.

Gynecologic oncologists must be trained and have skills in the pre- and postoperative care of their patients. It is not appropriate to try to outline all of these details here, but it is obvious that when one takes on the surgical responsibilities outlined above, one's knowledge of surgical principles and one's ability to care for complications must be as extensive as they are for all other surgeons caring for patients.

Radiation Therapy

The gynecologist and radiation therapist have long worked in close cooperation, and it is not surprising that this has remained so today. As a matter of fact, for many years many gynecologists used local radiation as an adjunct to their surgery without being part of a collaborative project with radiation therapists. We now know that the coordination of external therapy and intracavitary applications of radioactive sources is extremely complex. If the patient is to have the benefit of the best possible therapy, there must be good coordination among radiation therapists, radiobiologists or physicists, and gynecologic oncologists. This is also true in planning therapeutic programs that combine surgery and radiation therapy. To have a meaningful role in these cooperative efforts, the gynecologic oncologist must not only be skilled in the use or application of local radiation sources but must also know enough about radiation techniques, equipment, dosimetry, and control of complications so that effective collaboration can be carried out. One area of cooperation between radiation therapists and gynecologic oncologists which has developed quickly over the last few years has been in the use of a pretreatment planning laparotomy to surgically stage the disease to be treated by radiation therapy so that treatment fields can fit the actual extent of disease. Close cooperation between radiation therapists and gynecologic oncologists carrying out the operation is essential, since it has been shown that merely operating in a field to be irradiated can not only decrease the curability of the tumor, but increase the likelihood of a radiation-induced complication.

The involvement of gynecologic oncologists in the details of radiation therapy varies according to knowledge and skills and the cooperative programs worked out with the radiation therapists where they are working. In many institutions gynecologic oncologists have joint appointments in the Department of Obstetrics and Gynecology and in the Department of Radiation Therapy. In our own institution we have found it important for the gynecologic oncologist to see patients undergoing radiation therapy for gynecologic malignancies not only to give the patient the sense of continuity of care, but also because we have important contributions to make in the control of com-

follow-up and a willingness to direct or coordinate the next form of therapy if the initial treatment is not successful. Trying to teach students, residents, and fellows this approach is one of the most difficult tasks of education that we face.

Effect of Institutional Setting

Although trainees in a gynecologic oncology program may have shared similar experiences and have obtained the same skills and knowledge, where they choose to work will have an effect upon their functions. This has long been recognized and was the subject of a panel at the Fifth Annual Meeting of the Society of Gynecologic Oncologists in 1974. Dr. John Mikuta, who was then president of that organization, requested that three of us evaluate the role of gynecologic oncologists as affected by the nature of the institution in which they work: a university hospital with a core residency in obstetrics and gynecology, a cancer institute, and a community hospital (Mikuta 1974). The requirement that gynecologic oncologists work in a setting with all effective forms of therapy available clearly indicates that the place of work must be in some type of institution. Nothing prevents gynecologic oncologists from performing only surgery in an institution that does not have radiation therapy or the support facilities to give aggressive chemotherapy. If they do, however, they will not be functioning as gynecologic oncologists but as well-trained gynecologic surgeons who also happen to have been trained at one time in gynecologic oncology.

University Hospital

The effect of working in a university hospital with a core residency in obstetrics and gynecology was described at the 1974 meeting by Dr. Hervy Averette of the University of Miami. He used the particular experience of his own institution to point out some observations that must certainly be true for all gynecologic oncologists working in a university hospital setting (Averette 1974). There are unique characteristics of individual medical schools, and they must be taken into consideration when defining the role of the Department of Obstetrics and Gynecology or Division of Gynecologic Oncology within it. For example, the portion of the country in which the University of Miami is located has a very high ratio of elderly people and thus people at a high risk of developing cancer. For this reason, cancer is an important area of study and treatment for all departments within the medical school. In addition, University Hospital is owned by the county and therefore responsible for the medical care of many indigents. All university hospitals have independent characteristics that must have an effect on the programs they carry out.

Dr. Averette stated that one of the most significant developments in establishing a strong program in gynecologic oncology began with the establishment of an independent gynecologic oncology service within the Department of Obstetrics and Gynecology. By isolating a geographical unit, it was possible to concentrate efforts relating to gynecologic cancer in order to reduce competition and conflict with other programs within the department or the school. It was felt that rotation of medical students and trainees from the core residency program in obstetrics and gynecology enhanced the training of both categories of students. It was feared that the addition of a fellowship program in gynecologic oncology would raise the risk of conflicts with the core residency program regarding who was to perform certain surgical procedures, but this did not turn out to be a practical problem.

Several factors or potential problems unique to the university hospital setting were mentioned. The first was the support of the Chairman of Obstetrics and Gynecology for the development of gynecologic oncology as a division within the department and the necessity of this continued administrative support to handle some of the inevitable problems. One potential problem was the failure to delegate adequate authority to operate the division with necessary autonomy. It was also necessary that the chairman be willing to help enforce compliance with treatment protocols relating to gynecologic malignancies by all members of the faculty. Finally, the chairman's support would be necessary in jurisdictional disputes that could occur as a result of gynecologic oncologists working in anatomic areas or organ systems other than those in which the core resident in obstetrics and gynecology is trained to work.

A second problem involved convincing the hospital administration, Department of Nursing, and Department of Anesthesia that patients being cared for on a gynecologic oncology service need more intensive nursing and support activities than do patients on a regular gynecology service. Since most gynecologic surgery is elective and carried out in reasonably healthy patients, the needs of the gynecologic oncology patient could not be adequately met if special attention were not given to the problems they face.

Dr. Averette also pointed out the problems of the medical center as a tertiary care facility and the importance of the university in evaluating the general level of care within the community. He gave the interesting examples of a study of gynecologic cancer care in Florida and that of an innovative program developed to take a seminar series to individual hospitals. This was documented as not only improving the level of cancer care in the community but also increasing the likelihood that patients requiring complicated care would be referred to the medical center.

The greatest problem caused by functioning as a gynecologic oncologist in a university-based hospital was that of trying to allocate time successfully among all of the demands placed on such a faculty member. Because of the primary function of a medical center related to education, gynecologic oncologists in this setting are more involved with undergraduate medical school teaching and core residency teaching than are some others. In addition, if there are appropriate personnel, facilities, and patient load, it is likely that they will take on the added educational responsibility of a postresidency fellowship program in gynecologic oncology. Finally, the obligation of the university to lead in continuing medical education is becoming even more apparent. Similarly, the research activities of a unit within a medical school are under more scrutiny than are those in community settings. The difficulties in meeting clinical and teaching obligations while at the same time directing or carrying out basic research are great in any setting but may be more difficult in a university.

Cancer Institute

To describe the effect of working in a categorical institute dedicated to cancer alone, all of the members of the Society of Gynecologic Oncologists who worked in cancer institutes were polled and asked to describe what they did and did not do that was different from what people did in a university setting or community hospital setting (Lewis 1974). Responses indicated the advantages and disadvantages of functioning as a gynecologic oncologist in a cancer institute (defined as a categorical institute), which is goal oriented with a single focus of interest of all the personnel in the institution, be they clinicians, basic scientists, or supporting personnel. The goal of our institution is shared with all other cancer institutes: namely, to make progress in cancer care, education, and clinical and laboratory research. It is this dedication to a single disease process that makes cancer institutes unique. Given the primacy of interest in cancer, there is no need to waste time on matters that are unrelated to cancer. If one makes the assumption that cancer is the primary interest, then this is obviously a benefit. The patient load in a cancer institute represents important opportunities for clinical trials and the development of technical skills. It is not clear that this is a greater advantage in a cancer institute than in a university-based service that has enough patients, but more patients with gynecologic cancer tend to be in a cancer institute.

Another advantage seen by those responding to the questionnaire was that "there is a concentration of proper facilities including modern radiotherapy equipment, blood components, laminar flow rooms, operating rooms, special care units, and supporting laboratory facilities which gives the distinct advantage in treatment and supporting care." It was also thought that working in a cancer institute fostered closer interrelationships and collaboration with other oncology divisions, including basic and clinical sciences, which contributed to a speedy influx of new ideas necessary for the formulation and evaluation of new treatment methods. The setting of a cancer center was also seen as being more conducive to the development of training programs in gynecologic oncology and the ability to attract the best trainees. It was felt that in many institutions this allowed senior staff the freedom from day-to-day management of patients and gave them time to devise studies, carry out research, and teach.

A very important aspect of a cancer institute was that its status and reputation gave individual investigators more latitude in their clinical trials;

that is, they were able to be freer in their evaluation of possible changes in conventional therapy than someone would be in a smaller institution or private practice. Experimental therapy carried out in a cancer institute will have passed not only the review of the service or department in which it is being carried out but also a human subjects committee composed primarily of other people whose principal interest is cancer therapy and including as well the lay and paraprofessional representation required by law. It was suggested that these programs in cancer institutes may have more latitude than others. Finally, the mutual support that patients receive from each other and the feeling that they were in an institution in which everything was dedicated to their best interests gave them a degree of comfort not present in a general hospital or community hospital, where cancer patients might be segregated or treated with a sense of uniqueness or even despair.

Other observations were made by those responding to the letter of inquiry that pointed out the disadvantages of working as a gynecologic oncologist in a cancer institute as opposed to a university hospital or a community hospital. One of these was related to the nature of clinical care in a cancer institute, that is, a physician "never gets away from the cancer problem or cancer patient." This is obviously the reverse of the advantage of being able to concentrate one's time and effort on the cancer problem and involves the individual commitment and emotional needs of the oncologist. I have observed that this sense of commitment to a single group of patients can be determined fairly early in one's career, whereupon the decision may be made either not to select oncology as a specialty or to take a position in an institution in which one's time is not totally dedicated to the treatment of cancer patients.

A major problem was the physical separation from a general hospital or medical school faculty, resulting in the oncologist's working outside the mainstream of the discipline of obstetrics and gynecology as well as the first line of medical practice and education. For this reason, cancer centers have been characterized as academic cul-de-sacs. It is true that this has resulted in little mobility of personnel in cancer centers toward major academic positions elsewhere but it is not clear whether this represents lack of opportunity or the decision of these people to remain fully committed to the oncology effort.

Other disadvantages were seen as follows: objection to the full-time, salaried system of remuneration, rigid adherence to clinical study protocols resulting in loss of individualization of care and its inherent advantages; and a sense of never having completed one's obligations. This latter comment indicated that the problems of the cancer patient are so great and the amount of work to be done is so limitless that there is a sense of urgency from working in such an institution which invades leisure hours. In other words, there is always another paper to write, protocol to complete, or data to be analyzed. It is particularly noted that this places a hardship on the family structure and function. One respondent summarized it as follows: "On balance, I think a cancer institute provides a greater opportunity for most individuals to be functionally more productive in oncology than any other setting, although it does not necessarily assure their individual happiness."

Community Hospital

Evaluating the effect of working in a community hospital on the role of a gynecologic oncologist proved to be more difficult than evaluating any of the other settings in that there are few individuals doing this, and none who is a member of the Society of Gynecologic Oncologists. To obtain information concerning the possible or potential role of the gynecologic oncologist in a community setting, Dr. John Mikuta of the Hospital of the University of Pennsylvania sent a questionnaire to 75 practitioners who referred gynecologic oncology patients to the oncology unit where he works. The purpose of the questionnaire was to determine which patients were referred for care in an oncology unit and what was the potential for the development of a community-based gynecologic oncologist in their community or institution. This study had the obvious bias of eliciting answers from people who already utilized an oncology tertiary care center and therefore probably underestimates the local facilities. At the present time most of the patients referred are those judged likely to benefit from a radical hysterectomy and pelvic lymphadenectomy as treatment of early cancer of the cervix or radical vulvectomy and node dissection as treatment of carcinoma of the vulva. In addition, many patients with cancer of the cervix, vagina, or vulva were referred for secondary therapy. Significantly, patients with endometrial cancer and ovarian cancer were treated locally for both their primary care and secondary care after recurrences were experienced.

Of the 46 respondents to the questionnaire, the average number of gynecologic cancer patients per year per respondent was 60, with a range varying from 20 to 110. It was pointed out that they do have local radiation therapists and medical oncologists but no gynecologic oncologists to organize a team. Most felt that the local facilities were adequate to support a program involving all forms of radical surgery with the exception of exenterative surgery, adequate radiation therapy, and chemotherapy. There was general sentiment that a gynecologic oncologist would be utilized if locally based, since most of the gynecologic cancer patients in the regional area still received their primary therapy in their local community. A program was proposed in which gynecologic oncologists would develop a collaborative team within the community so that they could work with radiation therapists, medical oncologists, general surgeons, and urologists. Ideally, oncologists would be consultants to all gynecologic cancer care patients. For those patients in whom simple measures could be performed by the referring gynecologist, the oncologist would need to act only as a consultant, referring the patient back to the gynecologist for total management. Others would stay for primary surgery by the gynecologic oncologist or collaborative efforts, directed by the oncologist, with the radiation therapist and medical oncologist. The advantages to such a program were outlined. The objection of family and patient to traveling some distance for the latter's care, plus the associated socioeconomic and emotional problems, are overcome. Primary disease processes are more accurately identified, staged, and given appropriate initial therapy. Finally, it ensures the follow-up of all treated patients by maintaining a proper, up-to-date tumor registry. The goals and benefits of such a program are obvious, and only time will determine whether this ideal proposal is followed.

Persisting Controversies

Whenever a subspecialty such as gynecologic oncology develops rapidly, controversies will occur during the inception of the program. This was certainly true for the identification of gynecologic oncology as a subspecialty and the development of training programs and requirements for certification. Many of these controversies were heated at the time of evolution of this program, and many persist today. Fortunately, although they remain serious problems, they now can be discussed more on their merits than in the initial environment of inflammatory debate. I am not of the opinion that a slower development of the program would have avoided these controversies, since I find many of the discussions and arguments just as important and pertinent today, when reviewed coolly and rationally, as when they were presented. The list to follow certainly does not cover all of the important areas of discussion, but it does outline some of the remaining major considerations.

Radical Pelvic Surgery Program versus Gynecologic Oncology

When the question of subspecialization or specialized training in specific areas of the discipline of obstetrics and gynecology was first discussed, there were strong proponents for using the training period as a time to improve the level of general surgical competence of all trainees in obstetrics and gynecology. The identification of gynecologic oncology as an area of subspecialization requiring training not only in radical pelvic surgery but also radiation therapy and chemotherapy has not answered that problem, but it has clearly shown that gynecologic patients require surgical procedures that are not competently carried out by the average trainee in obstetrics and gynecology. The ability of gynecologic oncologists not only to perform radical pelvic surgery competently but to cooperate or collaborate in the complete care of gynecologic cancer patients has justified the approach taken, but it does not relieve these specialists of the obligation of all faculty members within our discipline, that is, to improve the training of all who specialize in obstetrics and gynecology. In many training programs in obstetrics and gynecology, the best teacher in surgical techniques and the principles of pre- and postoperative care is in the Division of Gynecologic Oncology. This commitment to improve training in surgery of the core residents in obstetrics and gynecology is important to those of us working in university-based hospitals with core residency programs and also those who will work in core residency programs that are not university based. It must be remembered that it is not enough for gynecologic oncologists to say that because they have knowledge and skills in chemotherapy and radiation therapy their surgery must not meet the exacting standards of anyone else who does complicated pelvic and abdominal surgery. It is my own opinion that those who wish to commit themselves to a career in gynecologic oncology might well benefit from the standard core residency in obstetrics and gynecology and two years of general surgery before beginning their two-year fellowship in gynecologic oncology. Rutledge (1972) has proposed that there might be advantages to altering the core residency program of those who decided to specialize in gynecologic oncology by requiring more surgical experience during their training. Most have felt, however, that it is important that gynecologic oncologists have shared the basic core training experience so that the choices of where they fit into the academic or practice community will not be limited. As will be noted later, there are only 25 to 30 trainees entering approved fellowship programs in gynecologic oncology in the United States each year, and when they finish they are in demand to fill positions in which they work essentially full time as gynecologic oncologists. When they work in academic institutions, this has resulted in rapid promotion through the academic ranks because of the small number of senior level people who have comparable training and experience. Thus I do not think it inappropriate for them to have longer training periods to allow for as much preparation as possible.

Which Gynecologic Cancer Patients Should Be Referred for Care?

Referral is one of the most difficult problems faced by the practicing obstetrician gynecologist and by the gynecologic oncologist. Stated simply, there are not enough facilities or personnel to care for all patients with gynecologic cancer in cancer institutes or in divisions of gynecologic oncology in university teaching centers. Thus for practical reasons it becomes important to work out reasonable schemes for determining who would benefit from referral. Mikuta has outlined a program for determining this, discussed earlier in this presentation. Ideally, he suggested that all practicing obstetrician gynecologists discuss the care of the gynecologic cancer patient with the local consultant prior to carrying out therapy. Then if the decision were made that care could be given just as well by the competent obstetrician gynecologist, there would be no need for that patient to be referred. In some states cancer is a reportable disease; in the ideas of some specialists, it should always be a referrable disease. Most of us, however, now feel that the greatest advantage would be to have it a consultable disease so that decisions regarding the benefits of referral could be made jointly by the practicing obstetrician gynecologist and the local gynecologic oncologist. A reasonable guideline is that the patient should be referred when the extent of the surgery or the need of coordination with other institution-based specialists is such that her care will be different and the outcome better. Secondary benefits from referral to an oncology service come from the ability to build up significant series of rare conditions or diseases, increased numbers of patients for entry into the essential randomized clinical trials, and the availability of special studies not available in local institutions. An example of this is the use of the soft agar stem cell colony inhibition assay to test chemotherapeutic sensitivity of an individual's ovarian cancer (Salmon et al. 1978). This assay requires that the tissue be placed into culture soon after surgery and, therefore, the patient must be in that institution.

Length of Training in Gynecologic Oncology

At the time the original members of the Division of Gynecologic Oncology proposed the contents and duration of training programs, the length of training was three years. For reasons related to the need to have practicing specialists enter the field as soon as possible, this was shortened to two years by the parent board, the American Board of Obstetrics and Gynecology. The end result was that this decreased the amount of time available for laboratory research and further clinical experience. This stipulation that training be of two years' duration does not preclude people from electing further training, but there is a tendency for training to be only as long as required. It is my view that the trainee and the training program director must agree on whether one's training is completed at the end of the two years, with the idea that where trainees go for their next position will be determined by whether it is a setting in which they can continue to have further on-the-job training by experienced gynecologic oncologists on the staff or whether they are ready to work independently.

Effect of Subspecialization on the Discipline of Obstetrics and Gynecology

One of the major objections to the identification of the three areas of subspecialization was that it would undermine the discipline of obstetrics and gynecology by creating an elite corps and making second-class citizens out of current practicing specialists in obstetrics and gynecology. A secondary consideration was that the presence of a fellowship training program in an institution which has a core residency program in obstetrics and gynecology would deplete the training experiences of the core resident. Not all of these objections are answerable at this time, but core residents have commented that the general level of surgical training in their institution improved with the development of a Division of Gynecologic Oncology and the recruitment of people trained in this area. In fact, in many residency programs in obstetrics and gynecology, the oncologist has become the specialist called in to help with complex surgical procedures whether they be in oncology patients or patients with obstetrical emergencies. A recent questionnaire sent to junior fellows of the American College of Obstetricians and Gynecologists elicited the view that gynecologic oncology was the "only important fellowship" and that "any well-trained obstetrician gynecologist from a decent residency should be well versed in perinatology and to a less extent endocrinology." The main reason that this development has not had a major splintering effect upon the discipline is that the numbers involved remain very small. This is done because the qualifications for a training program and the requirements for certification were organized in a demanding enough manner that the number of people wishing to devote this amount of time and energy to achieve this level of training remains low. Further consideration of the problem of numbers will be given in the last section.

Number of Gynecologic Oncologists Required

When the program was first outlined, there was great fear that the discipline of obstetrics and gynecology would be flooded with certified gynecologic oncologists. At the present time there have been 175 individuals certified by the American Board of Obstetrics and Gynecology as having special competence in gynecologic oncology. This includes not only those trainees who have finished approved training programs since 1972 but also all so-called grandfathers. My own personal view is that every residency program which trains core residents should have one gynecologic oncologist not only to care for patients but to teach the students and residents as part of their basic training. Since there are more than 200 training programs in obstetrics and gynecology, it is clear that this goal has not yet been met. This is particularly true since there are several centers that have as many as five or six trained gynecologic oncologists on their staff. The average number of trainees entering oncology programs for the last three years has ranged from 25 to 30 per year, and so I foresee a period of continuing need rather than one of oversupply. If Dr. Mikuta's proposal for developing a program of community-hospital–based oncologists is followed, it would seem that we need at least three times as many as are currently certified or in training.

References

Averette, H.A. The role of the gynecologic oncologist in a university hospital. Presented at fifth annual meeting of the Society of Gynecologic Oncologists, January 8, 1974, in Key Biscayne, Florida.

Bulletin of the Division of Gynecologic Oncology of the American Board of Obstetrics and Gynecology, 1979.

Lewis, J.L., Jr. The role of the gynecologic oncologist in a cancer institute. Presented at fifth annual meeting of the Society of Gynecologic Oncologists, January 8, 1974, in Key Biscayne, Florida.

Mikuta, J.J. The role of the gynecologic oncologist in the community. Presented at fifth annual meeting of the Society of Gynecologic Oncologists, January 8, 1974, in Key Biscayne, Florida.

Rutledge, F.N. The gynecologic oncologist. His responsibilities and training. *Obstet. Gynecol.* 40:749–754, 1972.

Salmon, S. E., et al. Quantitation of differential sensitivity of human tumor stem cells to anti-cancer drugs. *N. Engl. J. Med.* 298:1321–1327, 1978.

PERSPECTIVE:

The Role of the Gynecologic Oncologist

Richard C. Boronow

Contemporary gynecologic oncologists are a unique phenomenon in clinical medicine. They are a new breed of clinician whose training, experience, and practice extend beyond the confines of traditional gynecology and encompass clinical activities of a variety of other medical and surgical specialties. They are first and foremost clinicians. In many instances they are also administrators, educators, or investigators. But the degree to which these other activities are successfully handled should for the most part bear a direct relationship to the strength of their clinical competence.

This discussion will consider the role of the gynecologic oncologist in the context of the emergence of this new breed of clinician and the humane medical rationale for their emergence; a profile of the clinical and related activities of these physicians; and their responsibilities in helping respond to current challenges to the subspecialty itself.

The Emergence of the Subspecialty

The formal history of this neophyte specialty has been recorded in the foregoing section. My remarks will be confined to this specialty's emergence into the practical clinical arena (Boronow, 1979).

The surgical leaders in gynecology in the past have been mainly general surgeons who have devoted their practice primarily to gynecology. Among these have been the pioneers of gynecologic cancer surgery. In very recent decades the significant roles of radiotherapy and chemotherapy in the management of many gynecologic cancers have been more broadly appreciated. Certain physicians and institutional training programs incorporated these clinical areas into the education and practice of the physician treating gynecologic neoplasia. It was a unique departure from tradition.

Indeed, in medical communities of general surgeons, urologists, medical oncologists, radiotherapists, and even obstetrician-gynecologists, the emergence of this polygenetic subspecialty has received mixed reviews ranging from warm acceptance to tolerance to some instances of skeptical, even heated, disdain.

To many, we are a Trojan horse in the traditional hierarchy of organized medicine. This hierarchy is bred in the academic institution: territorial domain, teaching material, administrative control, and power are all at stake; that is how all but the youngest of today's practicing physicians were trained (fig. 1.1).

In this situation Ms. X with disease A is diagnosed by the family practitioner or gynecologist. A primary operation may be done (often appropriate, sometimes not), and then, or as an alternative, she is referred to a radiotherapist, or more likely, to a general radiologist, general surgeon, or chemotherapist. And, for various complications, she may be referred to a surgeon, a urologist, and occasionally to no one. Whether appropriate or not, this is consistent with the traditional hierarchy and its rigidly defined boundaries of care but elusive boundaries of responsibility.

If one were to consider the patient and her family, our existence would seem eminently justified. It is comforting as well as logical to have one physician sufficiently skilled to confirm the diagnosis, perform the necessary sur-

Figure 1.1

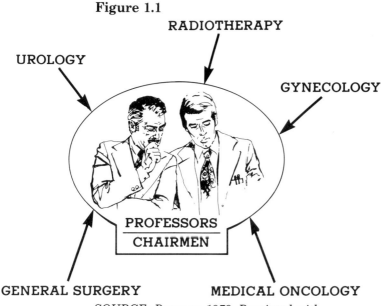

SOURCE: *Boronow 1979. Reprinted with permission.*

gery, participate in the planning and administration of radiotherapy, administer indicated chemotherapy, manage conservatively or operatively the complications of treatment and/or the disease, and also sufficiently sensitive and concerned to follow up carefully and provide, along with the family physician, continuity of support in the days, weeks, or months before death (fig. 1.2).

In my opinion, if we adhere to these responsibilities our survival can be assured, because the best ethics of medical practice are served, and the consumer will know it.

Nevertheless, skirmishes continue regarding territorial domain, as previously defined clinical lines are crossed. In addition, in the last decade or two, there has been an explosion of gynecologic oncologic investigation with clinical and pathologic correlations that, with the creation of a subspecialty division within obstetrics and gynecology, has contributed to the proliferation of postgraduate educational exercises. These are designated as "Oncology for the Practicing Gynecologist," and one may reasonably wonder if our specialty may be gradually decreasing its clinical utility.

This potentially superficial educational process, combined with the encroachment inherent in interspecialty struggles, allows some interesting speculation (table 1.1) regarding our future. Most practitioners, while eager to learn, are leery of mimeographed sheets. Most recognize that the succinct

Figure 1.2

GYNECOLOGIC ONCOLOGIST

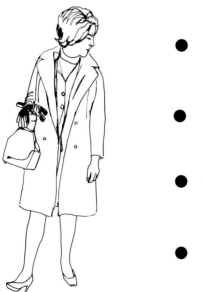

- **SURGERY**

- **RADIATION**

- **CHEMOTHERAPY**

- **CONTINUITY**

SOURCE: Boronow 1979. Reprinted with permission.

Table 1.1
The Diseases We Treat and Who Will
Treat Them

Cervix	
Cervical intraepithelial neoplasia (CIN)	General ob/gyn
Microinvasion	General ob/gyn
Invasive cancer	Radiotherapist
Favorable early cancer	Radical hysterectomy
Recurrence	Exenteration
Chemotherapy	Medical oncologist
Staging laparotomy	Abandon?

Endometrium	
Preinvasive lesion	General ob/gyn
Surgical pathologic staging or primary treatment	General ob/gyn and radiotherapist
Recurrence	Medical oncologist

Ovary	
Primary laparotomy	General ob/gyn
Chemotherapy	Medical oncologist
Radiotherapy	Radiotherapist
"Second look"	Abandon?

Vulva	
Preinvasive lesion	General ob/gyn
Invasive cancer	Radical vulvectomy

Vagina	
Preinvasive lesion	General ob/gyn
Invasive cancer	Radiotherapist

Trophoblast	
	General ob/gyn and medical oncologist

Related Procedures	
Urinary diversion	Urologist
Colostomy and closure	General surgeon
Small bowel obstruction	General surgeon
Complicated vaginal fistulas	Shared

SOURCE: *Boronow 1979.*

pages in the postgraduate course syllabi are inanimately devoid of seasoned clinical judgment and the capacity for individualization. In discussing the surgical oncologist within the field of general surgery, Lawrence (1979) stressed, ". . . his major contributions are his in-depth understanding of the natural history of the wide range of diseases we know as cancer and his ability to provide leadership to all of his colleagues in this general area."

Table 1.2 reflects American Cancer Society projections for new gynecologic cancers and gynecologic cancer deaths at the present time. It is self-evident that gynecologic cancer and its precursors constitute only a small segment of the average obstetrician-gynecologist's practice. By design or by default, our parent specialty education and training pertains more to obstetrics than gynecology; the gynecologic educational experience in most training programs is relatively light in terms of in-depth surgical experience in particular and gynecologic cancer education in general. These features have combined to make the acceptance of this new subspecialty quite satisfactory. While some regret the loss of a small segment of clinical material from their practice, it has been my experience that the majority are pleased to have the contemporary gynecologic oncologist available as a trained and educated resource person either for advice or for actual management of their cancer patients.

Clinical Profile of Gynecologic Oncologists

Utilizing the prerogatives of the tenth President of the Society of Gynecologic Oncologists, I had prepared a clinical activities profile to survey two identified groups of physicians practicing gynecologic oncology, to profile their individual clinical practice, their involvement in clinical activities of other medical and surgical specialties, their interrelationships with these specialties, and other related matters such as teaching responsibilities, scientific publications, and paramedical personnel with whom they work. It was hoped that an analysis of this material would provide a clearer picture both of the people and the problems of practicing gynecologic oncology today.

Table 1.2
Gynecologic Cancer—1979 Estimates of New
Cases and Deaths

Site	New Cases	Deaths
Cervix, invasive	16,000	7,400
Corpus, endometrium	37,000	3,300
Ovary	17,000	11,100
Other female genital	4,500	1,000

SOURCE: *American Cancer Society 1979.*

Of the 148 total members of the Society of Gynecologic Oncologists (SGO), questionnaires were not mailed to honorary members or to associate members, the vast majority of whom were general pathologists. The nine emeritus members did receive the questionnaire, but most declined to answer in view of the change of their current clinical activities. Of the 134 members who were surveyed, 128 (95.5%) responded. This first group was designated as members. The second group was comprised of 139 non-SGO members who have completed approved fellowship training in gynecologic oncology; 114 of these persons responded (82%). This second group was designated as nonmembers. The material was analyzed for each of these two groups (Boronow 1980).

The identifying features of the two groups are recorded in table 1.3. As expected the SGO member group is older: 36% are under age 45 versus 87% under age 45 in the nonmember group. Yet the nonmember group has at least an equal time commitment to gynecologic oncology, as would be expected from a group whose members are exclusively from current training programs. With increased age and experience among the SGO member group there was an increase in the department chairman designation (26% vs 7%), but there was only a slight edge in the chief—division of gynecologic oncology group. Obviously both groups are active in the work of the specialty.

Table 1.4 records responses to the breadth of surgical commitment. In both groups most felt that they operated within the full spectrum of gynecologic oncology surgery. Questions were then addressed to the gynecologic oncologist's personal involvement in related intestinal and urologic surgery or whether such related surgery is done with another surgical specialist or by another surgical specialist. Each response was to be to the closest 25th percentile. Analysis of the results suggests for both members and nonmembers that approximately 65% to 75% of related intestinal and urologic procedures are done by the gynecologic oncologist in the great majority of cases (75% to 100%); 1% to 4% of procedures are done by the other surgical specialists (in 75% to 100% of cases); the remaining cases (25 ± %) appeared to be done with the other surgical specialties, a conjoint effort, very likely shared or with alternating primary operating surgeons. Thus the gynecologic oncologist performs 90% of the spectrum of the surgery, but in some cases the surgical responsibility is shared.

To be sure it is known that among at least several established divisions of gynecologic oncology in this country, certain accommodations have been made: the pelvic exenteration, for example, is a shared (so-called team) effort with the gynecologist removing the specimen, the general surgeon performing the colostomy, and the urologist constructing the urinary diversion. These local situations have often existed for years, antedating contemporary training programs and will likely disappear, especially if the surgical competence of the new generation justifies the total spectrum of technical and critical care responsibilities.

In responding to the question on related vascular surgery it was evident

Table 1.3

Physician Information

	Members SGO, Total 128		Nonmembers, Total 114	
	Number	**Percentage**	**Number**	**Percentage**
Age (Years)				
30–35	1	0.78	44	38.60
36–40	13	10.16	38	33.33
41–45	32	25.00	17	14.91
46–50	26	20.31	9	7.89
51–55	25	19.53	5	4.39
56–60	14	10.94	1	0.88
61–65	10	7.81	0	0.00
66–70	4	3.13	0	0.00
Over 70	2	1.56	0	0.00
No response	1	0.78	0	0.00
Gynecologic oncology practice time (%)				
0–20	9	7.03	2	1.75
21–40	13	10.16	7	6.14
41–60	17	13.28	17	14.91
61–80	24	18.75	26	22.81
81–100	65	50.78	62	54.39
Job description				
Department chairman	33	25.78	8	7.02
Chief—Division of Gynecologic Oncology	63	49.22	39	34.21
Staff—Division of Gynecologic Oncology	16	12.50	47	41.23
Other full-time medical school faculty	5	3.91	2	1.75
Other	11	8.59	18	15.79

SOURCE: *Boronow 1980.*

that, beyond bleeding that can be controlled by packing or by simple suture technique, the majority called in a vascular surgeon or one with proficiency in this area. This area marked a notable deficit in the training and experience of the contemporary gynecologic oncologist.

The majority of both groups managed the majority of their patient's medical problems and the spectrum of medical complications, especially embracing critical care medicine; however, this is more positively reflected in the activities of the nonmember group, the new trainees.

Table 1.4
Gynecologic Oncology Surgery

	Members SGO, Total 128		Nonmembers, Total 114	
	Number	Percentage	Number	Percentage
Full spectrum of surgery	117	91.41	113	99.12
Major, nonradical surgery	5	3.91	1	0.88
Minor, operative gynecology	1	0.78	0	0.00
Little or no surgical time	5	3.91	0	0.00

SOURCE: *Boronow 1980.*

Most in both groups do most of their chemotherapy; however, the new trainees, the nonmembers, have a somewhat greater commitment. Approximately 33% of the member group do 50% or less of their chemotherapy, whereas the figure for the nonmember group is only 14%. Some of the collaboration (with or by medical oncologists) is a reflection of involvement in NCI study groups.

Similar trends exist in involvement with planning and implementing radiotherapy, with the majority of both groups involved in planning but fewer in the nonmember groups reflecting a negligible role (25% or less or never) than among the members. Yet a significant number in both groups (31% of members and 25% of nonmembers) reflect this negligible role in intracavitary applications.

The degree of compatibility or interspecialty friction was assessed by asking if there was (1) no problem with encroachment, (2) some problem, or (3) major problem. About one-quarter to one-third in both groups admit some problem with this encroachment or overlap of clinical work. For the most part this was not a major problem, although of the nonmembers 7% report a major problem with general surgery and 11% with urology (table 1.5).

As expected the member group had published more scientific papers, but the nonmember group was actively contributing to the literature. Table 1.6 reflects the commitment to teaching of both groups.

Challenges to the Subspecialty

Each gynecologic oncologist has a role in responding to the many challenges to our emerging, preadolescent subspecialty. While the list of challenges is broad and perceived differently by each of us, this section will address (1) further definition of the number and distribution of the gynecologic oncologists needed, (2) further improvement in the education and training of future gynecologic oncologists; (3) ecumenical efforts on the part of our several gynecologic oncology societies both for solidarity of our own purposes but also for expanded scientific interface with other medical and surgical specialists;

Table 1.5

Institutional Practice Relationships

	Members SGO, Total 128		Nonmembers, Total 114	
	Number	Percentage	Number	Percentage
Attitude of general surgeons				
No problem with encroachment	100	78.13	63	55.26
Some problem with encroachment	22	17.19	41	35.96
Major problem with encroachment	1	0.78	8	7.02
We voluntarily do not encroach	5	3.91	2	1.75
Attitude of medical oncologists				
No problem with encroachment	83	64.84	73	64.04
Some problem with encroachment	37	28.91	36	31.58
Major problem with encroachment	3	2.34	2	1.75
Encroachment not allowed by edict	1	0.78	0	0.00
We voluntarily do not encroach	4	3.13	3	2.63
Attitude of urologists				
No problem with encroachment	89	69.53	66	57.89
Some problem with encroachment	32	25.00	33	28.95
Major problem with encroachment	3	2.34	13	11.40
We voluntarily do not encroach	4	3.13	2	1.75
Attitude of internists				
No problem with encroachment	106	82.81	98	85.96
Some problem with encroachment	12	9.38	13	11.40
Major problem with encroachment	1	0.78	0	0.00
Encroachment not allowed by edict	1	0.78	0	0.00
We voluntarily do not encroach	8	6.25	3	2.63
Attitude of ob-gyn chairman				
No problem, I am the chairman	34	26.56	11	9.65
Full support from chairman	80	62.50	86	75.44
Chairman somewhat intimidated by others	4	3.13	12	10.53
Chairman significantly intimidated	3	2.34	2	1.75
No response	7	5.47	3	2.63

SOURCE: *Boronow 1980.*

and (4) education and organization of our paramedical personnel, especially nurses and enterostomal therapists.

Manpower Needs

In 1972–1973 a survey of certified obstetricians and gynecologists was conducted by the American Board and reported by Randall (1974). Of those responding 2.9% (274 physicians) indicated that gynecologic oncology was an area of particular interest "in which . . . you believe a majority of your practice time and efforts are now being devoted." A total of 1310 physicians or 14.1% indicated areas of special interest, and the board interpreted this as confirming its understanding that the developing provisions for certification of special competence in limited areas within the specialty were a desirable response to practice patterns already well established at that time.

More recently, with the implementation of these changes by the board and the three divisions, concerns of supply and demand have appropriately been raised. Pearse and Trabin (1977) considered a number of suggested mechanisms (number of major university medical centers, geographic regions and population densities, number of projected tertiary care centers for mothers and children) to determine future needs of the three new subspecialty groups (maternal-fetal medicine, reproductive endocrinology, and gynecologic oncology). All sources indicated similar projections, and these authors suggest a need of 350 gynecologic oncologists for the United States, an additional 350 physicians in reproductive endocrinology, and 750 in maternal-fetal medicine. Taken together this totals 10% of presently certified obstetrician-gynecologists. Of concern is a comprehensive survey of junior fellows of the American College of Obstetricians and Gynecologists indicating that fully 30% of present residents expect they will enter subspecialties.

Table 1.6
Teaching Activities

	Members SGO, Total 128		Nonmembers, Total 114	
	Number	Percentage	Number	Percentage
Fellows only	1	0.78	2	1.75
Residents only	4	3.13	7	6.14
Fellows, residents, students	71	55.47	54	47.37
Fellows and residents	0	0.00	5	4.39
Fellows and students	0	0.00	1	0.88
Residents and students	48	37.50	44	38.60
No specific teaching	4	3.13	1	0.88

SOURCE: *Boronow 1980.*

These authors caution that this expectation is far in excess of available fellowships and ultimate need.

In discussing the Pearse and Trabin paper, McElin (1977) verbalized the concerns of many: "The frightening aspect of the manuscript is the fearsome imbalance between the expectations and aspirations of the approximate one-third of our current trainees . . . and the projected national need. . . . For example, it is obvious that a superbly trained oncologist . . . will shortly desire and require a fellow to assist in the management of the complicated problems with which he will be confronted. This 'original' oncologist will then probably want a certified training program, and the spiral will geometrically escalate and could eventuate in a disproportion between supply and demand even greater than that which Dr. Pearse suggests."

As of late 1979, 143 physicians have been certified for special competence in gynecologic oncology. There are 35 approved training programs with 25 physicians entered in year one and 29 in year two. The projected number of 350 will likely be reached by the mid-1980s (Merrill 1979).

On the other hand, the federally contracted survey by Geomet, Incorporated, issued in late 1977 projects 811 gynecologic oncologists needed by 1980 and 863 by 1985. The term full time equivalent was used for these physicians working 80% of their time in patient care. These numbers were generated from an extensive data base of estimates of time needed for care of gynecologic cancer, exclusive of preinvasive lesions. Further, they are based on the premise that all invasive cancer is managed by the gynecologic oncologist.

Clearly the national needs may be reasonably projected somewhere between the estimates of Pearse and Trabin and of the Geomet study.

The clustering of gynecologic oncologists in medical school settings will change with time, as has, for example, the distribution of cardiovascular surgeons. It seems appropriate that most be in educational settings, however, as the academic environment remains in the forefront of new information and clinical trials. Nevertheless, high-quality work can and is being maintained in the private practice setting, and where the patient volume justifies it, this seems appropriate. I caution, however, that part-time gynecologic oncologists, like part-time cardiovascular surgeons, will soon lose their competency.

It is my personal view that entry into the private sector is best delayed for at least several years for our subspecialists for a number of reasons: (1) the requirement for advanced certification mandates an additional two years of clinical experience in an entirely suitable setting; (2) trainees can pay their dues by contributing much in terms of academic teaching responsibilities, participation in clinical studies, cooperatives, and the like, and the preparation of formal and informal talks and presentations, manuscripts, and other forms of scientific scholarship; (3) additional clinical experience inevitably matures and seasons the neophyte clinician.

Nevertheless, presently and for the future there are a great many sizable non-medical school communities (and medical school communities, for that matter) that not only can and will support, but desire, gynecologic oncologists in a strictly private setting. And contrary to McElin's concerns, we have personally established gynecologic oncology in a private setting without a training program, fellows, or residents but with a commitment from excellent gynecologic oncology nurses.

Education and Training

Further improvement in the education and training of the gynecologic oncologist is of practical as well as intellectual importance. Some changes could impact directly on the consideration of manpower needs as well.

It was stressed in an earlier section of this communication that, both in the context of rational medical and surgical considerations as well as humane and ethical considerations, the emergence of our specialty seems eminently justified. But as was emphasized elsewhere, justification alone is not enough. We must be unquestionably able to do this broad-based job. We have a highly legitimate place in medical practice. Our most valid answer to critics is to be certain that our training is unimpeachable. We must make our training programs even better than the ones from which we have come. We must be more than messenger RNA, replicating ourselves. We must be dynamic, in the best spirit of medical education, and work to produce trainees who are even better than their trainers. We do not need more graduates of our programs: we must strive for quality, not quantity. Terms of training should in my view be longer: three or four years rather than two. If requirements are tougher, examinations tougher, and training longer, the preparation will be better. And the graduates will be fewer, for only the most able and most motivated will pursue this more stringent track. And it is likely that a more limited number of fully comprehensive training programs than presently exist can be developed to fulfill these requirements. Both will effectively deal with concerns for oversupply while at the same time improving the clinicians entering the discipline.

One, preferably two years of surgical experience for the fellows (including some formal vascular surgical experience) will broaden the surgical and critical-care basis of our work. Then training programs will not have so much time consumed in "teaching the fellows to operate," and their remaining two years can more fully maximize their education and training in chemotherapy, radiotherapy, critical-care medicine, and the other essential tools of the trade. As competence is improved, concerns over so-called encroachment will be eased. If we possess and demonstrate the education and training for our broad-based job, we will have the respect of our interdisciplinary colleagues.

Cooperation among Societies

Even before the young specialty was formed, gynecologic oncology societies were begun. There are now five in North America. Initially, there was some sense of competitiveness as the individuality of each was becoming established, despite considerable overlap of memberships. Despite certain regional or institutional orientations of several, the overall commonality of all is recognized. Ecumenical efforts are underway, not in a structured, formalized sense, but in the shape of a combined meeting. The call for this conjoint meeting (GOALS I) was made, stressing our need to recognize our common purposes and the desirability of communication and cooperation (fig. 1.3). The twelfth annual meeting of the Society of Gynecologic Oncologists (January 1981) sponsored the first combined meeting of gynecologic oncology societies and included the Canadian Society of Gynecologic Oncologists, the Felix Rutledge Society, the Society of Memorial Gynecologic Oncologists, and the Western Association of Gynecologic Oncologists.

The ecumenical spirit under the common umbrella of gynecologic oncology is essential for the viability and growth of the specialty. This spirit should in no way detract from the individuality of the individual societies. As a small, young medical specialty, unity of purposes shared by all (GOALS) must be recognized and appreciated by all of us. The place to begin is to manifest unity among ourselves.

Then we should broaden our involvement with interspecialty opportunities to participate in such scientific forums as the American College of Surgeons, the American Radium Society, the American Society of Clinical On-

Figure 1.3

GYNECOLOGIC

ONCOLOGISTS

AMIABLY ALLIED FOR

LIAISON, LEGITIMACY, LEADERSHIP

SCIENCE, SOCIABILITY & SOLIDARITY

SOURCE: Boronow 1979. Reprinted with permission.

cology, and the Society of Surgical Oncology, to name a few. This allows us to enhance our professional and personal identities with interdisciplinary colleagues at a national level, to become more broadly conversant with the entire cancer field, and to do more than simply talk among ourselves.

Education and Organization for Nurses

As noted in the clinical activities profile many gynecologic oncology nurses have been identified. The precise job descriptions of these people have not been studied. Many are primarily chemotherapy nurses; others are actively involved in supervised patient care. Many also provide enterostomal therapy for their own services; some work as first assistants in surgery.

Our speciality should cultivate the thirst of those nurses for further education and identity. The registry of formal nursing associations is legion, and a wide range of backgrounds, training, and interests are reflected in but a representative sample of these organizations, as indicated in table 1.7. There is ample precedent. Already several specialty organizations of oncologic nurses exist. Our people deserve our support.

Unquestionably, effective implementation of responses to these and other challenges remains at the discretion of the leadership of the Division of Gynecologic Oncology, the American Board of Obstetrics and Gynecology, the American College of Obstetricians and Gynecologists, the Residency Review Committee, and other societies, especially those of our own subspecialty. But each of us has a role as an individual to make his or her views heard, for each of us has a personal and professional interest, not only in the viability, but in the continued growth and strength of gynecologic oncology.

Table 1.7
Representative Nurses Organizations

American Association of *Critical Care* Nurses
American Association of *Nephrology* Nurses and Technicians
American Association of *Neurosurgical* Nurses
American Association of *Nurse Anesthetists*
American College of *Nurse Midwives*
American *Urological* Association Allied
Association of *Operating Room* Nurses
Association of *Pediatric Oncology* Nurses
Association of *Rehabilitation* Nurses
Emergency Department Nurses Association
Gay Nurse Alliance
National *Black* Nurses Association
Orthopedic Nurses Association
Oncology Nursing Society

SOURCE: *Boronow 1979.*

References

American Cancer Society. *Facts and figures.* New York: American Cancer Society, 1978.

Assessment of manpower needs in selected clinical oncology specialties, Vol. 1. *Gynecologic oncology phase.* Final report submitted to National Institutes of Health, National Cancer Institute Research Contracts Branch. Geomet Incorporated, Gaithersburg, Maryland. November 1977.

Boronow, R.C. Odyssey of an endangered species: adjunct or archer? *Gynecol. Oncol.* 8:265–276, 1979.

Boronow, R.C. Clinical activities of gynecologic oncologists: report of a survey. *Gynecol. Oncol.* 9:310–323, 1980.

Lawrence, W. Is surgical oncology really a specialty? *Arch. Surg.* 114:659–661, 1979.

McElin, T.W. Discussion of Pearse and Trabin paper. *Am. J. Obstet. Gynecol.* 128:306–307, 1977.

Pearse, W.H., and Trabin, J.R. Subspecialization in obstetrics and gynecology. *Am. J. Obstet. Gynecol.* 128:303–306, 1977.

Randall, C.L. The current practices of board-certified obstetricians and gynecologists in the United States. *Am. J. Obstet. Gynecol.* 119:156–164, 1974.

PART I

CARCINOMA OF THE VULVA

Radical vulvectomy was described as the standard approach to the treatment of carcinoma of the vulva in 1912 by Basset. It remained, however, for Way to establish that improved survival was related directly to wide, deep removal of the entire vulva and the regional lymph nodes. Little in the past 30 years has altered the accepted treatment, which includes removal of the vulva to the external pelvic fascia, together with inguinal, femoral, and pelvic lymphadenectomy. Although recent advances in operative techniques have been described, the identification of features with both prognostic and therapeutic importance on which to base treatment modification has been relatively neglected.

One area of concern involves the identification of patients with early carcinoma who might achieve cure with more limited dissection of the vulva and/or regional lymph nodes. Unlike in situ epidermoid carcinoma of the cervix, the preinvasive stage of squamous carcinoma of the vulva is associated with a visible lesion and frequently is multifocal and diffuse. This has led to some reluctance on the part of surgeons to limit the breadth or depth of their excision. Recently, however, as younger women with intraepithelial neoplasia of the vulva have been identified, the cosmetic appearance of the vulva after operation and its psychosexual implications for the patient have been considered. Dr. Tamimi discusses a variety of approaches to this problem.

Of more critical importance is the woman with invasive carcinoma of limited extent. Several investigators have attempted to define the criteria for microinvasive carcinoma of the vulva and plan therapy accordingly. Drs. DiSaia and Rich discuss their innovative approach to this problem.

Although historically the initial attempt to modify the standard operative approach to invasive carcinoma of the vulva was to abandon the dissection of the pelvic lymph nodes, the controversy surrounding the need for this procedure continues. Dr. Curry bases his recommendations on the characteristics of the primary tumor and the status of the inguinal and femoral lymph nodes at the time of operation. Dr. Fuller, while defining a similar set of criteria, provides a detailed analysis of the cost and benefit of pelvic lymphadenectomy and sheds light on the pathophysiology and immunobiology of regional lymph nodes that contain metastatic tumor.

The message that each of these authors conveys is that although operative techniques for the management of patients with carcinoma of the vulva are easily learned, they must be applied in concert with an in-depth understanding of the natural history of the disease and the effect of treatment on the entire patient.

Chapter 2

*The Treatment of
Early Invasive Carcinoma
of the Vulva*

PERSPECTIVE:

Hisham K. Tamimi

Invasive carcinoma of the vulva represents approximately 5% of all gynecologic malignancies. It ranks fourth in incidence among female genital malignancies, being exceeded by endometrial, cervical, and ovarian cancer.

The standard therapy for invasive carcinoma of the vulva over the past 30 years has been radical vulvectomy with bilateral groin dissection, with or without pelvic lymph node dissection. The radical surgical approach has resulted in significant improvement in control of disease and patient survival (Way and Hennigan 1966; Franklin and Rutledge 1972; Krupp et al. 1975; Morley 1976). With the increased application of this radical approach in the past 30 years, two observations are relevant to this discussion:

1. The incidence of inguinal and femoral node metastases is directly related to the size of the primary tumor. Lesions smaller than 2 cm in diameter are noted to be less frequently associated with lymph node metastases.
2. Pelvic node involvement rarely occurs without involvement of the groin nodes.

Modifications of the standard surgical approach have resulted from these observations, particularly in the treatment of early invasive vulvar carcinoma.

Definition of Early Invasive Vulvar Carcinoma

In contrast to the staging system of the International Federation of Gynaecology and Obstetrics for carcinoma of the cervix, that for cancer of the vulva does not have a stage or substage for early disease. Consequently, individual authors and institutions have established their own criteria for this entity.

39

Figure 2.2

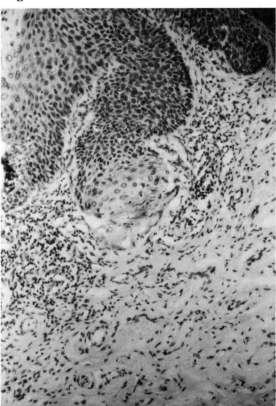

Photomicrograph of carcinoma in situ of the vulva with early stromal invasion. Note the pseudopearl formation.

and measurement of the depth of invasion requires thorough evaluation of the pathologic material with multiple sections of the involved area(s). Vascular channel involvement is sometimes difficult to establish, and adherence to specific criteria is necessary, namely, demonstration of endothelial lining and/or the presence of blood elements within the suspected vascular channel.

Treatment

With the increasing incidence of carcinoma in situ of the vulva in the younger age groups, simple vulvectomy is no longer considered the treatment of choice. Several modalities have been suggested. The use of topical 5-fluorouracil cream, laser vaporization, wide local excision, and skinning vulvec-

Table 2.1
Incidence of Lymph Node Metastases in
Microinvasive Carcinoma of the Vulva

Year	Author	Number of Patients	Depth of Invasion (mm)	Capillary Channel Involvement	Anaplasia	Positive Nodes
1974	Wharton, Gallagher, and Rutledge	25	5	0	?	0
1975	Parker et al.	58	5	2	1	3
1975	Dipaola, Gomez-Rueda, and Arrighi	11	5	?	?	3
1976	Jafari and Cartnick	6	3	0	?	1
1974	Nakao et al.	1	3	1	0	1
	Totals	101		3	1	8 (8%)

tomy with split-thickness skin graft have been advocated. The goal of each of these modalities is to decrease the psychosexual morbidity associated with simple vulvectomy without compromising the curability of the disease. This aspect of treatment, that is, decreasing the psychosexual morbidity, comes to be of great significance to the young patient concerned about her sexual function, body image, and feeling of femininity.

In selected cases of carcinoma of the vulva 2 cm or less in size, an operative approach suggested by Parker and colleagues includes (1) excisional biopsy of the vulvar lesion and careful inspection and cytologic evaluation of the cervix and vagina; (2) histopathologic evaluation of the biopsy with reference to depth of invasion, vascular channel involvement, and cellular anaplasia; (3) if invasion is present to 5 mm or less, without vascular channel involvement or cellular anaplasia, radical vulvectomy without lymphadenectomy should be adequate therapy; (4) if there is greater than 5 mm of invasion, or if at any depth vascular channel involvement or cellular anaplasia is seen, radical vulvectomy and lymphadenectomy is indicated; (5) if a patient is selected for radical vulvectomy only, and the operative specimen reveals the presence of residual disease, vascular channel involvement, or cellular anaplasia, the patient should have a staged lymphadenectomy. Wharton and associates (1974) reported on their experience with microinvasive carcinoma of the vulva and also concluded that its victims may be treated by radical vulvectomy alone.

Although this treatment plan has been curative and has eliminated the morbidity of groin dissection, it has certain disadvantages. The concept of radical vulvectomy with bilateral groin dissection was advanced to remove the vulva, the lymphatic channels, and the regional lymph nodes en bloc. Assuming that the regional lymph nodes are not involved, the advantage of performing a radical resection of the vulva is questionable, and a less radical excision may be as successful as the radical one.

Treatment should be individualized on the basis of several factors. Those related to the tumor itself should include size, location, number of lesions, depth of invasion, degree of differentiation, vascular channel involvement, and the status of the regional lymph nodes. Age, motivation, and patterns of sexual activity all must be considered before embarking on a specific plan of treatment.

Treatment of Carcinoma In Situ with Early Stromal Invasion

In young patients, carcinoma in situ is often multicentric. Early stromal invasion may be present in more than one focus, but in the majority of women it is unifocal. The upper vulva, particularly the clitoris, is rarely involved as the only site of disease. On the other hand, the lower part of the vulva and the perineum are frequently involved as the only disease sites.

Multicentric disease in a young patient is probably best treated by skinning vulvectomy with split-thickness skin graft. Wide local excision is probably satisfactory for unifocal lesions.

Other measures used in treatment of carcinoma in situ of the vulva should not be employed when there is evidence of early stromal invasion. Cryotherapy, laser vaporization, and topical chemotherapy are contraindicated in this situation. These nonoperative procedures do not provide tissue for histopathologic evaluation that might alter the treatment plan.

Table 2.2 outlines the treatment results in five patients with carcinoma in situ with early stromal invasion treated in our institution. All patients in this small series are without evidence of recurrent disease for a minimum of two and one-half years. The cosmetic and functional results of the split-thickness skin graft were excellent.

In summary, the treatment of vulvar carcinoma in situ with early stromal invasion is a surgical one and similar to the treatment of carcinoma in situ of the vulva. Longer periods of follow-up to detect recurrence are essential.

Treatment of Microcarcinoma

Table 2.1 clearly demonstrates that there are patients with early invasive cancer with less than 5 mm of invasion in whom both inguinal and pelvic lymph nodes contained metastatic disease; however, the incidence of positive nodes becomes infrequent when poorly differentiated lesions and those with vascular channel involvement are excluded. Until more data are available as

Table 2.2
Vulvar Carcinoma in Situ with
Early Stromal Invasion

Case Number	Age	Treatment	Results	
1	60	Simple vulvectomy	NED*	44 months
2	57	Partial vulvectomy	NED	30 months
3	17	Skinning vulvectomy with STSG†	NED	32 months
4	70	Simple vulvectomy	NED	30 months
5	67	Simple vulvectomy	NED	42 months

*NED = no evidence of disease.
†STSG = split-thickness skin graft.

to the prognostic value of these two criteria, regional lymph nodes in such patients are at risk for metastatic disease. Radical vulvectomy and bilateral groin node dissection are the treatment of choice. Pelvic lymph node dissection is added if metastatic disease is confirmed in the inguinal or femoral lymph nodes by frozen section.

Efforts should continue to define clearly a group of patients with microcarcinoma of the vulva in whom it is safe to employ operative procedure less extensive than radical vulvectomy and bilateral groin node dissection. This objective can be reached through cooperative efforts by gynecologic oncologists and pathologists. High-risk factors, such as depth of invasion, cellular differentiation, lymphatic and vascular channel involvement, and tumor volume should be investigated. The number of patients with microcarcinoma of the vulva treated by conservative approach is small, and the duration of the follow-up period has been short.

References

Dipaola, G.R.; Gomez-Rueda, N.; and Arrighi, L. Relevance of micro-invasion in carcinoma of the vulva. *Obstet. Gynecol.* 45:647–649, 1975.

Franklin, E.W., and Rutledge, F.N. Epidemiology of epidermoid carcinoma of the vulva. *Obstet. Gynecol.* 39:165–172, 1972.

Jafari, K., and Cartnick, E.N. Micro-invasive squamous cell carcinoma of the vulva. *Gynecol. Oncol.* 4:158–166, 1976.

Krupp, P.J. et al. Prognostic parameters and clinical staging criteria in epidermoid carcinoma of the vulva. *Obstet. Gynecol.* 46:84–88, 1975.

Kunschner, A.; Kaubour, A.I.; and David, B. Early vulvar carcinoma. *Obstet. Gynecol.* 132:599–606, 1978.

Morley, G. Infiltrative carcinoma of the vulva. *Am. J. Obstet. Gynecol.* 124:874–888, 1976.

Nakao, C.Y. et al. Microinvasive epidermoid carcinoma of the vulva with an unexpected natural history. *Am. J. Obstet. Gynecol.* 120:1122–1123, 1974.

Parker, R.T. et al. Operative management of early invasive epidermoid carcinoma of the vulva. *Am. J. Obstet. Gynecol.* 123:349–355, 1975.

Way, S., and Hennigan, M. The late results of extended radical vulvectomy for carcinoma of the vulva. *J. Obstet. Gynaecol. Br. Comm.* 73:594–598, 1966.

Wharton, J.T.; Gallagher, S.; and Rutledge, F.N. Micro-invasive carcinoma of the vulva. *Am. J. Obstet. Gynecol.* 118:159–162, 1974.

PERSPECTIVE:

The Treatment of Early Invasive Carcinoma of the Vulva

Philip J. DiSaia and
William M. Rich

Cancer of the vulva comprises about 3% to 4% of all female primary genital malignancies. It ranks fourth in incidence among female genital malignancies, being exceeded by endometrial, cervical, and ovarian cancer. Squamous cell carcinoma accounts for 95% of malignant vulvar lesions. The traditional therapy for squamous carcinoma of the vulva in the past 30 years has been radical vulvectomy with inguinal and pelvic lymphadenectomy, and this radical surgery approach has resulted in well-documented improved patient survivals (Collins et al. 1963; Franklin and Rutledge 1972; Way and Hennigan 1966).

In the last two decades this procedure has been applied to patients with greater skill and unprecedented support, resulting in a markedly diminished morbidity. Currently this procedure is being carried out in the ninth and tenth decades of life with surprising safety. On the other hand, one aspect of the morbidity has remained unaltered; this relates to the serious impact this procedure has both on sexual function and body image. It seems safe to assume that radical vulvectomy ranks with bilateral mastectomy in its impact upon the psychological state of a woman and her sexual response. This concern is particularly relevant in an era where reports would indicate that premalignant and early invasive neoplasia of the vulva are occurring in young age groups with increasing frequency (Forney et al. 1977; Hughes 1971).

Does all invasive squamous cell carcinoma of the vulva require the classical therapy of radical vulvectomy and bilateral inguinal lymphadenectomy? Wharton and associates (1974) recently reviewed their experience with microinvasive carcinoma of the vulva in an attempt to answer this question. In a study of 25 patients with lesions less than 2 cm in diameter and 5 mm or less of stromal invasion, they found neither positive lymph nodes in 10 patients who had lymphadenectomy nor any deaths due to cancer. They concluded from this that microinvasive carcinoma of the vulva is a definable stage and that this group of patients may be treated by conservative surgery consisting of radical vulvectomy alone. Their plea was to avoid a lymphadenectomy in this subset of patients and avoid the associated morbidity and prolonged hospitalization.

An opposite philosophy was heard in several reports of patients with early invasive disease (well within the criteria expressed by Wharton) who were noted to have metastatic disease to the lymph nodes (Nakao et al. 1974; Jafari and Cartnick 1976; Schwartz, personal communication; Lucas, personal communication; DiPaola et al. 1975; Yazigi et al. 1978). Clearly there are at least a small number of cases of early invasive cancer of the vulva with less than 5 mm of invasion where inguinal and pelvic lymphadenectomy would be beneficial in the patient's therapy. DiPaola and associates reported positive groin nodes in 3 of 11 patients with tumor invasion of 5 mm or less.

A review of 96 patients with stage I microinvasive squamous cell cancer of the vulva was reported by Magrina and associates (1979) from the Mayo Clinic. Nine percent of their patients studied had positive lymph nodes, and one patient had a positive deep pelvic node. In the group with 1 to 3 mm of invasion (68 patients) there were 2 patients (3%) with positive nodes. However, among 28 patients with 4 to 5 mm of invasion, 7 (or 25%) were found to have positive nodes. The incidence of positive nodes appeared to increase with microscopic confluence or lymphatic permeation.

Parker and associates (1975) attempted to delineate clinically the concept of early invasive epidermoid carcinoma of the vulva, to study the histopathologic criteria, and to select the proper operative procedure for each case. The clinical records and surgical specimens of 60 patients with squamous cell cancer of the vulva less than 2 cm in size were studied. Fifty-eight patients had stromal invasion 5 mm or less in depth. Three of the 60 patients (5%) had lymph node metastases; 2 of these 3 showed invasion of vascular channels; the third patient's tumor showed cellular anaplasia. They concluded that in selected patients who have a carcinoma of the vulva of 2 cm or less in size, an operative approach is suggested as follows: (1) excisional biopsy of the vulvar lesion and careful inspection and cytologic evaluation of the cervix and vagina; (2) histopathologic evaluation of the biopsy with reference to depth of invasion, vascular channel involvement, and cellular anaplasia; (3) if invasion is present to 5 mm or less without vascular channel involvement or cellular anaplasia, radical vulvectomy without lymphadenectomy should be adequate therapy; (4) if greater than 5 mm of invasion or if any depth vascular channel involvement or cellular anaplasia is seen, radical vulvectomy and lymphadenectomy are indicated; (5) if a patient is selected for radical vulvectomy only and the surgical specimen reveals the presence of residual disease with vascular channel involvement or cellular anaplasia, the patient should have a staged lymphadenectomy.

Wharton and Parker both considered radical vulvectomy a conservative approach. We suggest that for the young patient this is not a conservative approach but a devastating, mutilating procedure. Recently, DiSaia and associates (1979) reported a modified approach for early invasive carcinoma of the vulva, tailored to the known disease spread pattern of this neoplasm. The intent of this approach is to preserve vulvar tissue and sexual function where possible without sacrificing curability. All patients selected for this investigational approach met the following criteria: (1) an invasive cancer 1 cm or less in diameter confined to the vulva and/or perineum and (2) a lesion with focal invasion limited to 5 mm in depth. Only squamous carcinomas were accepted and the depth of invasion was measured from the base of the overlying epithelium. The specimens were reviewed histologically for confluency, defined as a mass of invading cancer which filled a 1 mm or greater field. Specimens were also carefully studied for vascular channel invasion by malignant cells and a high degree of anaplasia. Patients ranged in age from 34 to 58 years with a median of 46 years. All of the patients were multiparous. A previous history of intraepithelial neoplasia of the cervix or vagina was reported in six, or 33%, of the patients. Pruritus was the commonest presenting symptom, but this occurred in only 45% of the patients. In the majority of cases, the lesion had been recognized either by the patient or by a physician performing a routine pelvic examination. Eleven of the patients had lesions involving the posterior fourchette or the inferior poles of the labia minora. Nine of the patients had a lesion which involved the labium majus or the more superior aspect of the labium minus. In 10 of the patients, the lesion was rather centrally located on the posterior fourchette or perineal body whereas the remaining 10 patients had a lesion that had lateralized to one side or the other. None of the patients studied had lesions involving the clitoris or the tissue immediately adjacent.

Philosophy of Treatment

Lymphatic drainage of the external genitalia begins with minute papillae, and these are connected in turn to a multilayered meshwork of fine vessels. These layers, together with their numerous communicating branches, extend over the entire labia minora, the prepuce of the clitoris, the fourchette, and the vaginal mucosa up to the level of the hymenal ring. From the most anterior portion of the labia minora, there emerge three or four collecting trunks whose course is cephalic and anterior, bypassing the clitoris as they approach the mons veneris. Here they are joined by an anastomosis with vessels originating from the prepuce. The lymphatic capillary bed of the labia majora is appreciably more coarse in consistency than that of the labia minora. This difference becomes even more pronounced toward the lateral borders of the labia majora, where the lymphatic network terminates in a number of collecting trunks. The trunks emerge from the body of tissue at the anterior part of the labia majora, converging in an anterior, cephalad direction to the mons veneris, there joining the vessels of the prepuce and labia minora. Beyond this point of juncture, these lymphatic vessels abruptly change their direction and turn laterally and terminate in ipsilateral or contralateral femoral nodes. When this occurs it is usually limited to the medial upper quadrant of the femoral node group (Plentl and Friedman 1971). The nodes accepting the lymphatics which have traversed the mons veneris are reportedly located medial to the great saphenous vein above the cribriform fascia. These nodes in turn may freely drain secondarily through the cribriform fascia to the deep femoral group (Parry-Jones 1963).

The superficial inguinal lymph glands, placed immediately beneath the integument, are of large size and vary from eight to 10 in number. Some have divided these into two groups: an upper oblique set disposed irregularly along Poupart's ligament, which some authors feel receive the lymphatics from the integument of the vulva, clitoris, perineal and gluteal regions as well as the mucous membrane of the urethra and an inferior vertical set, two to five in number, which surround the saphenous opening in the fascia lata (*Gray* 1973). These same authors believe that this latter group receives the superficial lymphatics from the lower extremity. Thus, although there are some disagreements as to which nodes initially intercept the lymphatics from the vulva, all authors agree that the superficial inguinal lymph glands are the primary nodal group for the vulva and can serve as the sentinel lymph nodes of the vulva.

In a personal series of 79 cases of invasive squamous cancer of the vulva treated with radical vulvectomy and bilateral inguinal lymphadenectomy, DiSaia noted that the deep femoral group of lymph nodes was never positive in the absence of positive superficial inguinal lymph glands. In the last 20 cases of DiSaia's series, the inguinal lymphadenectomy specimen was carefully separated into two node groups: those lying superficial to the cribriform fascia and those beneath that layer. The observation stated above continued to be valid in a pathologic review of these surgical specimens. Recently, Cabanas (1977) reported an approach for penile carcinoma taking similar principles into consideration. In his report, the superficial inguinal lymph nodes in the area of the saphenous vein opening in the fascia lata were utilized as sentinel nodes in the therapy for penile carcinoma. When biopsies of these sentinel nodes were positive an inguinal lymph node dissection was carried out. When the biopsies of the sentinel nodes were negative for metastatic disease, a complete inguinal dissection was omitted and the patient was treated centrally with only an additional, partial, or complete amputation of the penis.

Our interest in a similar approach was stimulated in 1971 when a patient with early invasive epidermoid carcinoma of the vulva at age 33 presented with a lesion of the perineal body and absolutely refused radical vulvectomy. In long discussions with the patient concerning the disease and spread pattern, several issues came to light. First, removal of the superficial inguinal nodes would allow an assessment of those nodes for metastatic disease and thereby presumably would give some indication as to the biologic aggressiveness of the primary lesion. Second, satellite lesions on the vulva itself are quite rare in epidermoid carcinoma except in the so-called kissing lesions (Woodruff, personal communication). Every experienced gynecologic oncologist has seen lesions on the medial aspect of the labium minus with a corresponding lesion on the opposite labium where contact is frequent and prolonged. In the majority of cases, however (even with massive-sized lesions), one observes a primary lesion and then metastatic involvement in the regional lymph nodes with a clean, intervening skin bridge between them. Over the last several years, multiple random selections of this intervening skin bridge by our pathologists have revealed no evidence of disease trapped in communicating lymphatics. It would appear that the disease usually spreads by embolism from the primary lesion to the draining lymph nodes with little or no opportunity for metastatic sites to develop along the pathway. A third point which came from our discussions with this particular patient was the ease with which a recurrence could be detected in this preserved skin bridge, given an intelligent patient, one well motivated for follow-up care. Using the above set of hypotheses and observations, the treatment plan outlined below was first initiated.

Operative Technique

The patient is prepared for a radical vulvectomy with bilateral inguinal lymphadenectomy should the operative findings warrant a maximal surgical effort. An 8 cm incision is made parallel to the inguinal ligament 2 fingerbreadths (4 cm) beneath the inguinal ligament and 2 fingerbreadths (4 cm) lateral to the pubic tubercle (fig. 2.3). This allows access to the superficial inguinal lymph nodes of both the upper oblique and inferior vertical set. The incision is carried down through Camper's fascia and at this point skin flaps are bluntly and sharply dissected both superiorly and inferiorly, allowing access to the fat pad containing the superficial nodes. The sentinel nodes are located in the fatty layer of tissue beneath Camper's fascia anterior to the cribriform plate and the fascia lata (fig. 2.4). The dissection should be carried superiorly to the inguinal ligament and inferiorly to a point approximately 2 cm proximal to the opening of Hunter's canal. Laterally, the dissection should be taken to the sartorius muscle and medially to the adductor longus muscle fascia (fig. 2.5). Blunt dissection with the handle of the scalpel facilitates identification of the cribriform fascia, which is most easily identified just below the inguinal ligament or in the area of the saphenous opening. The cribriform fascia becomes one with the fascia lata and thus is contiguous with the fascia on the surface of the adductor longus and sartorius muscle;

Figure 2.3

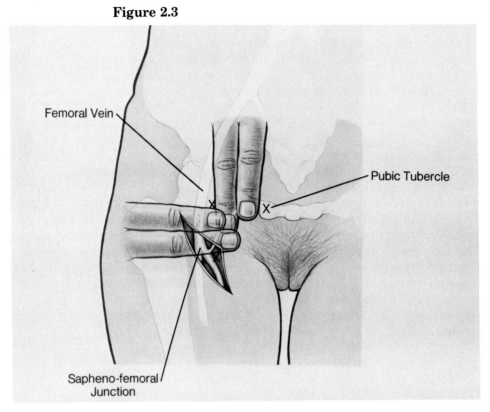

The incision can be made as demonstrated with easy access to all superficial inguinal glands and minimal risk of postoperative skin loss.

this may facilitate its identification. The portion of the fascia covering the femoral triangle is perforated by the internal saphenous vein and by numerous blood and lymphatic vessels; hence its name, the cribriform fascia. If the dissection is carried out properly, the adventitia of the femoral vessels should not be clearly seen except through the vessel openings mentioned above.

The superficial inguinal nodes were removed bilaterally in all instances, but a unilateral dissection with a lateralizing lesion is certainly something for future consideration as the incidence of contralateral metastases is very rare in the absence of ipsilateral involvement. The excised nodes are immediately sent for frozen section analysis, and the finding of positive nodes mandates a complete inguinal dissection including the deep femoral nodes as well as the pelvic nodes on the involved side. Absence of a report of metastatic disease is followed by simple closure of the incision with a subcuticular suture of polyglycolic acid (PGA) type over two medium-sized suction drainage tubes.

Figure 2.4

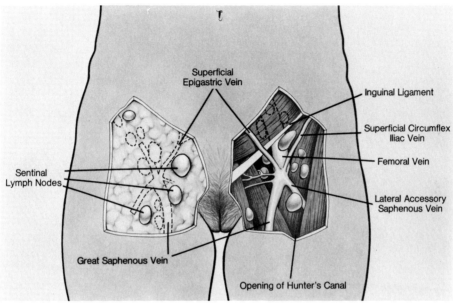

The area of dissection as seen beneath Camper's fascia is illustrated in the right groin, revealing the sentinel nodes (superficial inguinal nodes) at varying levels in the fat. The cribriform fascia has been removed in the left groin to illustrate the muscle boundaries of the dissection (modified from Cabanas 1977).
Acknowledgment: Illustrations by Jeff Fillbach, Huntington Beach, California.

A wide local excision of the vulvar skin is then performed, ensuring a margin of 3 cm of normal skin on all sides of the primary lesion. Adequate subcutaneous tissue should be taken, especially beneath the primary lesion. It has been our practice to submit both mucous membrane and skin margins as separate specimens.

Hemostasis having been established, a decision must be made as to primary closure of the defect versus the application of a split-thickness skin graft. Where a split-thickness skin graft is used, the graft is usually taken from the medial aspect of the right thigh at eighteen-thousandths of an inch thickness. Using an air-driven dermatome, this can be accomplished quite easily with minimal morbidity. The donor site is dressed with scarlet red gauze and an occlusive pressure dressing is applied. The skin graft is then sutured to the defect using 4-0 PGA suture and a pressure dressing is applied in a manner previously described (Rutledge and Sinclair 1968).

Figure 2.5

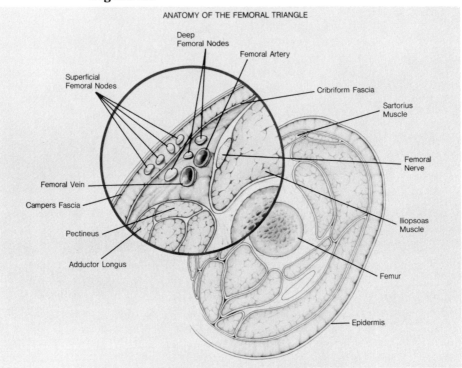

ANATOMY OF THE FEMORAL TRIANGLE

Deep
Femoral Nodes

Femoral Artery

Superficial
Femoral Nodes

Cribriform Fascia

Sartorius
Muscle

Femoral
Nerve

Femoral Vein

Campers Fascia

Iliopsoas
Muscle

Pectineus

Adductor Longus

Femur

Epidermis

*The lymph nodes of interest (sentinel nodes) lie
between Camper's fascia and the cribriform fascia,
as seen in this cross section through the femoral
triangle.*

In DiSaia's series, 18 of the 20 patients with stage I epithelial cancer of the vulva underwent the procedure outlined above. In 11 of the patients, the depth of invasion was between 1 to 3 mm and in the remaining nine patients the depth was between 3 to 5 mm (one patient on subsequent pathologic review had invasion between 6 to 7 mm). In 18 of the patients, the superficial inguinal nodes were found to be negative, and the primary lesion was treated with a wide local excision. These patients have been followed from 14 to 81 months (mean of 39) without evidence of recurrence. Two patients initially meeting the same histologic criteria (the patient with the 6 to 7 mm of invasion was included here) were observed with metastatic disease in the superficial inguinal nodes on the ipsilateral side and these two patients were treated with radical vulvectomy with complete bilateral inguinal and ipsilateral deep pelvic node dissection. Both of these patients had lesions 1 cm in size. One patient has been followed 44 months and the other patient 26 months without having evidence of recurrence. The deep pelvic node dissection on the ipsilateral side was negative in both patients. When these two patients were analyzed using the Parker criteria, both were found to have confluency greater than 1 mm in diameter and one patient had what was considered an anaplastic lesion. Of the 18 patients with negative nodes, 7 had confluency greater than 1 mm in diameter, 2 were anaplastic, and none had unequivocal vascular channel invasion.

Preservation of adequate sexual function in the 18 patients who underwent wide local excision has been complete. A questionnaire was distributed to all 20 patients and their replies are depicted in table 2.3. The patients were questioned concerning orgasmic response and dyspareunia. Those patients who underwent radical vulvectomy reported a significant change in sexual response, whereas this complaint was not elicited from a single patient who underwent a wide local excision. Preservation of the mons veneris with the clitoris as well as the majority of the superior aspect of the vulva obviously resulted in appreciably more satisfactory cosmetic result when patients who received modified surgery were compared with those who received radical vulvectomy.

None of the patients had palpable inguinal nodes of a suspicious variety prior to commencement of surgery. Eight of the patients had palpable inguinal nodes which were not suspicious and only one of the patients subsequently proven to have metastatic disease in the inguinal nodes was among this group. Morbidity from the modified procedure was limited to one patient who developed unilateral lymphedema after an episode of postoperative thrombophlebitis in that same leg. Skin loss occurred at the groin incision in two patients and was minimal.

Comment

It is generally believed that squamous carcinoma of the vulva, like carcinoma of the cervix, originates as an intraepithelial process, then extends laterally and invades deeply over an indeterminate period of time. That noninvasive vulvar carcinoma may be successfully managed by conservative surgery, such as local excision, has been well established. The concept presented here would tend to indicate that there is a category of invasive carcinoma of the vulva that also will respond to less than radical operations. Previous authors have suggested that the same subset of patients exists but they

Table 2.3
Sexual Function—Vulvar Carcinoma

	Number of Patients	Orgasmic Preoperative	Orgasmic Postoperative	Dyspareunia Postoperative
Radical vulvectomy	2	2	0	2
Wide local excision	18	17	17	0

SOURCE: *DiSaia, Creasman, and Rich 1979.*

have advocat d primarily a deletion of the inguinal lymph node dissection. While this certainly does diminish the morbidity for the patient in terms of prolonged hospital stay, skin loss in the groins, and subsequent lymphedema, the major long-term morbidity results from the radical vulvectomy itself. In addition, several case reports of lymphatic disease in inguinal lymph nodes originating from a primary lesion of microinvasive size make this approach less than optimal.

The approach outlined here attempts to gain optimum curability and preserve optimal cosmesis and sexual function. The dissection of the superficial inguinal nodes through small incisions in the groin allows a clearer categorization of patients between the high-risk and low-risk strata. Patients who have early invasive lesions of the vulva which are demonstrated as being vigorous or aggressive in their behavior must be treated by radical vulvectomy. Other early lesions can be suitably managed with a wide local excision and careful follow-up examinations of the remaining vulvar skin. This would allow preservation of many of the most erogenous zones of the female anatomy for more intact body image and apparently minimally altered sexual function.

References

Cabanas, R.M. An approach to the treatment of penile carcinoma. *Cancer* 39:456–466, 1977.

Collins, C.G. et al. Cancer involving the vulva. *Am. J. Obstet. Gynecol.* 87:762–772, 1963.

DiPaola, G.R.; Gomez-Rueda, N.; and Arrighi, L. Relevance of microinvasion in carcinoma of the vulva. *Obstet. Gynecol.* 45:647–649, 1975.

DiSaia, P.J.; Creasman, W.T.; and Rich, W.M. An alternate approach to early cancer of the vulva. *Am. J. Obstet. Gynecol.* 133:825–832, 1979.

Forney, J.P. et al. Management of carcinoma in situ of the vulva. *Am. J. Obstet. Gynecol.* 127:801–806, 1977.

Franklin, E.W. III, and Rutledge, F.N. Epidemiology of epidermoid carcinoma of the vulva. *Obstet. Gynecol.* 39:165–172, 1972.

Gray's Textbook of Anatomy. 29th ed. Philadelphia: Lea and Febiger, 1973.

Hughes, R.P. Early diagnosis and management of premalignant lesions and early invasive cancers of the vulva. *South. Med. J.* 64:1490–1492, 1971.

Jafari, K., and Cartnick, E.N. Microinvasive squamous cell carcinoma of the vulva. *Am. J. Obstet. Gynecol.* 125:274, 1976a.

Jafari, K., and Cartnick, E.N. Microinvasive squamous cell carcinoma of the vulva. *Gynecol. Oncol.* 4:158–166, 1976b.

Magrina, J.F. et al. Microinvasive squamous cell cancer of the vulva. Paper presented to Society of Gynecologic Oncology, Scottsdale, Arizona, January 1979.

Nakao, C.Y. et al. Microinvasive epidermoid carcinoma of the vulva with an unexpected natural history. *Am. J. Obstet. Gynecol.* 120:1122–1123, 1974.

Parker, R.T. et al. Operative management of early invasive epidermoid carcinoma of the vulva. *Am. J. Obstet. Gynecol.* 123:349–355, 1975.

Parry-Jones, E. Lymphatics of the vulva. *J. Obstet. Gynaecol. Br. Comm.* 70:751–765, 1963.

Plentl, A.A., and Friedman, E.A. *Lymphatic system of the female genitalia.* Philadelphia: W. B. Saunders, 1971.

Rutledge, F.N., and Sinclair, M. Treatment of intraepithelial carcinoma of the vulva by skin excision and graft. *Am. J. Obstet. Gynecol.* 102:806–818, 1968.

Way, S., and Hennigan, M. The late results of extended radical vulvectomy for carcinoma of the vulva. *J. Obstet. Gynaecol. Br. Comm.* 73:594–598, 1966.

Wharton, J.T.; Gallagher, S.; and Rutledge, F.N. Microinvasive carcinoma of the vulva. *Am. J. Obstet. Gynecol.* 118:159–162, 1974.

Yazigi, R.; Piver, M.S.; and Tsukada, Y. Microinvasive carcinoma of the vulva. *Obstet. Gynecol.* 51:368–370, 1978.

Chapter 3

*The Role of
Pelvic Lymphadenectomy
in the Treatment of
Invasive Carcinoma
of the Vulva*

PERSPECTIVE:

Arlan F. Fuller, Jr.

Since the time of Basset (1912) and his contemporaries, surgical treatment of carcinoma of the vulva has involved resection of the entire vulva, its lymphatics, and bilateral draining lymph nodes. Rigorous application of the tenets of en bloc resection of the primary site with its lymphatic watershed produced dramatic improvements in survival from this disease and general acceptance of the procedure for virtually all patients with invasive vulvar cancer.

As survival improved, particularly in patients with limited disease, recognition of the morbidity and mortality associated with radical surgery led to attempts at more conservative procedures, occasionally with unfavorable, even catastrophic, results. The contribution of pelvic lymphadenectomy to both morbidity and survival from the therapy of vulvar carcinoma has been a topic of some interest and deserves review from the standpoint of trends in the natural history of the disease and our understanding of the anatomy and pathophysiology of the vulva and its lymphatic system.

Historical Considerations

Evolution of the contemporary operative treatment of vulvar cancer began in the nineteenth century with radical vulvectomy and with recognition by Virchow and others of the role of lymphatics and lymphatic embolism in the dissemination of tumors (Hovnanian 1967). In 1912 Basset recommended en bloc resection of the regional nodes in both groins with resection of carcinoma of the clitoris. Taussig (1936) subsequently evaluated multiple procedures for vulvar carcinoma—radiation therapy, simple vulvectomy, vulvec-

59

tomy with removal of the superficial (inguinofemoral) nodes, and "vulvectomy with double-sided Basset operation." He established the superiority of en bloc lymphadenectomy in a group of 76 patients treated before 1929 with the report of 81% five-year cures with the Basset operation, compared to only 30% where only the superficial glands were removed, and no survivals with radiation therapy or simple vulvectomy. At that time he also reported on a larger, unselected series of 27 patients treated exclusively with the Basset operation. In the inclusive group of 43 patients, the operative mortality was only 4.7% and corrected 5- and 10-year survivals were 65% and 55%, respectively. The extensive nature of the disease in this group of patients was demonstrated by the high frequency of groin node metastasis: 26 of 43 patients (60%) had either one or both groins involved with metastatic carcinoma. He confirmed these results with additional patients in 1940 and established bilateral en bloc inguinofemoral and pelvic lymphadenectomy as the accepted therapy for vulvar cancer. In this later report, Taussig reviewed a number of problems which became foci of later controversy: the association of increasing operative mortality with advancing age and omission of lymphadenectomy in some aged patients, the use of three separate incisions for vulvectomy and node dissections, division of the inguinal ligament during pelvic lymphadenectomy, and limitation of the extent of pelvic lymphadenectomy to obturator and iliac nodes in light of the frequency and pattern of metastases encountered.

Anatomy of the Vulvar Lymphatics

Following the work of Taussig, Way (1951) based more extensive resection of lymphatics and node-bearing tissue upon a detailed review of the lymphatic anatomy of the vulva. He emphasized that the lymphatics arose from a fine network of freely intercommunicating channels which covered the vulva and coalesced laterally as collecting trunks on the lateral surface of the labia majora. Corresponding to the earlier studies described by Reiffenstuhl (Plentl and Friedman 1971), Way described drainage of the lateral trunks directly to the superficial femoral nodes.* Lymphatic drainage from the anterior vulva

---

*To standardize all of the descriptive classifications of lymph nodes, we will adhere to the following definitions:

1. Inguinofemoral (Groin) Nodes
   Inguinal—all nodes superior to the inguinal ligament and superficial to the external oblique fascia.
   Superficial Femoral—all nodes inferior to the inguinal ligament and superficial to the cribriform fascia at the femoral triangle.
   Deep Femoral—all the nodes about the femoral vessels that are deep to the cribriform fascia and inferior to the inguinal ligaments. These form part of the lymphatic drainage of the lower extremity. The "highest" group of these

and mons passed across the inferior aspect of the anterior abdominal wall and drained into the inguinal and superficial femoral nodes, while posterior lymphatic trunks ran along the medial aspect of the labiocrural fold to terminate in the superficial femoral nodes. Extensive anastomoses permitted bilateral drainage after unilateral injection.

The deviation from this pattern in cases of carcinoma of the clitoris has been emphasized by Plentl and Friedman, who have quoted Reiffenstuhl in delineating two pathways of direct metastasis to pelvic nodes. Indeed, of four specimens in which Reiffenstuhl (1964) studied the clitoral lymphatic drainage, the predominant channels drained to the medial superficial femoral nodes, while a secondary pathway of several delicate lymph vessels perforated through the urogenital diaphragm to terminate the pelvic nodes in one patient, and two deep channels ran over the superior border of the pubis to terminate in the deep femoral nodes in another. These secondary efferents from the clitoris could not subsequently be demonstrated with injection studies by Parry-Jones (1963), who did not conclusively demonstrate direct lymphatic drainage to the pelvic nodes at all. A logical explanation for this discrepancy is the source of material: Reiffenstuhl and others have dissected the lymphatics of stillborn children while Parry-Jones studied adults with vulvar cancer. Indeed, those "delicate lymph vessels" perforating the urogenital diaphragm may have become obliterated with age.

An analogous lymphangiographic study by Cabanas (1977) was carried out in men with penile carcinoma and in normal volunteers. He succeeded in demonstrating a sentinel node group in the medial superficial femoral nodes at the junction of the superficial epigastric vein and saphenous system. No direct efferent pathways to pelvic nodes were demonstrated in 100 patients (10 controls, 10 with benign disease, and 80 patients with cancer), and no patient had inguinofemoral metastases without involvement of the sentinel node group.

We may tentatively conclude from anatomic data that the lymphatic drainage from the vulva follows predictable pathways from the primary lesion to the groin. If the primary is unilateral and localized to the labia, the

---

nodes in the femoral canal are referred to as Cloquet's or Rosenmueller's node(s) and lie deep to the inguinal ligament. They represent an anatomically defined subgroup of deep femoral nodes and not necessarily a solitary node.

2. Pelvic Nodes

Iliac—all nodes associated with the external iliac vessels that are superior to the inguinal ligament.

Obturator—all nodes posterior to the iliac vessels, particularly those associated with the obturator vessels and nerves as these structures exit from the inferior pelvis.

Hypogastric—all nodes associated with the internal iliac or hypogastric vessels; these lie just superior to the obturator nodes.

ipsilateral nodes are usually the first to be involved. The superficial inguino-femoral nodes are the first echelon of draining nodes, although some lymphatics may penetrate the cribriform fascia to terminate at the second level, the deep femoral nodes. Lymphatics then pass from the primary and secondary inguinofemoral groups through the femoral canal (although also about the femoral vessels) to drain into the pelvic nodes. Exceptions to this pattern appear to occur only when the pelvic viscera themselves are involved, that is, upper urethra or vagina, where the lymphatic drainage from an advanced vulvar tumor may correspond to that of the organ affected.

Clinical Data

Answers to the following clinical questions should provide sufficient data to make a useful decision as to the costs and benefits of pelvic lymphadenectomy:

1. What is the incidence of inguinofemoral and pelvic lymph node metastases and how can they be expected to change over time?
2. What prognostic factors may delineate patients at increased risk for pelvic lymph node metastasis?
3. What clinical evidence exists that isolated pelvic node metastasis might occur in the absence of inguinofemoral node involvement?
4. What additional morbidity or mortality might be encountered as a result of pelvic lymphadenectomy?
5. What is the survival anticipated in patients with pelvic lymph node metastases and how can that be favorably affected?

To begin with the incidence of node metastasis, it becomes clear that this is closely related to the size and, hence, the stage of tumor; with earlier diagnosis there has been a progressive decrease in both. In the early data reported from the Massachusetts General Hospital (MGH) and Pondville State Cancer Hospital by Green and associates in 1958, 27% of patients seen from 1927 to 1950 could be offered only palliative treatment because of their extensive disease, while in the 25 years from 1951–1976, only 5% of patients were given palliative therapy. Both Basset and Taussig reported a 60% incidence of node metastasis in their early series of patients undergoing complete procedures. This has declined progressively during subsequent series (table 3.1). Moreover, within the two MGH-Pondville series, Green has documented a consistent diminution in the incidence of both groin and pelvic node metastasis (table 3.2), which is attributed to earlier diagnosis.

Examining the relationship between the prevalence of groin and pelvic node metastasis, one can conclude that roughly one-fifth of patients with groin node metastasis will have associated metastases to pelvic nodes. Review of 160 clitoral lesions by Way in 1972 disclosed a relative decrease in lymph node metastasis when these were compared with labial tumors of similar size. Review of patients with clitoral lesions at Roswell Park by Piver

Table 3.1
Incidence of Groin Node Metastasis by
Median Year of Study

Median Year	Author	Incidence (%)	Number of Patients
1925	Taussig	57	155
1942	Green	55	69
1943	Goplerud	46	68
1945	Way	51	100
1949	Way	45	146
1955	Morley	37	180
1956	Rutledge	38	127
1956	Boutselis	36	60
1957	House	26	35
1957	Benedet	28	120
1958	Collins	32	98
1963	Green	38	142

and Xynos (1977) revealed a 50% incidence of groin metastases and an estimate of the ratio of pelvic to groin node metastases of 0.27 from recurrence data: this ratio is not significantly different from those for all vulvar tumors (table 3.3). Piver's data reflected the preponderance of advanced stage lesions in the series rather than an increased risk related to clitoral involvement. Benedet (1979), on the other hand, noted that two of the four patients with pelvic node metastasis had clitoral lesions, but he did not state the extent of disease, noting only that the other two patients had extensive lesions involving the entire vulva. All patients had groin node metastasis as well. Figge (1974) described a 24% incidence of clitoral involvement and no change in the pattern of nodal spread.

Other risk factors predictive of groin node metastasis appear indirectly

Table 3.2
Incidence of Node Metastasis by Interval of
Study (MGH-Pondville Series)

Interval	Number of Patients with Groin Metastasis	%	Number of Patients with Pelvic Metastasis	%
1927–1950	38/69	55	16/69	23
1951–1959	25/47	53		
1960–1972	21/60	35	2/142	1.4
1973–1976	8/35	23		

Adapted from Green 1978.

Table 3.3
Relationship between Groin and Pelvic Node Metastasis

Year	Author	Number of Patients	⊕ Groin/ Number Dissected	⊕ Groin and ⊕ Pelvic/ Number Dissected	Ratio ⊕ Pelvis / ⊕ Groin	⊖ Groin but ⊕ Pelvis
1958a	Green, Ulfelder, and Meigs	238	38/69	16/69	0.42	None
1958b	Green, Ulfelder, and Meigs	142	54/142	2/142	0.04	None
1979	Magrina et al.	106	9/71	1/34	0.11	None
1979	Benedet et al.	204	34/120	4/51	0.12	None
1974	Wharton, Gallagher, and Rutledge	45	5/27	1/13	0.20	None
1968	House and Hester	34	9/34	0/9	0.00	None
1972	Boutselis	90	24/60	7/60	0.29	None
1960	Way	143	65/143	18/143	0.27	5/143
1976	Morley	165	50/157	6/23	0.12	None
1970	Rutledge, Smith, and Franklin	139	33/86	12/71	0.36	None
1978	Krupp and Bohn	195	39/195	9/195	0.23	1*/95
1974	Figge and Gaudenz	50	17/50	5/34	0.29	None

*Lowermost external iliac node in patient with 8 cm lateral vulvar lesion.
⊕ = metastatic involvement.
⊖ = no metastatic involvement.

predictive of pelvic node metastasis as well. The incidence of inguinal node metastasis, for example, ranges from 10% to 20% in most studies when the primary lesion is less than 3 cm in size, rising to 40% or more above 3 cm. Pelvic node metastasis is rare when the primary tumor is less than 3 cm, regardless of location. Anaplastic carcinomas in several series have been associated with an increased risk of node metastasis, but as these tumors are also associated with more advanced stage lesions, this relationship remains unclear.

The morbidity and mortality from the more extensive procedures that routinely extirpate the pelvic nodes are hard to evaluate. Some data in selective cases suggest, however, that the additional operative mortality and the long-term morbidity from leg edema is not inconsequential. The interruption of additional lymphatic collaterals through the pelvis appears to be associated with an increased frequency of leg edema. Parker and associates (1975) described leg swelling in 12 of 26 patients (47%) with groin and pelvic lymphadenectomies, in 3 of 14 patients (22%) with groin lymphadenectomies only, and in no patients with radical vulvectomy alone. Although postoperative regeneration of severed lymphatic channels has been postulated as the reason for resolution of the transient leg edema seen in the majority of patients, it is rather the development of the collateral circulation that is responsible. Although reestablishment of anatomic and functional continuity in transsected lymph vessels can be demonstrated experimentally, this is not true when such segments of lymphatic vessels are resected, as occurs with en bloc lymphadenectomy (Futrell and Pories 1975).

The mortality attributed to the addition of pelvic node dissection may be understated in many series in which it has been employed selectively, as only the better-risk patients would be considered candidates. Further support for this premise in such series comes from evidence for higher rates of death from intercurrent disease in patients undergoing less extensive procedures. Correspondingly, then, the mortality for patients undergoing only inguino-femoral dissection may be overstated, as these may be poorer risk patients. Figge and Gaudenz (1974) reported no operative mortality among 16 patients having only groin node dissections, while 3 of 33 patients having pelvic node dissections died postoperatively. Moreover, the incidence of major complications (27%) among the latter patients with pelvic node dissections was more than twice that of the former group (12.5%). Some of the significance of this data is lost in the recognition that it is a historical comparison, such that the most recent cases had been treated with inguinofemoral dissection alone, unless groin metastases were present. This observation of increasing mortality with more extensive surgery has been supported by Hill in discussion of Figge and Gaudenz's paper (1974) and by Morley (1976), who reported 4 of his 11 operative deaths occurred in the 23 patients undergoing pelvic lymphadenectomy, while only 7 deaths occurred in the other 255 patients not undergoing that procedure. He concluded that "the pelvic lymph node dissection added significantly to the operating time and the risk to the patient, without contributing significantly to the chance of survival." Indeed, in the early MGH-Pondville series, all five deaths among the 100 patients with adequate therapy occurred in those medically high-risk patients undergoing sequential vulvectomy and lymphadenectomy, while only 2 of the 16 patients with pelvic node metastases were cured (Green, Ulfelder, and Meigs 1958a). In the later series of 107 patients evaluated at five years, there were five postoperative deaths (4 occurring in the 44 patients with groin node metastases), and neither of the two patients with pelvic node metastases survived. All five patients who died postoperatively were more than 75 years old.

Based upon a cost benefit analysis, Morris codified his approach to pelvic lymphadenectomy. After noting only two cures in six patients with bilaterally positive groin nodes and an equal number of operative deaths, he advocated selective unilateral inguinofemoral lymphadenectomy in patients with unilateral lesions. Only if these groin nodes contained metastatic cancer would he then proceed to contralateral groin and bilateral pelvic lymphadenectomy. Comparison of patients with negative nodes treated selectively in this manner with those having bilateral groin and pelvic node dissections shows no significant difference in survival; however, the latter are historical controls. For a procedure to be considered beneficial, according to his formula, $a \times b$ must be greater than $c \times d$, where

> a = incidence of positive resectable nodes;
> b = cure rate if positive nodes are removed;
> c = increased operative mortality (applied only to negative node cases);
> d = estimated cure rate if procedure deferred or if radiotherapy employed.

Thus if one can assign arbitrary increases in mortality to more extensive procedures, one may calculate whether a benefit or debit in survival may accrue as a result. The formula emphasized only the therapeutic benefit, disregarding any diagnostic benefit of lymphadenectomy. In the context of research, however, even though the cure rate (b) may be low, identification of patients at increased risk for recurrence will provide an important means of improving survival through protocol studies. One cannot ignore easily obtainable data merely because a ready cure is not yet available; it should be the absolute incidence of node metastases, not necessarily the cure rate, that determines the potential benefit of lymphadenectomy.

Pathophysiology of the Regional Lymph Node and Metastasis

Future prospects for the treatment of the patient with pelvic and inguinofemoral node metastases from vulvar carcinoma merit a careful reassessment of the relationship of the primary draining nodes to a malignancy. Advances in our understanding of the experimental immunobiology of the regional

66

lymph node may have considerable influence upon the management of patients with node metastases.

The traditional concept of the regional lymph node as a passive filter had been fathered by Virchow (1863) in the nineteenth century and emphasized in vulvar cancer by Way, who noted that the nodes formed "very efficient filters capable of holding up structures larger than 2 mm in diameter." He stated that although lymph may bypass one or more nodes in a given group, it never bypasses a complete group of nodes. Anatomically, it appeared impossible for lymph to reach the bloodstream without traversing at least one node; the afferent vessels entered the cortical sinus of the node and passed through its substance, exiting via medullary sinuses to the efferents at the hilum leading to the next group of nodes. The regional draining nodes anatomically and functionally separated the lymphatic and venous systems. They provided a barrier to tumor cells which had invaded lymphatic channels within the primary tumor and then embolized to the subcapsular cortex. The propensity of epithelial tumors for lymphatic rather than venous dissemination was poorly understood.

Fisher and Fisher (1966, 1967a, 1967b) demonstrated for the first time that, although lymph nodes did filter inanimate particles, they did not provide a barrier to the passage of tumor cells. They suggested that early hematogenous dissemination of tumor did occur and concluded that the absence of node metastases was not due to lack of anatomic contact with the tumor cell but rather represented a physiologic state of tumor immunity (1971). Our present understanding of the relationship between the primary tumor and its draining regional nodes in the experimental animal suggests that sensitization to the incipient tumor begins as contact with shed antigen or viable cells occurs. Intact tumor cells presumably do pass into the venous circulation but either fail to implant or are destroyed by host factors. Having processed the antigen and acquired specific cytotoxicity, the regional node then appears to mediate systemic immunization, even as its own cytotoxicity begins to wane (Goldfarb and Hardy 1975).

In squamous cancers of the head and neck in man, evidence suggests that progressive tumor growth is accompanied by a fall in the T:B lymphocyte ratio in all nodes, particularly those draining the tumor; moreover, the lowest T:B ratio is seen in tumor-bearing nodes (Saxon and Portis 1977). Decreasing cytotoxicity in the regional lymph node has been attributed in the past to blocking antibody, or antigen-antibody complexes, but recently Herr has demonstrated that the regional lymph node cells from some patients with bladder cancer inhibit the reactivity of normal and autologous peripheral blood lymphocytes in mixed lymphocyte culture. Putative suppressor cells appeared to be associated with tumor extension beyond the bladder, and their presence was attributed to induction by a high concentration of tumor-related products, possibly antigens or antigen-antibody complexes.

As the tumor progresses, characteristic histologic changes may occur in the draining node which are predictive of the host's prognosis in many carcinomas (Tsakraklides, Anastassiades, and Kersey 1973; Van Nagell et al. 1977). The outlook is best for the patient with a pattern of lymphocyte predominance in the lymph nodes, less satisfactory for the patient with an unstimulated pattern or germinal center predominance, and still worse with the pattern of lymphocyte depletion. Only those patients with actual node metastases have a poorer prognosis.

Both experimental data and an ever-increasing body of clinical evidence suggest that the presence of metastatic carcinoma in the regional lymph nodes mirrors the physiologic state of host immunity rather than the anatomic extent of intralymphatic tumor spread. Recognition of this fact may explain our failure to improve survival in patients with node metastases and such enigmas as the lack of improved survival after lymphadenectomy and irradiation for stage I and II_a carcinoma of the cervix (Fuller et al., in preparation). As recently reviewed by Israel (1978), the tumor-bearing node indicates failure of the host immune control and merits systemic rather than local therapy. In early cases lymphadenectomy may remove tumor bulk and perhaps favorably alter the immune status of the host; but as increasing numbers of nodes become involved with metastatic carcinoma, survival progressively diminishes.

Conclusions and Recommendations

It has become clear that the appearance of node metastases from primary carcinoma follows a consistent pattern which may not be related as much to true anatomic spread of tumor as to localized immunosuppressive effects of the tumor which facilitate local tumor growth. Tumors confined to one labium spread predominantly to the ipsilateral femoral nodes, beginning with the medial superficial femoral nodes and subsequently to deep femoral nodes and, by way of the femoral canal, to iliac and obturator nodes. Bilateral or central lesions may involve either one or both regions. Clitoral lesions are not associated with any variation in the normal pattern of node metastases; lymphatic pathways delineated in the newborn do not appear to function in the adult. Isolated pelvic lymph node metastases are a distinct rarity and should prompt pathologic review of inguinofemoral specimens. Approximately 20% to 25% of patients with inguinofemoral metastases will have pelvic node metastases; these will be rarely associated with tumors less than 3 cm in size. Undifferentiated tumors may be associated with node metastases only insofar as they are associated with large tumors and advanced stage.

It would appear appropriate, first of all, to limit pelvic lymphadenectomy only to patients demonstrating inguinofemoral metastases at frozen section examination of the specimen. As the trend toward earlier diagnosis, and hence earlier stage at diagnosis, continues, fewer patients will require this procedure. In light of increased mortality from the addition of pelvic lymphadenectomy to the treatment of women over 75 years of age, this procedure should be withheld for the high-risk patients until better survival can be demonstrated among younger women with pelvic node metastases. Restating the Morris formula, for the good-risk individual, the modest cost of morbidity easily is justified by the potential benefits of successful treatment that might accrue to all women with pelvic node metastases. An inclusive group at suitable risk appears to be those patients with groin metastases, of whom 20% to 25% will have pelvic node metastases. In light of anecdotal success with Adriamycin (Deppe, Bruckner, and Cohen 1977) and bleomycin (Yahia, Fuller, and Cloud 1978), further experience with an agent active against advanced or recurrent disease might also prove beneficial in an adjuvant setting for patients at high risk of recurrence. Acceptable drug toxicity and activity in patients with pelvic node metastases would then justify subjecting all patients with node metastases to such a protocol.

In 1963 Taussig referred to the indications for radical lymphadenectomy in carcinoma of the breast as the basis for his therapy of vulvar cancer; so, too, should our present understanding of the concepts of adjuvant therapy and regional lymph node biology now be extended to treatment of pelvic lymph node metastases from vulvar carcinoma.

References

Basset, A. Traitement chirurgical opératoire de l'épitheliome primitif du clitoris. *Rev. Chir.* (Paris). 46:546–552, 1912.

Benedet, J.L. et al. Squamous carcinoma of the vulva: results of treatment 1938–1976. *Am. J. Obstet. Gynecol.* 134:201–207, 1979.

Boutselis, J.G. Radical vulvectomy for squamous cell carcinoma of the vulva. *Obstet. Gynecol.* 39:827–836, 1972.

Cabanas, R.M. An approach for the treatment of penile carcinoma. *Cancer* 39:456–466, 1977.

Collins, C.G.; Lee, R.Y.L.; and Roman-Lopez, J.J. Invasive carcinoma of the vulva with lymph node metastasis. *Am. J. Obstet. Gynecol.* 109:446–452, 1971.

Deppe, G.; Bruckner, H.W.; and Cohen, C.J. Adriamycin treatment of advanced vulvar carcinoma. *Obstet. Gynecol.* 50:13s–14s, 1977.

Figge, D.C., and Gaudenz, R. Invasive carcinoma of the vulva. *Am. J. Obstet. Gynecol.* 119:382–395, 1974.

Fisher, B. Present status of the management of regional lymph nodes and planned clinical trials. *Am. J. Roetgenol.* 111:123–129, 1971.

Fisher, B., and Fisher, E.R. Transmigration of lymph nodes by tumor cells. *Science* 152:1397–1398, 1966.

Fisher, B., and Fisher, E. R. The barrier function of the lymph node to tumor cells and erythrocytes. I. Normal nodes. *Cancer* 20:1907–1913, 1967a.

Fisher, B., and Fisher E.R. The barrier function of the lymph node to tumor cells and erythrocytes. II. Effect of x-ray, inflammation sensitization, and tumor growth. *Cancer* 20:1914–1919, 1967b.

Fuller, A.F., Jr. et al. Lymph node metastases from carcinoma of the cervix stages I_b and II_a: implications for prognosis and treatment. In preparation.

Futrell, J.W., and Pories, W.J. Physiologic and immunologic considerations of the lymphatic system in tumors and transplants. *Surg. Gynecol. Obstet.* 140:273–292, 1975.

Goldfarb, P.M., and Hardy, M.B. The immunologic responsiveness of regional lymphocytes in experimental cancer. *Cancer* 35:778–783, 1975.

Goplerud, D.R., and Keetel, W.C. Carcinoma of the vulva. *Am. J. Obstet. Gynecol.* 100:550–553, 1968.

Green, T.H. Carcinoma of the vulva, a reassessment. *Obstet. Gynecol.* 52:462–469, 1978.

Green, T.H.; Ulfelder, H.; and Meigs, J.V. Epidermoid carcinoma of the vulva: an analysis of 238 cases. I. Etiology and diagnosis. *Am. J. Obstet. Gynecol.* 75:834–847, 1958a.

Green, T.H.; Ulfelder, J.; and Meigs, J.V. Epidermoid carcinoma of the vulva: an analysis of 238 cases. II. Therapy and end results. *Am. J. Obstet. Gynecol.* 75:848–864, 1958b.

House, T.E., and Hester, L.L. Radical vulvectomy for carcinoma of the vulva. *Obstet. Gynecol.* 31:739–745, 1968.

Hovanian, A.P. The evolution and present status of pelvi-inguinal lymphatic excision. *Surg. Gynecol. Obstet.* 124:851–865, 1967.

Israel, L. An immunologic look at the TNM classification: therapeutic implications and strategies. *Cancer Treat. Rep.* 62:1177–1182, 1978.

Krupp, P.J., and Bohm, J.W. Lymph gland metastases in invasive squamous cell carcinoma of the vulva. *Am. J. Obstet. Gynecol.* 130:943–952, 1978.

Magrina, J.F. et al. Stage I squamous cell cancer of the vulva. *Am. J. Obstet. Gynecol.* 134:453–459, 1979.

Morley, G.W. Infiltrative carcinoma of the vulva: results of surgical treatment. *Am. J. Obstet. Gynecol.* 124:874–888, 1976.

Morris, J. McL. A formula for selective lymphadenectomy: its application to cancer of the vulva. *Obstet. Gynecol.* 50:152–158, 1977.

Parker, R.T. et al. Operative management of early invasive epidermoid carcinoma of the vulva. *Am. J. Obstet. Gynecol.* 123:349–355, 1975.

Parry-Jones, E. Lymphatics of the vulva. *J. Obstet. Gynaecol. Brit. Comm.* 70:751–765, 1963.

Piver, M.S., and Xynos, F.P. Pelvic lymphadenectomy in women with carcinoma of the clitoris. *Obstet. Gynecol.* 49:592–595, 1977.

Plentl, A.M., and Friedman, E.A. *Lymphatic system of the female genitalia.* Philadelphia: W.B. Saunders, 1971.

Reiffenstuhl, G. *Lymphatics of the female genital organs.* New York: Lippincott, 1964. Translation of *Das lymphsystem des weiblidren genitare.*

Rutledge, F.; Smith, J.P.; and Franklin, E.W. Carcinoma of the vulva. *Am. J. Obstet. Gynecol.* 106:1117–1130, 1970.

Saxon, A., and Portis, J. Lymphoid subpopulation changes in regional lymph nodes in squamous head and neck cancer. *Cancer Res.* 37:1154–1158, 1977.

Taussig, F.J. Late results in the treatment of leukoplakic vulvitis and cancer of the vulva. *Am. J. Obstet. Gynecol.* 31:746–754, 1936.

Taussig, F.J. Cancer of the vulva. *Am. J. Obstet. Gynecol.* 10:764–779, 1940.

Tsakraklides, V.; Anastassiades, O.T.; and Kersey, J.H. Prognostic significance of regional lymph node histology in uterine cervical cancer. *Cancer* 31:860–868, 1973.

Van Nagell, J.R. et al. The prognostic significance of pelvic lymph node morphology in carcinoma of the cervix. *Cancer* 39:2624–2632, 1977.

Virchow, R. *Cellular pathology* London: J.A. Churchill, Ltd., 1863.

Way, S. *Malignant disease of the female genital tract.* Philadelphia: The Blakiston Co., 1951.

Way, S. Carcinoma of the vulva. *Am. J. Obstet. Gynecol.* 79:692–697, 1960.

Way, S. Anatomic pathology of vulvar cancer. In *Aspects and treatment of vulvar cancer, first international symposium, Madrid, 1971.* Basel: Karger, 1972.

Wharton, J.T.; Gallagher, S.; and Rutledge, F.N. Microinvasive carcinoma of the vulva. *Am. J. Obstet. Gynecol.* 118:159–162, 1974.

Yahia, C.; Fuller, A.F., Jr.; and Cloud, L.P. Successful longterm palliation of Stage IV vulvar carcinoma with operation and bleomycin sulfate. *Am. J. Obstet. Gynecol.* 130:360–361, 1978.

PERSPECTIVE:

The Role of Pelvic Lymphadenectomy in the Treatment of Invasive Carcinoma of the Vulva

Stephen L. Curry

Since the beginning of this century surgery has been the primary therapy of invasive carcinoma of the vulva. To date there are no effective chemotherapeutic agents, and radiotherapy is of limited value because of the nature of the vascular supply of the vulva and the severe local necrosis that results with cancerocidal radiation doses. Thus surgery is the only valid therapeutic alternative.

The major controversy over the last decade has concerned the extent of the surgical procedure necessary in a given stage and cell type of vulvar cancer to ensure the highest chance of cure with the least complications. All concur that radical vulvectomy should be part of every operation for cure of invasive cancer of the vulva. Surgeons such as Taussig (1940), Collins and associates (1963), and Way and Hennigan (1966) realized that the spread of disease was primarily lymphatic and advocated bilateral groin and deep pelvic node dissection in all cases because they observed numerous patients with both groin and deep pelvic node metastases. Their survival statistics were impressive when compared with previous results; however, the operative mortality and long-term morbidity were also significant. With the advent of improved postoperative care including intravenous fluids, blood transfusions, better understanding of fluid and electrolyte management, antibiotics and prophylactic use of anticoagulation, the operative mortality and morbidity have been greatly reduced. Major problems remain, and recent authors have become more aware of the necessity of tailoring surgical treatment adequately to treat the disease with the least number of complications (Rutledge, Smith, and Franklin 1970; Morris 1977).

The lymphatics of the vulva are described in Plentl and Friedman's textbook (1971). The anatomic studies would indicate that direct extension to the pelvic lymph nodes is likely not only for lesions located in the clitoral region but also in those where the lower third of the vagina or the perineal region is involved. These studies are used by many authors to justify the need for deep pelvic node dissection in all cases of vulvar carcinoma. According to recent clinical data, however, no positive correlation exists between the potential spread as indicated by anatomic findings and the actual spread as revealed by histopathologic findings (Morris 1977; Piver and Xynos 1977; Curry, Wharton, and Rutledge 1980).

A review of the literature identifies two opinions in regard to the usefulness of deep pelvic node dissection in all cases of invasive carcinoma of the vulva: the traditional teaching that all patients with invasive carcinoma of the vulva should have a radical vulvectomy with inguinal, femoral, and deep pelvic node dissection (Gusberg and Frick 1978), and the more recent recommendation that deep pelvic node dissection should only be included when the perineum, vagina, clitoris, or inguinal lymph nodes are histologically proven to be involved (McGowan 1978). The latter group would also include any patient with melanoma of the vulva regardless of size or area of involvement.

Although no conclusive data exist establishing definite increased morbidity with bilateral pelvic node dissection, many authors believe that prolonged surgical time with all of its inherent problems and severe lower extremity lifelong lymphedema are directly related to this part of the operation (Rutledge, Smith, and Franklin 1970; Morris 1977; McGowan 1978). In table 3.4 a review of the data from the M. D. Anderson Hospital and Tumor Institute showed a two-fold increase in both mild and severe lower extremity lymphedema when pelvic lymphadenectomy was added to the procedure (Curry, Wharton, and Rutledge, 1980).

Because there are no prospective studies that adequately answer the question of the need for pelvic lymphadenectomy in all patients, retrospective analysis of data in the literature will be used. In addition, the need for pelvic lymphadenectomy is assessed as it pertains to the histology, the site of the primary lesion, and the involvement of groin lymph nodes.

Table 3.4
M. D. Anderson Hospital and Tumor
Institute Incidence of Lymphedema Following
Surgery for Vulvar Carcinoma

	With Deep Nodes Removed (No./%)	**Without Deep Nodes Removed (No./%)**
Total patients	112	78
Mild edema	25/23%	6/8%
Severe edema	35/31%	13/16%
Total edema	60/54%	19/24%

SOURCE: *Curry, Wharton, and Rutledge 1980.*

Histology of the Primary Lesion

Recent data by Wharton, Gallagher, and Rutledge (1974) and Parker and associates (1975) indicate that squamous lesions of less than 2 cm in diameter with less than 5 mm of invasion and no evidence of vascular channel invasion have no risk of lymph node metastases and therefore can be treated with radical vulvectomy alone. Although not pertinent to the immediate problem discussed in this chapter, one must keep in mind that others have indicated that there is a more significant risk of lymph node metastasis than that reported by Wharton, thus, whether or not groin node dissection is carried out may depend not only on the size of the lesion and depth of invasion but also on the overall medical status of the patient (DiPaola, Gomez-Rueda, and Arrighi 1975).

There are data in the literature to indicate that the differentiation of a primary squamous carcinoma of the vulva is predictive of lymph node involvement. Anaplastic lesions tend to be larger and endophytic rather than exophytic, thus giving a higher incidence of groin node metastasis than do well-differentiated lesions. They do not, however, show abnormal patterns of histologic spread (Way 1960).

The dictum that all patients with melanoma of the vulva should have bilateral inguinal and pelvic node dissection as part of their treatment is based on a single case reported in the literature of Way. He discusses a patient with melanoma with deep pelvic node metastases and negative inguinal nodes. It became commonly accepted that since melanoma is an extremely virulent malignancy, extensive surgical extirpation of lymphatics is necessary for cure to be achieved. In fact there is evidence in the literature that vaginal melanoma, either primary or from vulvar extension, has an extremely poor prognosis, indicating a high probability of widespread disease at the time of treatment (DiSaia and Morrow 1975). Vulvar melanoma, on the other hand, especially in localized lesions, has a prognosis similar to squamous lesions with the standard surgical treatment (Morrow and DiSaia 1976). Since no prospective data are available, one is left to assume that the more extensive surgery usually performed is a function of the single case report by Way and the individual surgeon's anxiety upon learning the natural history of the disease. As in other sites, melanoma of the vulva can spread not only lymphatically but subdermally and hematogenously, and extensive lymph node metastases occur early in the course of disease. Recent data indicate that classification of depth of invasion can be applied to the vulva and thus be useful in predicting the amount of surgery necessary for cure (Chung, Woodruff, and Lewis 1975). Thus there is no strong evidence that direct spread to the deep pelvic nodes is a problem unless the vagina or the groin nodes are involved. Consequently need for pelvic node dissection should be a function of Clarks classification, extravulvar extension, or positive groin nodes rather than the histologic diagnosis of melanoma alone.

Site of the Primary Lesion

Morris recently reviewed the entire literature on the surgical approach to carcinoma of the vulva and found only three papers in which direct metastases to the pelvic lymph nodes without inguinal lymph node involvement were noted. None of the three reports mentions any data as to the size, location, or histologic presentation of the primary lesion (Collins et al. 1963; Way 1960; Merrill and Ross 1961). In a subsequent paper Collins's group further discussed his patients and showed diagrams grossly depicting the area of the vulva involved (Collins, Leww, and Roman-Lopez 1971). One is left with the impression that vaginal involvement was present in the majority of lesions.

Recent textbooks (McGowan 1978; DeSaia, Morrow, and Townsend 1975) continue to recommend that clitoral involvement should remain as an indication for deep pelvic node dissection. The report of Piver and substantiating data from a recent review by this author of cases of carcinoma of the vulva treated at the M. D. Anderson Hospital and Tumor Institute in Houston, Texas indicate that clitoral involvement alone is associated neither with direct extension to the deep pelvic nodes without groin involvement nor with an increased incidence of pelvic node involvement when compared with other sites on the vulva, even when the groin nodes are involved.

Other anatomic sites often mentioned as indication for pelvic node dissection include vaginal and/or perineal lesions. Again there is no conclusive evidence that this parameter alone is associated with a different spread pattern. In the M. D. Anderson series no patients had pelvic node metastases unless the groin nodes were involved. Therefore it appears that location per se of the vulvar lesion is not an indicator of the need for pelvic node dissection.

Involvement of the Inguinal Lymph Nodes

Morris (1977) has long been an advocate of selective lymphadenectomy in carcinoma of the vulva. His data indicate that the size of the lesion, its location in the vulva, and the involvement of the inguinal lymph nodes, along with an assessment of the general medical status of the patient, should dictate the extent of surgical treatment of vulvar carcinoma. Following statistical analysis he discouraged routine bilateral inguinal lymphadenectomy in unilateral vulvar disease which had not crossed the midline. In his opinion such extensive surgery may result in an actual loss of life, to say nothing of the unnecessary swollen legs and prolonged hospitalization in elderly women. He concluded that if superficial ipsilateral dissection shows no positive nodes, further dissection is ill advised.

Green's data (1978) showed that if one evaluates the location and number of positive lymph nodes it can be shown that patients with less than three unilaterally positive groin nodes have a much better prognosis than those with greater than three positive nodes in one groin, bilateral groin nodes, or deep pelvic node metastases. He cautioned, however, that a significant percentage of patients with histologically reported negative lymph nodes may in fact have microscopic disease undetected by the pathologist. He quotes figures of up to 20% in his report for false negative nodes in vulvar cancer. This paralleled recent data from breast cancer studies where multiple sections of lymph nodes increase the incidence of microscopic nodal involvement (Fisher et al. 1978).

The author's recently published paper on lymph node status in vulvar cancer indicates that finding three or less positive nodes in one groin portends to 68% survival, whereas greater than three unilaterally positive nodes was uniformly fatal. None of those patients reported in table 3.5 had positive pelvic nodes. More importantly, no patient had positive pelvic nodes where three or less positive nodes were found in one groin. When four or more unilateral nodes were present, however, 50% of the patients had positive pelvic nodes. Similarly positive groin nodes bilaterally, regardless of the number, were associated with a 26% incidence of deep pelvic node involvement. The survival when deep pelvic nodes were present was 22%, which is consistent with other series reported in the literature (Way and Hennigan 1966; Morris 1977; Green 1978). Both patients who survived five years, however, had a single microscopically positive pelvic node, and both died of recurrent disease after five years.

Recommendations

All data pertaining to the efficacy of pelvic node dissection as a part of the primary treatment of invasive carcinoma of the vulva are retrospective. A large prospective study is presently being conducted by the Gynecologic On-

Table 3.5
Survival by Number of Unilateral
Positive Groins

Number Positive Nodes in Groin	Total Number	Survivors	Percentage
1	16	11	69
2	5	3	60
3	4	3	75
>3	5	0	0
Totals	30	17	57

SOURCE: *Curry, Wharton, and Rutledge 1980.*

cology Group, and more accurate information should be available as to the likelihood and prognosis of pelvic lymph node metastases in squamous cell carcinoma of the vulva.

In the meantime, retrospective literature reviews indicate that regardless of histology, area of vulvar involvement, or status of the inguinal lymph nodes, no clinical data exist indicating that pelvic lymphadenectomy should be a part of the operative procedure for all patients with invasive carcinoma of the vulva. Recent data from M. D. Anderson and Piver report that clitoral involvement alone is not necessarily a primary indication for pelvic lymphadenectomy. Green and Curry's reports suggest that the number of inguinal lymph nodes involved and the location of the positive nodes, unilateral versus bilateral, can give a definite indication of the risk of positive deep pelvic nodes.

With present knowledge it is recommended that patients with squamous lesions less than 2 cm in diameter, with less than 5 mm of invasion, and no vascular involvement, be treated with radical vulvectomy alone. All patients with invasive carcinoma of the vulva, either squamous or melanoma, undergo a radical vulvectomy as primary treatment for cure of their disease. Unless life-threatening medical indications intervene, bilateral inguinal lymphadenectomy should also be carried out. If histologically positive nodes are present on frozen section at the time of surgery, then one must either perform pelvic node dissection or postoperative radiation of the pelvis. Should the final histology report indicate more than three unilaterally positive nodes or bilaterally positive nodes, either reoperation for bilateral pelvic node dissection or radiation to the whole pelvis should be considered. The role of postoperative irradiation is yet to be determined in patients with three or less positive lymph nodes unilaterally and unsuspected at the time of surgery.

References

Chung, A.F.; Woodruff, J.N.; and Lewis, J.L. Malignant melanoma of the vulva, a report of 44 cases. *Obstet. Gynecol.* 45:638–646, 1975.

Collins, C.G. et al. Cancer involving the vulva: a report on 109 consecutive cases. *Am. J. Obstet. Gynecol.* 87:762–772, 1963.

Collins, C.G.; Leww, F.Y.L.; and Roman-Lopez, J.J. Invasive carcinoma of the vulva with lymph node metastasis. *Am. J. Obstet. Gynecol.* 109:446–452, 1971.

Curry, S.L.; Wharton, J.T.; and Rutledge, F. Positive lymph nodes in vulvar squamous carcinoma. *Gynecol. Oncol.* 9:63–67, 1980.

DiPaola, G.R.; Gomez-Rueda, N.; and Arrighi, L. Relevance of micro-invasion in carcinoma of the vulva. *Obstet. Gynecol.* 45:647–649, 1975.

DiSaia, P.J.; Morrow, C.P.; and Townsend, D.E. *Synopsis of gynecologic oncology.* New York: John Wiley and Sons, 1975.

Fisher, E.R. et al. Detection and significance of occult axillary node metastasis in patients with invasive breast cancer. *Cancer* 42:2025–2031, 1978.

Green, T.H. Carcinoma of the vulva, a reassessment. *Obstet. Gynecol.* 52:462–469, 1978.

Gusberg, S.B., and Frick, H.C. *Corscaden's gynecologic cancer.* Baltimore: Williams & Wilkins, 1978.

McGowan, L. *Gynecologic oncology.* New York: Appleton-Century-Crofts, 1978.

Merrill, J.A. and Ross, N.L. Cancer of the vulva. *Cancer* 14:13–20, 1961.

Morris, J.M. A formula for selective lymphadenectomy, its application in cancer of the vulva. *Obstet. Gynecol.* 50:152–158, 1977.

Morrow, C.P., and DiSaia, P.J. Malignant melanoma of the female genitalia: a clinical analysis. *Obstet. Gynecol. Surv.* 31:233–271, 1976.

Parker, R.T. et al. Operative management of early invasive epidermoid carcinoma of the vulva. *Am. J. Obstet. Gynecol.* 123:349–355, 1975.

Piver, M.S., and Xynos, F.P. Pelvic lymphadenectomy in women with carcinoma of the clitoris. *Obstet. Gynecol.* 49:592–595, 1977.

Plentl, A.A., and Friedman, E.A. *Lymphatic system of the female genitalia.* Philadelphia: W.B. Saunders, 1971.

Rutledge, F.; Smith, J.P.; and Franklin, E.W. Carcinoma of the vulva. *Am. J. Obstet. Gynecol.* 106:1117–1130, 1970.

Taussig, F.J. Cancer of the vulva: an analysis of 155 cases. *Am. J. Obstet. Gynecol.* 40:764–779, 1940.

Way, S. Carcinoma of the vulva. *Am. J. Obstet. Gynecol.* 79:692–697, 1960.

Way, S., and Hennigan, M. The late results of extended radical vulvectomy for carcinoma of the vulva. *J. Obstet. Gynaecol. Br. Comm.* 73:594–598, 1966.

Wharton, J.T.; Gallagher, S.; and Rutledge, F.N. Microinvasive carcinoma of the vulva. *Am. J. Obstet. Gynecol.* 118:159–162, 1974.

PART II

DES:
WHAT ARE THE
EFFECTS?

During the 1940s many physicians prescribed synthetic, nonsteroidal estrogens (diethylstilbestrol) to pregnant women with histories of spontaneous abortion, diabetes, or toxemia of pregnancy. In 1971, a link was reported between maternal diethylstilbestrol (DES) therapy during pregnancy and the occurrence of clear cell adenocarcinoma of the vagina in females exposed to this drug in utero. In all cases of malignancy for which precise information is available, the drug was initiated before the eighteenth week of gestation. As little as 1.5 mg of DES administered daily throughout pregnancy has been associated with subsequent cancer in female offspring.

The number of pregnant women treated with DES or chemically-related compounds during pregnancy has been estimated at about 2 million, but only 200 to 300 cases of adenocarcinoma of the vagina have been reported in the female offspring of these women. The risk of adenocarcinoma in an exposed woman under 30 years of age appears to be minimal in view of the large exposed population and the low incidence of the disease reported. Because women have developed adenocarcinoma of the vagina without exposure in utero to synthetic, nonsteroidal estrogens, other factors must play a role in the etiology of these tumors.

Recent attention has focused on the nonneoplastic developmental abnormalities associated with in utero exposure to DES. A variety of benign changes of the uterus, cervix, and vagina have been cataloged. The fate of men exposed in utero also recently has been addressed. Dr. Sandberg provides an analysis of the abnormalities encountered in a large population of exposed females examined regularly for almost a decade. Recommendations for appropriate screening intervals, the examination of exposed males, and the medicolegal aspects of the problem are discussed. Of particular importance is a description of the wide variety of changes observed in the cervix and vagina of exposed women.

The complementary discussion by Dr. Nordqvist includes a detailed discussion of the embryology of the female reproductive apparatus together with an analysis of the effect of a variety of hormones administered to pregnant laboratory animals. An attempt is then made to correlate the laboratory data with observed changes in the human population.

These effects of DES, unknown a decade ago, have surfaced after painstaking observation and description of women exposed in utero. Although the ultimate consequences of exposure are unknown, an increasing awareness of the potential results of hormonal manipulation during pregnancy already exists.

Chapter 4

DES Exposure in Utero: What Are the Effects?

PERSPECTIVE:

Eugene C. Sandberg

During the last decade a number of uncommon conditions, including a few never previously described, have been found in the reproductive tract of many women born in the United States since 1940. The majority are benign and appear to have only a limited effect on sexual and reproductive function. One, however, is malignant and appears in the form of clear cell adenocarcinoma. Both the benign and malignant conditions have been found most often in individuals embryologically exposed to diethylstilbestrol (DES). Not every exposed woman is affected, however, nor can all women affected be shown to have been exposed. On this basis it is apparent that a direct cause-and-effect relationship does not exist. Nonetheless, an association between exposure to DES in utero and the presence of these conditions has been accepted as incontrovertible. The effects purported to result from exposure to DES in utero are outlined in tables 4.1 through 4.5. (The social, political, psychological, and economic effects of exposure to DES in utero will not be examined, although their importance equals or transcends many of the effects listed in these tables.) Information relative to each is developed in the notes. In addition, many of the teratologic effects are pictured in figures 4.1 through 4.4.

The conditions reputed to be associated with exposure to DES in utero have appeared only in women. (The single and contradicted report to the contrary is described in table 4.2, note‡.) These conditions have been restricted to organs derived from the Müllerian duct, the vagina, cervix, uterus, and tubes. Neither benign nor malignant conditions have been found in the appendix testis or the prostatic utricle, remnants of the Müllerian ducts in the male. Although unproved, it is generally accepted that all the benign conditions have been embryologically, and not postnatally, derived. All malignancies have developed many years following birth.

Clear cell carcinoma is an uncommonly occurring cancer. In unexposed

Figure 4.1

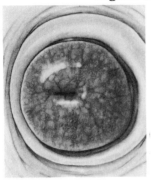

A
Type I Cervix (36%)*

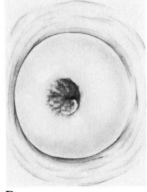

B
Type II Cervix (7%)†

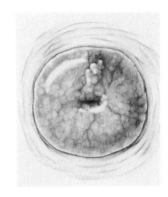

C
Type III Cervix (7%)‡

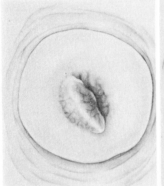

D
Sessile Polyp (5%)§

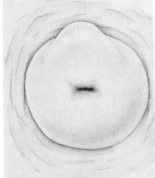

E
Anterior Cervical
Protuberance (14%)||

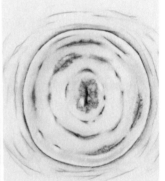

F
Concentric Sulci (1%)#

Types and approximate incidence of
cervical changes seen in women exposed to
DES in utero. (Stippled areas represent
columnar epithelium and are red in color
on gross examination.) (Sandberg 1976.
Reprinted by permission.)

*An arclike or completely circular sulcus separates the central periorificial area from the outer exocervical rim. Surfaces may be covered with either squamous or columnar epithelium.

†A recessed periorificial area is present which resembles a conically patulous lower endocervical canal. The exocervix may be covered with either squamous or columnar epithelium.

‡The exocervix is totally covered with columnar epithelium from external os to cervicovaginal junction.

§A broad-based and localized hypertrophy of endocervical tissue arises at the margin of the external os.

||A localized hypertrophy of exocervical tissue is inexplicably limited to the anterior exocervix. The form may be smooth (as shown) or irregular.

#Arclike depressions are arranged in a manner suggesting several circular sulci of differing diameters.

84

Figure 4.2

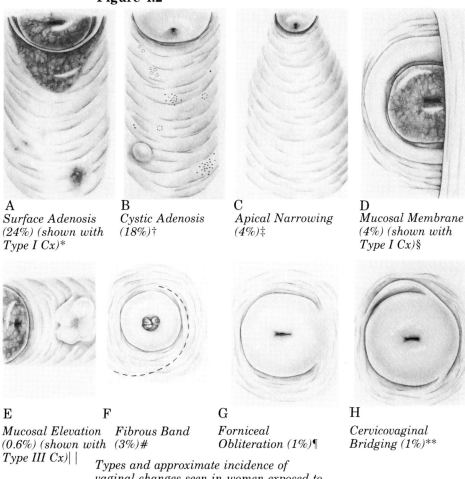

A
Surface Adenosis
(24%) (shown with
Type I Cx)*

B
Cystic Adenosis
(18%)†

C
Apical Narrowing
(4%)‡

D
Mucosal Membrane
(4%) (shown with
Type I Cx)§

E
Mucosal Elevation
(0.6%) (shown with
Type III Cx)| |

F
Fibrous Band
(3%)#

G
Forniceal
Obliteration (1%)¶

H
Cervicovaginal
Bridging (1%)**

Types and approximate incidence of
vaginal changes seen in women exposed to
DES in utero. (Stippled areas represent
columnar epithelium and are red in color
on gross examination.) (Sandberg 1976.
Reprinted by permission.)

*Areas of the vaginal surface are covered with columnar, mucus-producing epithelium. This is most commonly seen in the anterior and posterior fornices. The earlier the embryonic exposure to DES, the higher the incidence of adenosis (e.g., ≤ 8 weeks, 73%; 9 to 12 weeks, 49%; 13 to 16 weeks, 29%; and after 17 weeks, 7% [Herbst et al. 1975]).

†Cystically dilated, mucus-producing glands beneath the vaginal epithelium range from one millimeter to several centimeters in diameter.

‡The proximal end of the vagina is conically constricted.

§A veil-like strip of anteroposteriorly oriented vaginal mucosa hides the fornix and often a portion of the exocervix. Nearly all are seen on the left.

| |A raised area in the form of a bowl or corolla appears exclusively on the lateral vaginal wall close to the cervix and is covered by squamous epithelium.

#An invisible, circular or semicircular, wirelike stand of fibrous tissue can be detected beneath the mucosa upon spreading the examining fingers intravaginally.

¶A broad band of squamous mucosa attaches the crown of the exocervix to the adjacent vaginal surface, obliterating a portion of the fornix.

**A narrow, arclike bridge of squamous mucosa connects the cervix to the nearby vaginal wall.

85

women it has been reported to develop in the vagina, cervix, uterine fundus, and ovary. Among women exposed to DES in utero, however, it has been described only in the vagina and cervix. Clear cell carcinoma has not been seen to develop in the fallopian tubes or to occur in males, either exposed or unexposed.

In 1939 Schiller introduced the term mesonephroma to describe an ovarian tumor the architecture of which he considered to recapitulate mesonephric glomeruli. It was later convincingly shown (Teilum 1959) that Schiller had described two tumors, one a true mesonephroma and the other a tumor of germ cell origin now referred to as an endodermal sinus tumor or embryonal carcinoma. Histologically, the true mesonephroma is characterized by hobnail-shaped tumor cells arranged in the form of cysts and tubules, plus solid masses of clear cells resembling those of renal cell carcinoma. In a few such tumors, a histologic transition from benign mesonephric epithelium has been demonstrated (Hart and Norris 1972). Nonetheless, the currently pre-

Figure 4.3

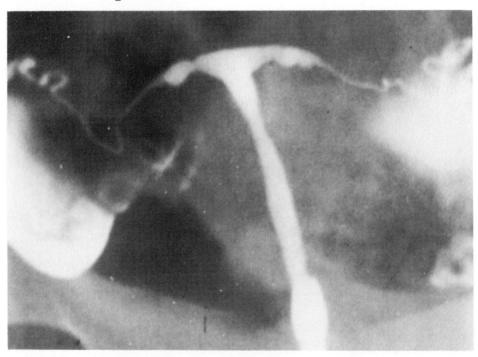

Hysterosalpingogram from exposed patient showing T-shaped uterine cavity. The uterine fundus is linearly narrowed, and vertically arranged constrictions are noted in the uterine horns (Kaufman et al. 1977. Reprinted by permission.)

dominant opinion is that the majority of tumors with this histologic appearance are derived from Müllerian, not mesonephric, epithelium.

It was on the basis of the supporting evidence for this conclusion that Scully and Barlow (1967) suggested that tumors of this histologic description which could not be clearly shown to arise from mesonephric remnants be called clear cell carcinomas. They noted that pelvic endometriosis had been found in 53% of their series of 17 unselected cases of ovarian mesonephroma but was present in only 7% of patients with other types of ovarian cancer. Additionally, in nearly a dozen cases they were able to demonstrate that the tumor arose from the lining of benign endometrial cysts. Some tumors were mixed with endometrioid carcinoma, and frequent examples of histologic transition between mesonephroma and endometrioid adenocarcinoma were seen. Additional evidence of origination from endometrial epithelium was found in an endocervical mesonephroma in which a histologic transition from "glands of endometrial type" could be demonstrated. Tumor with the same

Figure 4.4

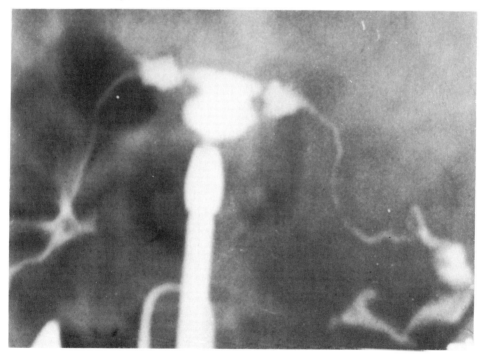

Hysterosalpingogram from exposed patient showing narrow, transversely arranged constriction in the upper uterine fundus and vertically arranged constrictions in the uterine horns (Kaufman et al. 1977. Reprinted by permission.)

87

histologic appearance has also been seen to arise in endometrial implants outside the reproductive organs (Goldberg et al. 1978).

In a recent study of 21 clear cell cancers of the endometrium, Kurman and Scully (1976) described several tumors in which typical endometrial adenocarcinoma (with small foci of benign squamous epithelium) was mixed with clear cell carcinoma. Moreover, 3 of the 21 tumors were confined to the endometrium, 2 within otherwise benign endometrial polyps.

Scully and Barlow (1967) pointed out, however, that the tubular and cystic architecture noted in these tumors is a frequent finding in epithelial tumors of diverse origin and is not pathognomonic of histogenesis. Clear cells are also nonspecific and have been demonstrated in tumors of the salivary gland, lung, skin, parathyroid, thyroid, stomach, epididymis, and kidney. Consequently, evidence for origination of the histologic pattern of clear cell carcinoma from both mesonephric remnants and Müllerian tissues should not be disconcerting.

Clear cell carcinomas originating in the vagina, cervix, endometrium, and ovary are indistinguishable from one another on both light microscopy and ultrastructural examination (Silverberg and DeGiorgi 1972; Puri et al. 1977). No difference is noted in clear cell tumors occurring in exposed and unexposed individuals.

Not all tumors reported to the Registry for Research on Transplacental Carcinogenesis (previously the Registry of Clear Cell Adenocarcinoma of the Genital Tract in Young Females) have been of the classical clear cell variety. In some, the characteristic clear cells and hobnail-shaped cells have been absent or difficult to find. As might be anticipated from the observations above, these tumors have had the appearance of poorly differentiated carcinoma or have resembled in "various degrees the classical adenocarcinoma of the uterine corpus" (Scully, Robboy, and Herbst 1974). One of the tumors in the eight patients described in the original report linking vaginal cancer to DES exposure in utero was regarded as an endometrioid carcinoma (Herbst, Ulfelder, and Poskanzer 1971).

Vaginal adenosis is a condition in which glandular epithelium of Müllerian origin is present either in or on the wall of the vagina. (Some investigators have expanded the definition to include the presence in or below the vaginal epithelium of mucin or metaplastic squamous epithelium. They argue that mucin in this area can only have been derived from previously existing cells of adenosis. Moreover, as squamous metaplasia is the physiologic process by which ectopically located endocervical epithelium is eliminated, squamous metaplasia will be seen only in areas where this epithelium previously existed. While intuitively appealing, these definitional assumptions remain unproved.) When subepithelial in location and not distended with mucin, the glands of adenosis are hidden and impalpable, as are similar glands in the substance of the exocervix. When on the wall of the vagina, the glandular epithelium forms the vaginal surface; a single layer of adenomatous cells takes the place of the usual stratified squamous epithelium. This

88

one-cell-thick layer of mucin-producing cells is grossly invisible and is identical to the surface of cervical ectropion in all regards. The gross appearance in both situations is that of the color and texture of the underlying capillary bed.

The incidence of occult adenosis approximates 40% in unexposed postpubertal women (Sandberg 1968). The incidence of occult adenosis in exposed women has not been determined. Surface adenosis is detected in fewer than 1% of unexposed women (Gunning and Ostergard 1976; Ng et al. 1975; Herbst et al. 1975) but is present in at least 25% to 40% of those exposed (Sandberg 1976; Herbst et al. 1975; Wu et al. 1980).

Among tumor-free exposed patients undergoing screening examinations, surface adenosis is found with greatest frequency anteriorly and posteriorly in the upper one-third of the vagina. Most vaginal clear cell cancers have developed in these areas. Furthermore, histologic evidence of adenosis has been found in examinable adjacent vaginal tissues in nearly all exposed patients whose clear cell carcinoma has been treated surgically (Herbst et al. 1974). For these reasons, many have considered adenosis to be the progenitor of clear cell carcinoma.

Adenosis is most commonly composed of mature endocervical cells. Cancer arising from this epithelium would be expected to be of the classical mucin-producing endocervical variety. In fact, histologic transition from benign vaginal adenosis to typical endocervical adenocarcinoma has been demonstrated (Sandberg et al. 1965). In the case reported, primary and metastatic tumors were histologically identical, and both were mucin-secreting. On the other hand, Hill (1973) has reported a patient about whom he described a transition from benign adenosis to a tubuloacinar variety of clear-cell carcinoma. The histologic appearances of the patient's vaginal recurrence (papillary pattern) and cervical lymph node metastasis (adenomatous pattern) were different, and different from that in the original tumor. Clear cells were not described, and the presence or absence of mucin or glycogen was not mentioned. No other histologic transition from benign adenosis to invasive tumor has been described. A transition from benign to malignant epithelium in a single gland of adenosis has recently been reported, however, in a patient with papillary adenocarcinoma of the vagina (Ballon et al. 1979).

Scully, Robboy, and Herbst (1974) have described what they consider at the light microscopy level to be endometrial and tubal epithelial cells in some areas of adenosis. Fenoglio and associates (1976) appear to have confirmed this observation by electron microscopy. In 2 of 32 specimens of adenosis (6%), they observed glands containing a mixture of endocervical cells and cells identical to those in the endometrium. They failed, however, to note any cells of the tubal variety.

In a recent report of findings in 3339 exposed patients being followed in the National Cooperative Diethylstilbestrol Adenosis (DESAD) Project (Robboy et al. 1979), histologically defined tuboendometrial cells were diagnosed in 21% of all biopsy specimens of adenosis. The incidence varied with location of the adenosis. For example, tuboendometrial cells were seen in 20% of biopsies of adenosis obtained from the upper vagina, in 31% of those from the mid-vagina, and in 100% of those from the lower vagina. Tuboendometrial cells were seen in 28% of biopsies of adenosis from the anterior wall, in 18% and 14% from the lateral walls, and 12% from the posterior wall. (Among cervical biopsies positive for ectropion, tuboendometrial cells were found in only 3% of specimens.) Tuboendometrial cells were present in 40% of biopsies in which adenosis was present in the subepithelial tissues but were only rarely found in adenosis confined to the vaginal surface.

If adenosis is the progenitor of clear cell carcinoma in exposed patients, the endometrial component is currently felt to be the most likely cell of origin (Scully, Robboy, and Welch 1978). Atypical versions of these cells have been described in surgical specimens from patients with clear cell carcinoma (Robboy et al. 1977) and may represent a transitional stage. To date, however, a transition from adenosis to clear cell carcinoma has not been demonstrated in any of the 389 cases reported to the Registry. Additional evidence against this theory of origination is the observation that while some endometrial cancers are responsive to hormonal therapy, clear cell carcinoma is not. At least none of the nine clear cell tumors treated exclusively with progestational agents has shown regression (Herbst et al. 1979a).

Only a small fraction of exposed female offspring develop clear cell carcinoma. It is apparent from this that factors other than DES exposure are required for tumor development. That these factors are nongenetic in character and extrauterine in location is implied by the report of two sets of exposed identical twins discordant for this cancer (Richmond 1979; Sandberg and Christian 1980). Moreover, approximately one-fourth of patients with cervicovaginal clear cell carcinoma whose mothers' prenatal records are available for review cannot be shown to have been exposed to DES or similar agents (Herbst et al. 1979b). This strongly implies that the stilbene molecule is not essential for clear cell cancer formation and that some other agent or condition may, in a significant proportion of circumstances, be an adequate substitute.

Major Concerns for the Future

The most commonly asked questions regarding the future of exposed individuals are the following:

1. Will men develop effects from DES exposure in utero? The results of the studies of Gill and associates (1979) (table 4.2, note‡) describing abnormalities in the gonads and mesonephric duct derivatives of exposed men have caused many to believe that the question has already been answered in the affirmative. The inability, however, of Andonian and Kessler (1979) to confirm these observations is unsettling, as is the apparent restriction of both

teratologic and oncologic changes in exposed women to tissues of Müllerian origin.

As previously mentioned, the currently predominant opinion is that clear cell carcinoma arises from endometrial or endometrioid cells, either normally or ectopically placed. In exposed women, these cells are thought to be commonly available in the epithelium of vaginal adenosis. Estrogenization of these cells as a requirement for oncogenesis is strongly implied by the infrequent occurrence of clear cell cancer in prepubertal girls. It is also implied by the fact that the peak incidence of cervicovaginal clear cell cancer occurs shortly after puberty and by the absence of clear cell carcinoma in Müllerian remnants in the man (exposed or unexposed). Ectopically located Müllerian epithelium (the counterpart of vaginal adenosis) has not been described in men. This and the lack of significant levels of estrogen may explain the absence of an oncogenic effect from DES exposure on Müllerian cells in men to date.

Mesonephric remnants are not known to be affected in exposed women, and the incidence of carcinoma in mesonephric tissues is no greater in exposed than unexposed offspring, male or female. These observations imply that any oncogenic influence that may derive from embryonic exposure to DES is not directed at mesonephric derivatives.

Clear cell carcinoma in women occurs in organs having the same embryologic derivation as those in which teratologic changes have developed. By analogy, if mesonephric structures are not subject to the oncologic effects of DES exposure, it is equally unlikely that they will be subject to the teratologic effects. Similarly, gametogenesis, gamete maturation, and gamete release have not been demonstrated to be abnormal in exposed women. By analogy, gamete abnormalities would not be expected in exposed men. While such reasoning is intuitive and may seem excessively simplistic, only the unconfirmed report of Gill and associates (1979) contests its accuracy.

In summary, only two studies of exposed men have been recorded, and these offer opposite conclusions. Acquisition of additional information is obviously required. Using analogies drawn from the effects on women and noting the paucity of descriptions of abnormalities in exposed men despite nearly a decade of opportunity for their development and discovery, it seems reasonable to conclude that exposed men in whom Müllerian duct regression has been normal are unlikely to develop either teratologic or oncologic effects.

2. Will many more women develop clear cell carcinoma? Using material reported to the Registry from 1972 through the first two months of 1976, Herbst and associates (1977) noted that the age of peak incidence of cervicovaginal clear cell carcinoma for all patients recorded was 19 years. The age at peak incidence appeared to be similar for subgroups arranged according to year of birth, implying that this age of peak incidence represented a characteristic of the tumor rather than merely a reflection of the frequency of use

of the drug. A sharp decline in incidence was noted through at least age 22. Estimating that between 1% and 10% of all pregnant women in the period studied had taken DES, it was calculated that the rate of development of clear cell carcinoma through age 24 would range from 1 per 700 to 1 per 7000 exposed female offspring.

Data regarding sales of 25 mg tablets of DES (Herbst et al. 1977) suggest that there was a sharp national increase in the use of DES during pregnancy in the late 1940s, culminating in a peak period of use between 1950 and 1952, with a steady decline in use through 1961. Heinonen (1973) has estimated that 100,000 to 160,000 exposed female offspring were born in the United States between 1960 and 1970. (Approval of the drug for use in pregnancy was withdrawn by the Food and Drug Administration in 1971.)

Using the estimated range of the rate of clear cell cancer development noted above, between 14 and 224 clear cell carcinomas would be expected to develop in exposed women born between 1960 and 1970. Accepting momentarily that all those born before 1957 (each now 22 years of age or older) are beyond the age of serious risk for clear cell cancer development, it could reasonably be anticipated that no more than 400 additional cases will develop. It is also possible that there will be as few as one-tenth that number. These figures, of course, are based on the concept that there will be only a single period of increased incidence of this cancer during the lifetime of exposed individuals. The most recent report from the Registry (Herbst et al. 1979) implies that this concept should be accepted with caution. Though the authors clearly state that the new expanded age incidence curve is unstable beyond the age of 24, the curve now suggests the possibility of continuing incidence through the middle twenties and a second elevation in incidence beyond that age range. Consequently, while a decline in the annual number of patients developing clear cell carcinoma and an age limit to the cancer's appearance are pleasing to contemplate, the reality of these hopeful anticipations remains uncertain. The acquisition of additional information will be required to resolve this question.

3. Will exposed women have a higher incidence of cervicovaginal squamous cell carcinoma than those in the unexposed population? It appears that the answer to this question will become apparent only after a sufficient number of exposed patients have reached the age where the possibility of this effect can reasonably be assessed. The results of the studies published to date relative to the incidence of squamous dysplasia and squamous carcinoma in the exposed population (table 4.1, note†) are too discrepant to allow one to believe that a trend has been detected or that a rational basis for prediction has evolved. The uncertainty and confusion regarding squamous epithelial changes in exposed patients are underscored by the commonly noted but unexplained lack of correlation between histologic findings and those from cytologic examinations (Robboy et al. 1978) and between histologic findings and colposcopic observations (Welch et al. 1978; Mangan et al. 1979).

Whether or not squamous dysplasia develops at the same rate and has the same natural history and the same potential for neoplastic change in vaginal adenosis as it does in cervical ectropion is unknown. Consequently, predictions based on the anticipation that information derived from the study of cervical metaplasia can be applied directly to metaplasia occurring in vaginal adenosis, and that exposed patients with adenosis are at an increased risk of developing vaginal squamous carcinoma, are unsupported to date.

4. Will the reproductive abilities of exposed women be impaired? The available information relating to this topic is contained in table 4.3, note‡ and in table 4.4. In brief, fertility appears to be comparable to that of the unexposed population but the incidence of both tubal gestation and pregnancy loss seems to be accentuated.

The Continuing Care of Exposed Female Offspring

Screening Examinations

It has become the common feeling in both medical and lay circles that all exposed female offspring, 14 years of age and older, should have recurrent prophylactic examinations for the early discovery of clear cell and squamous carcinomas of the vagina and cervix. Social and emotional attitudes have been stirred to the extent that numerous lobbying and action groups have been formed and are operating at local, state, and national levels. Many are closely allied with the women's movement, a sociopolitical phenomenon occurring contemporaneously with the development of clear cell tumors in exposed women. These groups have publicized and politicized the DES problem and have disseminated information and advice to readers, listeners, and viewers of national public media. They have solicited involvement of health associations and other public institutions in the problem, have promoted screening examinations for those exposed and potentially exposed, have pressed for the establishment of training courses in screening procedures for medical and paramedical personnel, have encouraged litigation against former and present DES manufacturers, and, most recently, have secured legislation in the states of New York, Maine, Illinois, and California to enforce and subsidize some of these activities. This newly secured legislation also prevents disqualification by medical insurance carriers of DES-related claims from exposed individuals. The concerns of these activist groups are embraced by the American populace, whose sympathy for young women who develop cervicovaginal cancer is easily and justifiably aroused.

It would be highly unpopular stance at present to question publicly whether such screening examinations are economically sound on a cost/benefit basis. It would be equally brash to inquire whether the energy and attention given to detection of this cancer are appropriate when compared to the

93

energy and attention extended to detection of more commonly occurring cancers to which the American population (including the DES-exposed individual) is heir. Nonetheless, it should be noted that only 5 of nearly 400 cases of cervicovaginal clear cell carcinoma reported since 1971 are stated to have been detected during regular screening examinations in centers organized for this purpose (Anderson et al. 1979; Mangan et al. 1979; Robboy et al. 1979). The first instance of such, occurring approximately six years following widespread inauguration of screening examinations, was sufficiently important and uncommon to warrant publication as a case report (Anderson et al. 1979). It appears that most of the tumors have been discovered on examination occasioned by the development of symptoms. Pain, bleeding, and/or discharge were present at the time of diagnosis in 84% of the first 170 patients reported to the Registry (Herbst et al. 1974). The circumstances leading to the discovery of tumors in the other patients are not described. From the information available it is apparent that very few women have been shown to achieve early detection of their clear cell cancer as a consequence of repetitive, prophylactic examinations.

At a minimum, examinations consist of a gynecologic evaluation and a cytologic smear. Colposcopic examination and iodine staining are frequently included, and biopsies, incurring additional cost for histologic preparation and interpretation, are commonly obtained. If all the charges for these services at the office and clinic visits of the thousands of exposed women undergoing recurrent screening examinations throughout the United States during the past six or seven years could be determined, and the cost per cancer discovered could be calculated, it is likely that the latter figure would be astronomical. Moreover, to this cost must be added the charges for the numerous and dubiously beneficial procedures performed on many of these patients (for example, cauterization, cryotherapy, laser vaporization, biopsy ablation, conization, and even partial vaginal excision), none of which can be shown to have reduced the incidence of cancer development.

Defenders may cite as evidence of the value of these examinations the fact that 57% of the tumors reported to the Registry were stage I (Herbst et al. 1979a). They may also cite the fact that the 5-year actuarial survival of patients with clear cell tumors (78%) is higher than that for patients with other types of vaginal and cervical cancer (30% and 55%, respectively), suggesting that early detection of clear cell carcinoma is the basis for these results. The cynic would counter with the contention that similar results might have been obtained by an equally widespread admonition to exposed individuals to seek attention not prophylactically, but upon the appearance of symptoms, a guideline apparently spontaneously followed by the majority of those who contributed to the statistics.

Defenders might also cite as justification for the costs entailed the discovery and elimination of ultimately life-threatening squamous dysplasia and in situ carcinoma in a number of these patients. The majority of investigators, however, find the incidence of these squamous atypicalities in exposed patients to be no greater than that anticipated in the unexposed population (Robboy et al. 1978), implying no greater or lesser need for regular screening examinations in either group.

The major benefit from screening examinations has been the accumulation of information concerning the nature of the teratologic effects resulting from embryonic exposure to the stilbene molecule, the natural history of these anatomic changes, and the effects of these changes on organ function. Only by perpetuating recurrent screening examinations of large numbers of exposed individuals can we continue to accumulate information at the current rate. For the investigator, continued support for the principle of screening is justified on this basis alone.

For the exposed individual, the most compelling argument favoring continuation of screening examinations is lessening of fear. These individuals have been frightened by unexpectedly finding themselves in a group uniquely heir to an uncommon cancer. They have become nervously aware of the lack of knowledge about the future of their predicament and must also live with the uneasy feeling that additional unanticipatable crises may develop. They absorb the anxious concern of others, regardless of source, and see much of this confirmed by the intense interest of their physicians. Their fear, having real but unquantifiable justification, is easily and, on occasion, manipulatively stimulated. Their families and friends share their burden.

In summary, despite certain persuasive arguments to the contrary, continuation of recurrent examinations of exposed female offspring is recommended for psychological, social, and political, as well as medical, reasons.

Methods for the Early Detection of Clear Cell Carcinoma

There is no evidence at present to suggest that any type of examination beyond systematic and meticulous visualization and palpation of the entire vaginal wall and cervix (Sandberg and Hebard 1977), together with a cytologic smear, are effective in the early detection of clear cell carcinoma. In fact, the smallest invasive clear cell carcinoma reported ($2 \times 2 \times 2.5$ mm) (Chambers, Rogers, and Julian 1978) was found on routine vaginal examination.

It has been amply confirmed that clear cell carcinoma can be detected by cytologic examination. The results, however, are inconsistent, and the method is unreliable. For example, among the first 95 cases of clear cell carcinoma reported to the Registry (Taft et al. 1974), the cytologic smear had been positive or suspicious in only half of the 21 patients from whom smears had been obtained before the tumor was grossly detected. Among patients with grossly observable tumor, the smear had been positive or suspicious in only 80% of cases. With this information, it obviously would be inappropriate to rely on cytologic examination as an efficient screening method. It should be pointed out, however, that cytologic examination is the only method employed to date that has detected clear cell carcinoma indiscernible by inspection or palpation.

Cervicovaginal staining with an iodine solution continues to be recommended (Herbst 1978; Richmond 1978) although the method has not been demonstrated to detect clear cell cancer not already detected by inspection or palpation. Nor has the recommendation to biopsy all nonstaining areas of the vagina in the quest of otherwise undetectable clear cell carcinoma (Herbst et al. 1974; American College of Obstetricians and Gynecologists 1973) been reported to be fruitful.

Colposcopic examination for early diagnosis of this tumor (Herbst et al. 1974; Gunning and Ostergard 1976; Burkman 1978) has also been widely touted, more vigorously in the past than at present. To date, however, there are no reports of discovery by colposcopy of clear cell carcinoma that was undetectable by gross visualization or palpation. In addition to the fact that no specific colposcopic changes compatible with clear cell carcinoma have been described, "small carcinomas that were easily palpable have not been visible in several patients examined by experienced colposcopists, usually because of their location submucosally or behind an obstructing fibrous ridge" (Herbst 1978).

There are two reports of patients in whom colposcopic visualization of white epithelium led to biopsy and the discovery of hidden and completely subepithelially located clear cell carcinoma (Puri et al. 1977; Shefren, personal communication regarding case reported by Hill, E.C., in discussion of Sandberg and Hebard 1977). The discovery was fortuitous in both circumstances as white epithelium has not been demonstrated to be associated with or to be a characteristic of clear cell carcinoma. In fact, white epithelium has been seen by Emens and associates (1979) in 96% of 51 exposed patients and has been shown invariably to represent squamous metaplasia and to disappear spontaneously in 3 to 4 years. Similar observations have been reported by Burke and associates (1981). In one patient, recurrence of clear cell carcinoma is said to have been discovered on colposcopically-directed biopsy (Mangan et al. 1979).

An exciting and potentially valuable but unconfirmed method for clear cell carcinoma detection is the determination of the serum concentration of cathepsin B1. Cathepsin B1 is a lysosomal proteinase which is present at or near the surface of human tumor cells but which is absent from their benign counterparts. Its specific function is unknown but its average concentration has been found to be 47 times greater than normal in five patients with clear cell carcinoma (Pietras et al. 1978). In two patients studied serially, serum levels fell to normal within seven to twelve days following excision of the tumor. The enzyme is not specific for tumor type, and elevated serum concentrations have also been noted in patients with cancers of the breast, lungs, bladder, and pancreas. Whether this assay can be developed into an inexpensive and reliable cancer detection tool for use in exposed patients remains uncertain.

Methods for the Early Detection of Squamous Cell Carcinoma

Systematic and meticulous visualization and palpation of the entire vaginal wall and cervix are fundamental. Additionally, cytologic examination should be particularly useful for the detection of dysplasia and squamous cell carcinoma of the cervix in exposed patients inasmuch as it has been effective in detecting identical abnormalities of the cervix in unexposed patients since its introduction to clinical use. The reliability of cytologic examination in the detection of squamous cell carcinoma of the vagina has received little attention, but there is no compelling reason to believe that it will be any less reliable in exposed than in unexposed individuals.

In the event of discovery of an abnormal cytologic smear in an exposed patient, the response need be no different from that occasioned by a similar discovery in an unexposed patient (that is, colposcopic examination with endocervical curettage and biopsy as indicated). Iodine staining may be used to direct the examiner to a potentially fruitful area for colposcopic evaluation. It has not been demonstrated, however, that exposed patients need or benefit more from this exercise than unexposed individuals. In patients with normal cytologic smears, random biopsy of nonstaining areas for the purpose of ruling out the presence of squamous cell atypicalities or squamous carcinoma is of little benefit as squamous abnormalities rarely have been detected in such individuals. Iodine staining as a method for the detection of squamous carcinoma of the vagina or cervix was discarded decades ago. There is no evidence that its reinitiation will be beneficial either to exposed or unexposed women.

In the presence of a normal cytologic smear, the use of colposcopy routinely to evaluate the cervix and/or vagina of exposed patients for squamous cell carcinoma or dysplasia has not been demonstrated to be either necessary or advantageous. Neither carcinoma nor dysplasia has been proved to occur with any greater frequency in exposed than in unexposed patients (table 4.1, note†), and few investigators recommend routine colposcopic examination for the latter. Moreover, colposcopic abnormalities appear to be associated with less severe histologic change and to be less consequential in exposed than in unexposed women. Similar discrepancies between cytologic and histologic diagnoses in exposed patients have also been pointed out (see Major Concerns for the Future, this chapter).

In summary, an appropriate recommendation for the early detection of both clear cell and squamous cell carcinoma of the cervix or vagina in exposed women is visualization and palpation of the cervix and vagina, together with cytologic examination. This should be followed by colposcopic evaluation and biopsy if cytologic abnormality or a lesion suspected to be malignant is detected. Additional procedures have not proved to be either economically or medically advantageous.

Methods for the Detection of Vaginal Adenosis

Because of its exceptionally high incidence in patients with clear cell carcinoma (table 4.1, note *) and its frequent presence in exposed patients at risk for the development of that disease, vaginal adenosis is viewed in many quarters with suspicion and apprehension. Despite the fact that histologic transition from benign adenosis to clear cell carcinoma has not been confirmed in any of the 384 cases reported to the Registry, the feeling that adenosis is involved with the histogenesis of clear cell carcinoma and is perhaps the direct progenitor of this cancer is unshakable. As a consequence, detection of adenosis has been considered to be important, and methods to accomplish this have been eagerly sought.

Surface adenosis is said to be detectable cytologically in 76% to 98% of biopsy-proved cases (Ng et al. 1975; Hart et al. 1976). Colposcopic identification has been reported to have a 7.5% to 9% false positive rate (Burke and Antonioli 1976; Gunning and Ostergard 1976) and a 9.5% false negative rate (Burke and Antonioli 1976). Iodine staining appears to be less reliable. Although complete excision of nonstaining areas has revealed adenosis in 97% of 188 exposed patients (Sherman et al. 1974), random biopsies of nonstaining areas in exposed patients have been positive in only 15% to 61% of instances (Herbst et al. 1975; Gunning and Ostergard 1976). In these reports of the incidence of adenosis in nonstaining areas, no distinction was made between adenosis found on the vaginal surface and that restricted to the subepithelial tissues. Inasmuch as there is no reason to believe that subepithelial adenosis can be detected by epithelial staining, the figures in these studies for the frequency of detection of adenosis by staining can be expected to have been overstated by the number of patients whose adenosis was limited to the subepithelium.

Vaginal surface adenosis may also be detected by gross visual examination in the same manner that ectropion or erosion may be visualized on the exocervix. The two are substantially identical in gross appearance and undergo the same process of squamous metaplasia.

Determination of the presence of adenosis by assay of serum levels of cathepsin B1 is currently under investigation. Experience to date has shown that 68 exposed patients with adenosis and 15 exposed patients with adenosis plus concomitant squamous dysplasia have had average serum levels 10 and 27 times greater than normal, respectively (Pietras et al. 1978). The assay, however, is not specific for adenosis. Moreover, a significant proportion of patients with uncomplicated adenosis had normal values, implying incomplete diagnostic reliability. Adenosis detected by this assay must be localized by inspection or the use of one or more of the other methods described.

Detection of adenosis has been useful in permitting an academic detailing of its natural history but has not served a clinically practical purpose, except possibly to suggest a history of DES exposure in utero. Adenosis is rarely symptomatic and, except for a single unconfirmed exception (Hill 1973), has not been shown to transform into clear cell carcinoma or to have a greater propensity for neoplastic change than any other vaginal tissue. Exceptionally few investigators currently consider medical or surgical treatment of vaginal adenosis (or its prophylactic ablation) to be either necessary or desirable.

Management of Benign Teratologic Changes

None of the teratologic changes is known to be harmful to life or health or to progress or change spontaneously or deleteriously (table 4.2, note*). Areas of columnar epithelium on the vagina and cervix may be expected to undergo squamous metaplasia. When present, the circular sulcus on the exocervix may be expected to fill in (that is, become shallower and disappear). Nodulations in the vaginal wall that remain stable in size or regress may be safely assumed to be cystic adenosis and not to require treatment. Enlarging submucosal nodules, excrescences from the vaginal surface, ulcerations, and areas of subepithelial induration may represent neoplastic growth and require investigation by biopsy.

Any of the constrictive vaginal changes (apical narrowing, fibrous band, or partial vaginal septum) may lead to dyspareunia. If the complaint is not spontaneously alleviated by continuing coital activity, surgical relaxation may be required.

The presence of constrictive vaginal changes, nearly all of which are located in the upper vagina, may hinder both the fitting and contraceptive use of the diaphragm. Discomfort associated with vaginal distension is the common complaint in such individuals and may or may not be relieved by persevering in use of the diaphragm or switching to a different type or size. Forniceal obliteration may lead to a similar problem, especially if it involves the posterior fornix.

The teratologic changes in the uterine fundus (table 4.2, note †) are not known to cause complaints or to require treatment. Two-thirds of exposed patients, however, have been shown to have abnormalities of the uterine cavity with even a higher incidence in the presence of cervicovaginal changes. All abnormalities are associated with constrictions of the cavity and many distort its outline considerably. Because of this situation it is intuitively reasonable to recommend that hysterography be performed before selecting and inserting intrauterine devices in exposed patients.

99

Exposed women, with or without teratologic changes, should be observed closely during pregnancy (table 4.3, note ‡ and table 4.4)

Optimal Interval between Screening Examinations

To determine rationally the most appropriate interval between cancer screening examinations, it is necessary to know the rate and characteristics of growth of the cancer to be detected. Specifically, how rapidly will the malignancy, present but undetectable on current examination, become diagnosable? Greater intervals simply allow a diagnosable tumor to progress needlessly. Unfortunately, so few clear cell cancers have been detected during repetitive screening examinations to date that the observations required to determine the speed and characteristics of tumor growth have not been made. As a consequence, the intervals recommended have been intuitively derived.

By common accord, a 6-month interval was arbitrarily accepted when screening examinations were initiated nationally approximately eight years ago. A year-long interval has since been suggested for patients without cervical erosion or other abnormalities (Herbst et al. 1974), although no evidence has been offered to justify the longer interval by showing that clear cell cancers in these patients are slower growing or more readily detectable. Nor is there evidence that patients without these abnormalities have a lower incidence of clear cell cancer, a feature which might be used to argue for an increased interval on the basis of an improved cost/benefit ratio. On the other hand, if lowering the cost/benefit ratio is to be the basis for recommendations, greater interexaminational intervals should also be recommended for exposed women at either end of the age incidence curve for clear cell cancer. Greater intervals should also be recommended for women exposed only during the second half of pregnancy, no more than one of whom has been reported to have developed clear cell carcinoma (Herbst et al. 1979b). Basically, however, if the cost/benefit ratio is to be used to determine the most appropriate examination interval, the entire concept of performing screening examinations for the discovery of clear cell cancer can be seriously questioned.

Whenever recommendations are made for patients having no clinically detectable adenosis, it should be remembered that the absence of visible, surface adenosis does not guarantee absence of the subepithelial, occult variety. In fact, occult adenosis is generally considered to be the more common form. Moreover, if the tuboendometrial cells in adenosis are the progenitors of clear cell carcinoma, as has been suggested, the odds regarding point of origin would favor subepithelial over surface adenosis. Robboy and associates (1979) found cells of the tuboendometrial type in 40% of patients with adenosis in whom glands were present in the subepithelial tissues but only rarely in individuals in whom the adenosis was confined to the vaginal surface. This confirmed a similar observation made earlier (Sherman et al. 1974).

In short, while the original choice of 6-month intervals for screening examinations for clear cell carcinoma was wholly arbitrary, no evidence has accumulated to discredit or to improve upon that selection.

The Continuing Care of Exposed Male Offspring

There is no conclusive evidence that men would benefit from periodic screening examinations performed solely because of DES exposure in utero. Gill and associates (1979) point to the possibility of an increased potential for the development of testicular carcinoma as a consequence of their observation of an increased incidence of cryptorchidism in exposed men. The authors cite three unreported cases of testicular carcinoma associated with cryptorchidism and DES exposure in utero. The association awaits confirmation. Apart from this potentiality, no life-threatening effect from such exposure has been detected.

Table 4.1
Oncologic Effects Purported to Result
from Exposure to Diethylstilbestrol (DES)
in Utero

In Female Offspring	In Male Offspring
Vagina–cervix	None reported
Clear cell adenocarcinoma*	
Squamous cell carcinoma†	

*The Registry for Research on Hormonal Transplacental Carcinogenesis has accessioned 384 patients with clear cell carcinoma diagnosed between 1961 and 1978 (Herbst et al. 1979b). Fifty-five percent were embryologically exposed to DES or its congeners. For 24% there was no historical evidence of maternal hormone usage. Exposure to DES in the remainder is unknown or uncertain.

Age at diagnosis ranged from 7 to 29 years, with a median of 18.9 years (Herbst et al. 1979b). Five percent of patients were less than 14 years of age. Only two were older than 26. The risk of development of clear cell carcinoma in exposed women through age 24 has been estimated to be between 1 in 700 and 1 in 7000 (Herbst et al. 1977). The risk is greatest for those exposed in the first trimester and least for those exposed later than the seventeenth week of gestation. The median time of first exposure to DES was 9.2 menstrual weeks. No direct relationship with maternal DES dosage has been noted.

Fifty-five percent of tumors have originated in the vagina; 42% have developed in the cervix (Robboy et al. 1977). The organ of origin of the remainder has been indeterminable. Vaginal tumors have been found most commonly in the upper one-third with the anterior wall being the predominant site. Cervical tumors principally have involved the exocervix. Only rarely has the endocervix appeared to be the site of origin.

The tumors have ranged in size from 2.6 mm to 10 cm in greatest dimension (Chambers, Rogers, and Julian 1978; Robboy et al. 1977). Most have been nodular and exophytic. Some have been flat or ulcerative. On rare occasion the tumor has been hidden beneath intact vaginal epithelium. The depth of penetration has varied widely.

Histologically clear cell carcinoma may show a solid pattern of large clear cells with vacuolated or clear cytoplasm, a papillary pattern with cross sections of papillae within gland lumina, or a tubulocystic pattern with hobnail-shaped cells or naked nuclei lining tubules and small cysts. Combinations of these patterns are common. On occasion the tumor may be confused with the Arias-Stella reaction or with benign microglandular hyperplasia (Wilkinson and Dufour 1976; Robboy and Welch 1977).

Among specimens suitable for examination, microscopic evidence of benign adenosis has been found in normal vaginal tissue about the tumor in 97% of surgically treated patients with vaginal cancer and 52% of those with cervical cancer (Herbst et al. 1974). At present this association appears to be coincidental rather than etiologic as histologic transition from adenosis to clear cell carcinoma has not been demonstrated in any of the 384 tumors (Herbst et al. 1979b).

Primary therapy most commonly has consisted of radical tumor excision and pelvic lymphadenectomy with or without preservation of the ovaries and with or without vaginal reconstruction. Irradiation has also been used in the primary treatment of stage I disease as well as for treatment of advanced and recurrent tumors. The optimal method for primary treatment has not been determined but the lowest rate of recurrence has been noted in patients treated by radical hysterectomy (Herbst et al. 1979a).

Lymph node metastases have been observed in one-sixth of patients with stage I vaginal tumors and in one-third of patients with stage I and stage II_a cervical tumors (Robboy et al. 1977). Lymph node metastases have been found with tumors as small as $2 \times 2 \times 2.6$ mm (Chambers, Rogers, and Julian 1978).

Recent evaluation regarding the follow-up of 346 patients recorded in the Registry shows an overall actuarial five-year survival of 78% (Herbst et al. 1979a). For women with stage I tumors the rates are 87% for those with vaginal tumors and 91% for those with cervical tumors. For women with stage II vaginal and stage II_a cervical tumors, the rates are 76% and 77%, respectively. Survival for patients with stage II_b cervical tumors is 60%, while that for those with stage III tumors is 30%. Only one patient among the five with stage IV disease has survived.

The actuarial five-year survival of patients ages 15 and under, 16 to 18, and 19 and above at time of diagnosis are 71%, 78%, and 83%, respectively (Herbst et al. 1979b). The accentuated survival in the eldest group is associated with the highest incidence of both stage I lesions and of tumors with the tubulocystic histologic pattern. At all ages tumors showing a solid or papillary pattern are associated with a lower survival than those with the tubulocystic form (Herbst et al. 1979a).

The actuarial five-year survival is greater for users than for nonusers of oral contraception (Herbst et al. 1979b). This is most readily explained by the higher incidence of stage I tumors in the user group, a probable consequence of more frequent vaginal examinations. Being pregnant at the time of diagnosis has had no apparent effect on survival following treatment.

The overall recurrence has been 23% at five years with the first recurrence being detected an average of 17 months after initial therapy (Herbst et al. 1979a). Most recurrences have been diagnosed within three years. The most common site of recurrence has been within the pelvis. In approximately 40% of patients with recurrence, however, the tumor had metastasized to the lungs and/or the supraclavicular nodes. This incidence is three times greater than that noted in unexposed patients with squamous cell carcinoma of the vagina and cervix. In 26 patients with recurrence confined to the pelvis, the five-year survival following treatment of the recurrence was 40%. In eight patients with recurrence confined to the lungs, the five-year survival following therapy was 11%.

Pelvic recurrence has been most effectively treated by surgical excision (Herbst et al. 1979a). In one patient multiple pulmonary metastases have been effectively and recurrently resected. The patient is free of disease two years following the last operation and 92 months after primary therapy. In two other patients with pulmonary metastases, complete tumor regression followed whole lung irradiation (1800 rad at 150 rad per day) plus weekly administration of actinomycin D. Both succumbed to subsequent tumor recurrence, however, one after 20 months and the other after 34 months.

Various chemotherapeutic regimens have been utilized, and objective response has been noted in about 25% of patients (Herbst et al. 1979a). In none, however, was a total remission observed. Progestational agents were regularly ineffective.

†Invasive squamous cell carcinoma of the cervix is reported to have developed in three exposed patients (Herbst 1978). Invasive squamous cell carcinoma of the vagina in exposed patients has not been described.

The results of the studies by nine groups of investigators regarding the incidence of biopsy-diagnosed carcinoma in situ and lesser degrees of squamous cell abnormality in exposed patients have been compiled by Robboy and associates (1978). For all grades of dysplasia of the vagina and cervix combined, the incidence figures ranged from 18%, reported by Mattingly and Stafl (1976) (231 patients) to 2% reported by Robboy and associates (1400 patients). For seven of the nine groups, embracing 3622 patients, the incidence was 4% or below. For the more severe atypicalities (moderate dysplasia to carcinoma in situ), the figures reported by Mattingly and Stafl and Robboy and associates were 5% and 1%, respectively. For the same seven groups, the incidence of these more severe atypicalities was 2% or below.

Among 3339 patients enrolled in the DESAD project, 21 patients (0.6%) have been shown to have squamous dysplasia of the vagina (Robboy et al. 1979). This was mild to moderate in all but one. Thirty-eight patients (1%) have been shown to have squamous dysplasia of the cervix. This was mild to moderate in all but six. Serial examination of 1125 exposed patients by Robboy and associates (1978) has revealed an incidence of development of cervicovaginal squamous dysplasia of 0.85 per 100 women-years of follow-up.

Table 4.2
Teratologic Effects Purported to Result from
Exposure to DES in Utero

In Female Offspring	In Male Offspring
Vagina* Numerous, benign (see fig. 4.1.)	Epididymis‡ Uncertain, contradicting reports
Cervix* Numerous, benign (see fig. 4.2.)	Testes‡ Uncertain, contradicting reports
Uterine cavity† Constrictions (see figs. 4.3. and 4.4.)	Penis‡ Uncertain, contradicting reports
Uterine tubes† Constrictions, interstitial portions (see figs. 4.3. and 4.4.)	Seminal fluid‡ Uncertain, contradicting reports

*The teratologic changes in the vagina and cervix pictured in figures 4.1. and 4.2. have been reported to be present in one-third (Kaufman and Adam 1978) to two-thirds (Sandberg 1976) of exposed female offspring. All changes are benign and essentially asymptomatic. Adenosis is more common in patients exposed early in gestation and in those exposed to higher doses of DES (Herbst et al. 1979b). Correlation of the incidence of the other cervicovaginal changes with dosage and time of initial exposure has not been undertaken.

Cervical ectropion and surface adenosis, both of which are more common and more extensive in exposed than in unexposed patients, spontaneously undergo metaplastic squamous epithelialization. Observations to date suggest that squamous metaplasia of cervical ectropion in exposed patients progresses linearly with time and becomes complete in a projected overall mean time of 5.6 years (Antonioli, Burke, and Friedman 1980). The rate at which squamous metaplasia of surface or occult adenosis progresses has not been determined. Cystic adenosis, while most often stable, may spontaneously subside and revert to the occult form.

The circular sulcus of the type I cervix also appears to resolve spontaneously and linearly with time. The sulcus becomes progressively shallower to the point of disappearance. The projected average time to completion has been calculated to be 11 years (Antonioli, Burke, and Friedman 1980). Filling in of the recessed ectropion of the type II cervix has also been observed (Sandberg, personal observation), but its rate of progress has not been determined. The remainder of the conditions are stable and do not appear to undergo change spontaneously.

†Hysterosalpingographic studies by Kaufman and associates (1980) revealed abnormalities of the form of the uterine cavity in 69% of 267 exposed patients. An association of these abnormalities with teratologic changes in the cervix and vagina was evident. The incidence of abnormalities in patients without changes was 50%, while in those exhibiting cervical and vaginal changes the incidence was 86% and 82%, respectively. Abnormalities were present three times more commonly in patients exposed in the first trimester than in those exposed later in gestation. No correlation between the incidence of these changes and total maternal dosage of DES was noted (Kaufman et al. 1977).

A T-shaped cavity was the most frequently observed abnormality. Other less specific variations of contour were also noted. The feature common to published photographs of these uterine cavity abnormalities (Kaufman et al. 1977) appears to be a constrictive reduction of normal width. The constriction associated with the T-shaped cavity is broad, as noted in figure 4.3., extending from the upper fundus to the internal os. In other uteri (fig. 4.4.) the constriction appears to be narrow and localized. It is possible that the anteroposterior diameter of the uterine cavity has also been modified, but this dimension has not been radiologically evaluated. Constrictions at right angles to those described in the fundus are noted in the cornual portions of some uteri. On occasion the constrictions appear to involve the interstitial portion of the tubes, but their precise locations have not been defined. Neither histologic nor gross anatomic correlation with radiographic findings has yet been possible. No structural abnormalities of the remaining areas of the tubes have been detected, and all published photographs appear to demonstrate bilateral tubal patency. No differences in hysterographic findings have been noted in the few patients studied before and after pregnancy.

There are no published reports on the external appearance of the uterus or the tubes in exposed patients, with or without hysterographic abnormalities.

In a separate radiologic study, Haney and associates (1979) compared the average dimensions of various portions of the uterine cavities of 13 exposed and 22 unexposed (infertile) patients. Statistically smaller mean values were found in the exposed group for the length of the upper segment, the total area of the endometrial cavity, and the widest diameter of the endocervical canal. No significant differences were noted between the two groups in values for the circumference of the endometrial cavity, the length of the lower segment, the diameter of the internal os, the intercornual distance, or the diameters of either the isthmic or interstitial portions of the tubes. Twelve of the 13 patients in the study group had teratologic changes in the cervix or vagina plus one or more of the constrictive hysterographic changes previously described.

‡Among 308 exposed and 307 unexposed adult males, Gill and associates (1979) noted a statistically elevated incidence in the exposed group of epididymal cysts (21% vs. 5%), hypoplastic testes (8% vs 2%), and microphallus (1.3% vs 0%). Among patients with testicular hypoplasia, 17 of 26 in the exposed group had a history of cryptorchidism as compared to one of six in the unexposed group. Cytologic examinations of urine and prostatic fluid were negative for all patients. Gill and co-workers refer to four studies of the effects on male mice and rats of exposure (as newborns or in utero) to DES. Large numbers of the animals developed abnormalities essentially identical to those described in their study of exposed human males.

Andonian and Kessler (1979), in their examination of 24 exposed men and an equal number of controls, failed to confirm these findings. They found no significant differences in the incidence of epididymal, testicular, or penile abnormalities between the two groups.

Gill and associates evaluated the semen of 43% (134) of their exposed and 28% (87) of their unexposed subjects. The basis for the selection of these patients from the larger groups was not stated. They noted that the average sperm count was lower in the exposed than in the unexposed group with a sperm count below 20 million per ml being found in 15% of the former and 9% of the latter. An Eliasson score designating severely pathologic semen was observed in 24% of exposed men but in only 8% of the controls, a statistically significant difference.

Andonian and Kessler (1979) examined semen from each of the patients in their study, except one, and failed to find any significant differences between the two groups. Severely pathologic semen was found in 17% of the exposed and 20% of the unexposed men.

Henderson and associates (1976), in a study by questionnaire, received responses from the mothers of 225 exposed and 111 unexposed men. The authors concluded that from maternal recollections the two groups of men appeared to be comparable in their histories of genitourinary problems. The one exception was that a larger proportion of the exposed men were said to have experienced problems in passing urine. This was considered by the investigators to result primarily from unexplained urethral stenosis. Neither Gill and colleagues nor Andonian and Kessler mention the presence of complaints of this nature in the history of either exposed or unexposed patients.

The study of prepubertal males by Yalom, Green, and Fisk (1973) purported to show that exposed individuals were less aggressive, less assertive, and had fewer athletic skills than those unexposed. These results have been neither confirmed nor extended.

In summary, information regarding teratologic effects in exposed men is sparse and for the most part contradictory.

Table 4.3
Effects on Function Purported to Result from
Exposure to DES in Utero

In Female Offspring	In Male Offspring
Hormonal*	Hormonal§
None verified	None reported
Sexual†	Sexual
Dyspareunia	None reported
Reproductive‡	Reproductive‖
Deficiencies suggested (see table 4.4.)	Deficiencies suggested

*The possibility that embryonic exposure to DES might affect the developing hypothalamic-pituitary axis and cause disturbance of cyclic gonadotropin release has been suggested. Among 15 exposed patients, Pomerance (1973) noted a "high incidence of anovulatory bleeding." In separate groups of identical size, both Williamson and Satterfield (1976) and Haney and colleagues (1979) found that 7 of 15 exposed patients (46%) had menstrual abnormalities. Among a larger group of exposed patients (114), Wu and colleagues (1980) noted an incidence of menstrual irregularity of only 6.7%.

Bibbo and associates (1977), working with a portion of the daughters born to women involved in a DES study 27 years ago at the Chicago Lying-in Hospital (Dieckmann et al. 1953), obtained a history of irregular menstrual cycles (oligomenorrhea) from 18% of 229 exposed patients compared to 10% of 136 control patients. In a recent evaluation of exposed women from the same patient pool, Herbst and colleagues (1980) observed a 10% and a 4% incidence of menstrual infrequency among 226 exposed and 203 unexposed patients, respectively. On the other hand, among patients in Boston, Herbst and colleagues (1975) noted no difference in age at menarche or in menstrual frequency between 110 exposed and 82 unexposed subjects. Also in Boston, Barnes (1979a) made the same observation in a study of 218 exposed and 158 control patients. The incidence of menstrual irregularity at the time of the report was 12% and 13% for the two groups.

Reports of the evaluation of large numbers of exposed patients, for example, 830 (Mangan et al. 1979) and 3339 (O'Brien et al. 1979), make no mention of the existence of a higher (or lower) incidence than expected of menstrual or endocrine abnormalities.

Wu and colleagues (1980) found slightly higher serum levels of testosterone (T) in the postovulatory and perimenstrual phases of exposed patients, as well as in exposed patients with irregular menses. They found no differences, however, in serum levels of follicle-stimulating hormone (FSH), luteinizing hormone (LH), estradiol, estrone, androstenedione, or progesterone between exposed and unexposed individuals. These results correlate with the lack of differences in serum FSH and LH values between exposed and unexposed patients reported earlier (Bibbo et al.).

Both Bibbo and co-workers and Cousins and associates (1980) have observed significantly shorter menses in exposed than in unexposed patients. If true for exposed patients at large, this may be explained by the smaller mean endometrial surface area noted in hysterographic studies of exposed individuals (Kaufman et al. 1977; Haney et al. 1979).

†The only reported anatomic interference with normal sexual activity in exposed patients has been deep dyspareunia present in about one-third of the patients with apical narrowing of the vagina (Sandberg 1976). With continuing coitus, this has resolved spontaneously in essentially all patients. In the uncommon circumstance in which a fibrous band extensive enough to warrant the diagnosis of partial vaginal septum is present, dyspareunia accompanying the condition may require surgical correction. Adenosis and the other conditions noted in these patients are rarely related to coital complaints.

‡In a study of 229 exposed and 136 unexposed female offspring, Bibbo and colleagues (1977) noted a history of pregnancy in 18% of the exposed patients in contrast to 33% of the control group. More recent figures for women from the same patient pool at the Chicago Lying-in Hospital (Herbst et al. 1980) show that 67% of 226 exposed and 86% of 203 unexposed patients have become pregnant. These figures imply that fecundity is lower in exposed than in unexposed women. However, neither Cousins and associates (1980) (71 exposed vs. 69 unexposed patients) nor Barnes (1979b) (381 exposed vs. 381 unexposed patients) noted any difference in fertility between study and control subjects. Additionally, Barnes (1979b) noted that the age at first pregnancy was similar for the groups and that there was no substantial difference in their cumulative pregnancy rates.

Available information regarding the outcome of pregnancies in exposed patients is contrasted with that in unexposed-control women in table 4.4. This is a compilation of the results of all pregnancies among these women (some women having contributed more pregnancies than others). The results of almost all studies suggest that the incidence of ectopic pregnancy, spontaneous abortion, and pre-term delivery is higher in exposed than in unexposed-control women. (The incidence of term deliveries and surviving infants is lower.) An important consideration in evaluating these figures, however, is the fact that none of the differences noted was statistically significant, with the exception of that relating to pre-term deliveries reported by Cousins and co-workers (1980). As may be seen, two-thirds of all pregnancies in exposed patients that were not electively aborted resulted in a surviving infant, as opposed to 87% in control subjects.

When the experiences of individual women were compiled, rather than the results of all pregnancies, Herbst and associates (1980) and Barnes and colleagues (1980) found that slightly over 80% of exposed parous women whose pregnancy outcome was not restricted to elective abortion had one or more surviving infants. The incidence was over 90% for comparable unexposed parous subjects.

The number of ectopic pregnancies in each reported study has been too low to allow comparative evaluation of incidence between exposed and unexposed-control women. Upon summation of the results of all studies, however, it can be noted in table 4.4 that exposed patients experienced one ectopic pregnancy for every 16 deliveries (term or pre-term). If all pregnancies are considered (including those that resulted in spontaneous or elective abortion), the incidence was 1 of 33. These figures, if confirmed, are sufficiently above standard incidence rates to safely consider ectopic gestation as the most common physical hazard resulting from DES exposure in utero.

Information regarding the possible effects of teratologic changes in the vagina and cervix on pregnancy outcome is limited because each group of authors chose to evaluate the effects of a different combination of changes (Sandberg et al., in press). Nevertheless, statistically significant differences in results were rarely observed. Only Kaufman and associates (1980) have reported on the association of abnormalities of intrauterine contour in exposed patients with pregnancy outcome. They noted a higher incidence of ectopic pregnancy, spontaneous abortion, and pre-term delivery (and a lower incidence of term delivery and surviving infants) among exposed patients with hysterographic abnormalities than among those without. Inadvertent bias in patient selection, however, was evident. Nonetheless, only the difference in incidence of term deliveries was statistically significant.

Cervical incompetence during pregnancy has been reported in at least 20 women among a collective total of 229 exposed parous patients (Singer and Hochman 1978; Nunley and Kitchin 1979; Berger and Goldstein 1980; Schmidt et al. 1980; Cousins et al. 1980; Herbst et al 1980). It is likely, however, that this represents a grossly overstated incidence of this abnormality. Kaufman and associates (1980) and Barnes and co-workers (1980) have reported on the pregnancy outcome of 210 and 289 exposed parous women, respectively. Neither group mentioned the occurrence of cervical incompetence among their patients. It is impossible to determine from reported studies whether the incidence of cervical incompetence during pregnancy is greater in exposed or in unexposed women.

§Gill and associates (1979) measured serum levels of FSH, LH, and T in 271 exposed and 244 unexposed men. Results were within the normal range for all patients, including those with "hypoplastic testes."

‖Studies of the fertility of exposed men have not been undertaken. The results of studies of their semen are contradictory (table 4.2, note ‡) and induce opposing expectations.

105

Table 4.4
Outcome of Pregnancies in DES-Exposed and Unexposed-Control Women

Year	Reference	Exposed or Unexposed	Number of Women	Number of Pregnancies	Elective Abortions	Ectopic Pregnancies	Spontaneous Abortions	Pre-Term Deliveries	Term Deliveries	Surviving Infants
1980	Cousins et al.	Exposed	24	43	16	2	5	8	12	15
		Unexposed	32	56	17	0	8	0	31	31
1980	Herbst et al.	Exposed	82	137	21	4	25	30	57	76
		Unexposed	112	201	42	0	20	10	129	137
1980	Kaufman et al.	Exposed	210	344	84	9	58	28	165	193
		Unexposed	87	147	37	0	9	5	96	101
1980	Berger and Goldstein	Exposed	46	80	18	3		8	21	26
1980	Schmidt et al.	Exposed	75	127*	36	7	22	15	47	58
1980 in press	Sandberg et al.	Exposed	167	255	91	8	36	27	93	113
	Totals	Exposed	604	986	266	33	176(24%)	116(16%)	395(55%)	481(67%)
		Unexposed	231	404	96	0	37(12%)	15(5%)	256(83%)	269(87%)

NOTES:
Percentages relate to evaluable pregnancies, i.e., those not electively aborted.

Results of study of pregnancy outcome in 289 exposed and 310 unexposed-control women by Barnes and associates (1980) not included, as data are not described in a manner applicable to this table.

*Excludes two molar pregnancies—the only molar pregnancies reported in DES-exposed women.

106

Table 4.5

Legal Effects Resulting from Exposure to
DES in Utero

Female Offspring	Male Offspring
Suits filed	None known
Numerous	
Suits dismissed or withdrawn	
Many	
Suits settled out of court	
Several	
Judgments for the plaintiff	
Three	

Note: The legal effects of DES exposure have not been recorded in the medical literature and have been described with only spotty and incomplete reference in the lay press. A collective account of these effects has not
been published. From gathered information, however, it appears that over 200 suits have been filed against
present and past manufacturers of DES by women who claim to have been exposed to DES. A number of suits
have been withdrawn because of the plaintiffs' inability to demonstrate that DES was administered and others have been withdrawn because of a defendant's ability to demonstrate that it was not.

A number of suits have involved legal questions arising from the inability of the plaintiff to identify the
manufacturer of the DES taken by her mother. In Detroit in 1977 approximately 144 women and 40 of their
husbands were labeled as plaintiffs in the case of *Abel* v. *Abbott Laboratories et al.* The plaintiffs who could
not identify the manufacturer of the DES to which they were exposed were dismissed by the Wayne County
Circuit Court. The Michigan Court of Appeals has since reversed this ruling, and the case is now on appeal to
the Supreme Court in that state.

At least a dozen suits have been settled out of court for amounts ranging from $1000 to $350,000, depending on the circumstances of the various cases. Specifically, the case of *Conway* v. *Carnrick Laboratories*
was settled out of court in Newark, New Jersey in 1978 following a three-week trial but before the initiation
of jury deliberation. The sum was confidential but is presumed to have approximated $100,000. In San Diego
in 1979 the case of *Gompf* v. *Eli Lilly and Company* was settled out of court before trial for a sum of $125,000.
In Philadelphia in 1980 the case of *Harris* v. *Abbott Laboratories* was settled out of court before trial for
$350,000. In several unpublicized settlements payment has been shared by as many as 15 defendants.

In three recent court actions, juries have found in favor of the plaintiff and have awarded sums of
$500,000 (*Bichler* v. *Eli Lilly and Company*, 1979), $800,000 (*Needham* v. *White Laboratories*, now Schering-
Plough Corporation, 1979) and $350,000 (*Zucker* v. *Eli Lilly and Company*, 1980). The results in the case of
Bichler v. *Eli Lilly and Company*, tried in the state of New York, are unique. It was the first suit won by a
DES plaintiff. The award was made to the plaintiff even though it was never established that the drug consumed by the plaintiff's mother was manufactured by the defendant company. The court's ruling held that Eli
Lilly and Company (one of over 300 manufacturers of DES at the time) had acted in concert with other manufacturers in the production and marketing of the drug and were jointly liable on the basis of alternative
liability, a legal theory never before successfully argued in a case of product liability. Eli Lilly and Company
has the option to seek apportionment of the award among the other manufacturers. The ruling in this case is
under appeal, as are essentially all others handed down to date.

Following opposite rulings by trial and appellate courts, the premise of alternative liability in another
suit involving DES use (*Sindell* v. *Abbott Laboratories, et al.*, 1980) was heard by the California Supreme
Court. The court ruled (4 to 3) that individuals may sue any or all of the major manufacturers of DES when
the specific manufacturer of the DES ingested cannot be identified. The United States Supreme Court subsequently reviewed this ruling and let it stand. These decisions could have broad implications, as establishment
of this premise could affect all manufacturers of identical or similar products, regardless of their nature,
throughout the United States.

Suits against physician-prescribers have been rare and unpublicized. Joyce Bichler filed suit against the
obstetrician who had prescribed DES for her mother. The case was settled out of court for $30,000.

In many of the suits filed, the plaintiff's health and life have been jeopardized by the development of cer
vicovaginal clear cell carcinoma. A larger number of suits have been filed by cancer-free patients complaining
of the presence of benign adenosis. The first of such suits (*Kelly* v. *Eli Lilly and Company*, 1980) was recently
decided by a jury in a United States District Court in Detroit. The jury ruled in favor of the defendant, saying
that the company was not negligent for marketing DES. In August 1979 a Boston jurist gave class-action
status to a case filed by 27 exposed women in Massachusetts for damages allegedly due simply to fear and
anguish occasioned by their potential to develop a life-threatening condition. This case has not yet been heard.

Considering the number of exposed women who have developed clear cell carcinoma (table 4.1, note*), the immensely larger number of exposed women who have benign adenosis (table 4.2, note*), and 1 or 2 million exposed women who are at risk for development of fear and anguish, it is clearly evident that DES litigation has far-reaching potential, and that the results may have immense effects on both legal principles and future business activities.

References

American College of Obstetricians and Gynecologists. Technical Bulletin #22. *Maternal stilbestrol—genital adenocarcinoma—and follow-up of exposed young women*. Chicago: American College of Obstetricians and Gynecologists, 1973.

Anderson, B. et al. Development of DES-associated clear cell carcinoma: the importance of regular screening. *Obstet. Gynecol.* 53:293–299, 1979.

Andonian, R.W., and Kessler, R. Transplacental exposure to diethylstilbestrol in men. *Urology* 13:276–279, 1979.

Antonioli, D.A.; Burke, L.; and Friedman, E.A. Natural history of diethylstilbestrol-associated genital tract lesions: cervical ectopy and cervicovaginal hood. *Am. J. Obstet. Gynecol.* 137:847–853, 1980.

Ballon, S.C. et al. Primary adenocarcinoma of the vagina. *Surg. Gynecol. Obstet.* 149:233–237, 1979.

Barnes, A.B. Menstrual history of young women exposed in utero to diethylstilbestrol. *Fertil. Steril.* 32:148–153, 1979a.

Barnes, A.B. The effect of in utero diethylstilbestrol (DES) exposure on fecundity and fertility in women: preliminary findings from the DESAD project. Paper read at the 35th Annual Meeting of the American Fertility Society, San Francisco, February 1979b.

Barnes, A.B. et al. Fertility and outcome of pregnancy in women exposed in utero to diethylstilbestrol. *N. Engl. J. Med.* 302:609–613, 1980.

Berger, M.J., and Goldstein, D.P. Impaired reproductive performance in DES-exposed women. *Obstet. Gynecol.* 55:25, 1980.

Bibbo, M. et al. Follow-up study of male and female offspring of DES-exposed mothers. *Obstet. Gynecol.* 49:1–8, 1977.

Burke, L., and Antonioli, D. Vaginal adenosis. Factors influencing detection in a colposcopic evaluation. *Obstet. Gynecol.* 48:413–421, 1976.

Burke, L. et al. Evolution of diethylstilbestrol-associated genital tract lesions. *Obstet. Gynecol.* 57:79–84, 1981.

Burkman, R.T. How to help daughters exposed to DES. *Female Patient* 3:41–43, 1978.

Chambers, J.; Rogers, L.W.; and Julian, C.G. Minute clear cell carcinoma of vagina with early metastasis to pelvic lymph nodes. *Am. J. Obstet. Gynecol.* 131:223–225, 1978.

Cousins, L. et al. Reproductive outcome of women exposed to diethylstilbestrol in utero. *Obstet. Gynecol.* 56:70–76, 1980.

Dieckman, W.J. et al. Does the administration of diethylstilbestrol during pregnancy have therapeutic value? *Am. J. Obstet. Gynecol.* 66:1062–1081, 1953.

Emens, J.M.; Allen, J.M.; and Jordan, J.A. The significance of white epithelium on the cervix and vaginas of diethylstilbestrol exposed young women. *Obstet. Gynecol. Surv.* 34:874–875, 1979.

Fenoglio, C.M. et al. Scanning and transmission electron microscopic studies of vaginal adenosis and the cervical transformation zone in progeny exposed in utero to diethylstilbestrol. *Am. J. Obstet. Gynecol.* 126:170–180, 1976.

Gill, W.B. et al. Association of diethylstilbestrol exposure in utero with cryptorchidism, testicular hypoplasia and semen abnormalities. *J. Urol.* 122:36–39, 1979.

Goldberg, M.I. et al. Clear cell adenocarcinoma arising in endometriosis of the rectovaginal septum. *Obstet. Gynecol.* 51 (suppl.):38s–40s, 1978.

Gunning, J.E., and Ostergard, D.R. Value of screening procedures for the detection of vaginal adenosis. *Obstet. Gynecol.* 47:268–271, 1976.

Haney, A.F. et al. Diethylstilbestrol-induced upper genital tract abnormalities. *Fertil. Steril.* 31:142–146, 1979.

Hart, W.R. et al. Cytologic findings in stilbestrol exposed females with emphasis on detection of vaginal adenosis. *Acta Cytol.* 20:7–14, 1976.

Hart, W.R., and Norris, H.J. Mesonephric adenocarcinomas of the cervix. *Cancer* 29:106–113, 1972.

Heinonen, O.P. Diethylstilbestrol in pregnancy. Frequency of exposure and usage patterns. *Cancer* 31:573–577, 1973.

Henderson, B.E. et al. Urogenital tract abnormalities in sons of women treated with diethylstilbestrol. *Pediatrics* 58:505–507, 1976.

Herbst, A.L. Newsletter, Registry for Research on Hormonal Transplacental Carcinogenesis. Chicago, 1978.

Herbst, A.L. et al. Clear cell adenocarcinoma of the vagina and cervix in girls: analysis of 170 Registry cases. *Am. J. Obstet. Gynecol.* 119:713–724, 1974.

Herbst, A.L. et al. Prenatal exposure to stilbestrol. A prospective comparison of exposed female offspring with unexposed controls. *N. Engl. J. Med.* 292:334–339, 1975.

Herbst, A.L. et al. Age-incidence and risk of diethylstilbestrol-related clear cell adenocarcinoma of the vagina and cervix. *Am. J. Obstet. Gynecol.* 128:43–50, 1977.

Herbst, A.L. et al. An analysis of 346 cases of clear cell adenocarcinoma of the vagina and cervix with emphasis on recurrence and survival. *Gynecol. Oncol.* 7:111–122, 1979a.

Herbst, A.L. et al. Epidemiologic aspects and factors related to survival in 384 Registry cases of clear cell adenocarcinoma of the vagina and cervix. *Am. J. Obstet. Gynecol.* 135:876–886, 1979b.

Herbst, A.L. et al. A comparison of pregnancy experience in DES-exposed and DES-unexposed daughters. *J. Reprod. Med.* 24:62–69, 1980.

Herbst, A.L.; Ulfelder, H.; and Poskanzer, D.C. Adenocarcinoma of the vagina. Association of maternal stilbestrol therapy with tumor appearance in young women. *N. Engl. J. Med.* 284:878–881, 1971.

Hill, E.C. Clear cell carcinoma of the cervix and vagina in young women. *Am. J. Obstet. Gynecol.* 116:470–484, 1973.

Kaufman, R.H. et al. Upper genital tract changes associated with exposure in utero to diethylstilbestrol. *Am. J. Obstet. Gynecol.* 128:51–59, 1977.

Kaufman, R.H. et al. Upper genital tract changes and pregnancy outcome in offspring exposed in utero to diethylstilbestrol. *Am. J. Obstet. Gynecol.* 137:299–308, 1980.

Kaufman, R.H., and Adam, E. Genital tract anomalies associated with in utero exposure to diethylstilbestrol. *Isr. J. Med. Sci.* 14:347–362, 1978.

Kurman, R.J., and Scully, R.E. Clear cell carcinoma of the endometrium. An analysis of 21 cases. *Cancer* 37:872–882, 1976.

Mangan, C.E. et al. Six years' experience with screening of a diethylstilbestrol-exposed population. *Am. J. Obstet. Gynecol.* 134:860–865, 1979.

Mattingly, R.F., and Stafl A. Cancer risk in diethylstilbestrol-exposed offspring. *Am. J. Obstet. Gynecol.* 126:543–548, 1976.

Ng, A.B.P. et al. Cellular detection of vaginal adenosis. *Obstet. Gynecol.* 46:323–328, 1975.

Nunley, W.C., and Kitchin, J.D. Successful management of incompetent cervix in a primigravida exposed to diethylstilbestrol in utero. *Fertil. Steril.* 31:217–219, 1979.

O'Brien, P.C. et al. Vaginal epithelial changes in young women enrolled in the National Cooperative Diethylstilbestrol Adenosis (DESAD) Project. *Obstet. Gynecol.* 53:300–308, 1979.

Pietras, R.J. et al. Elevated serum cathepsin B1 and vaginal pathology after DES exposure. *Obstet. Gynecol.* 52:321–327, 1978.

Pomerance, W. Post-stilbestrol secondary syndrome. *Obstet. Gynecol.* 42:12–18, 1973.

Puri, S. et al. Clear cell carcinoma of cervix and vagina in progeny of women who received diethylstilbestrol: three cases with scanning and transmission electron microscopy. *Am. J. Obstet. Gynecol.* 128:550–555, 1977.

Richmond, H. Vaginal clear cell adenocarcinoma and adenosis in monozygotic twins. *J. Clin. Pathol.* 32:416, 1979.

Richmond, J.B. (Surgeon-General). *Physician advisory.* Washington, D.C.: Department of Health, Education and Welfare, Office of the Assistant Secretary for Health, October 1978.

Robboy, S.J. et al. Intrauterine diethylstilbestrol exposure and its consequences. *Arch. Pathol. Lab. Med.* 101:1–5, 1977.

Robboy, S.J. et al. Squamous cell dysplasia and carcinoma in situ of the cervix and vagina after prenatal exposure to diethylstilbestrol. *Obstet. Gynecol.* 51:528–535, 1978.

Robboy, S.J. et al. Pathologic findings in young women enrolled in the National Cooperative Diethylstilbestrol Adenosis (DESAD) Project. *Obstet. Gynecol.* 53:309–317, 1979.

Robboy, S.J., and Welch. W.R. Microglandular hyperplasia in vaginal adenosis associated with oral contraceptives and prenatal diethylstilbestrol exposure. *Obstet. Gynecol.* 49:430–434, 1977.

Sandberg, E.C. The incidence and distribution of occult vaginal adenosis. *Am. J. Obstet. Gynecol.* 101:322–333, 1968.

Sandberg, E.C. Benign cervical and vaginal changes associated with exposure to stilbestrol in utero. *Am. J. Obstet. Gynecol.* 125:777–789, 1976.

Sandberg, E.C. et al. Adenosis vaginae. *Am. J. Obstet. Gynecol.* 93:209–222, 1965.

Sandberg, E.C. et al. Pregnancy outcome in women exposed to diethylstilbestrol in utero. *Am. J. Obstet. Gynecol.,* in press.

Sandberg, E.C., and Christian, J.C. Diethylstilbestrol-exposed monozygotic twins discordant for cervicovaginal clear cell adenocarcinoma. *Am. J. Obstet. Gynecol.* 137:220–228, 1980.

Sandberg, E.C., and Hebard, J.C. Examination of young women exposed to stilbestrol in utero. *Am. J. Obstet. Gynecol.* 128:364–370, 1977.

Schiller, W. Mesonephroma ovarii. *Am. J. Cancer* 35:1–21, 1939.

Schmidt, G. et al. Reproductive history of women exposed to diethylstilbestrol in utero. *Fertil. Steril.* 33:21–24, 1980.

Scully, R.E., and Barlow, J.F. "Mesonephroma" of ovary. Tumor of Müllerian nature related to the endometrioid carcinoma. *Cancer* 20:1405–1417, 1967.

Scully, R.E.; Robboy, S.J.; and Herbst, A.L. Vaginal and cervical abnormalities, including clear cell adenocarcinoma, related to prenatal exposure to stilbestrol. *Ann. Clin. Lab. Sci.* 4:222–233, 1974.

Scully, R.E.; Robboy, S.J.; and Welch, W.R. Pathology and pathogenesis of diethylstilbestrol-related disorders of the female genital tract. In *Intrauterine exposure to diethylstilbestrol in the human,* ed. A.L. Herbst. Chicago: American College of Obstetricians and Gynecologists, 1978.

Sherman, A.I. et al. Cervical-vaginal adenosis after in utero exposure to synthetic estrogens. *Obstet. Gynecol.* 44:531–545, 1974.

Silverberg, S.G., and DeGiorgi, L.S. Clear cell carcinoma of the vagina. A clinical, pathologic, and electron microscopic study. *Cancer* 29:1680–1690, 1972.

Singer, M.S., and Hochman, M. Incompetent cervix in a hormone-exposed offspring. *Obstet. Gynecol.* 51:625–626, 1978.

Taft, P.D. et al. Cytology of clear cell adenocarcinoma of genital tract in young females: review of 95 cases from the Registry. *Acta Cytol.* 18:279–290, 1974.

Teilum, G. Endodermal sinus tumors of the ovary and testis. Comparative morphogenesis of the so-called mesonephroma ovarii (Schiller) and extraembryonic (yolk sac-allantoic) structure of the rat's placenta. *Cancer* 12:1092–1105, 1959.

Welch, W.R. et al. Comparison of histologic and colposcopic findings in DES-exposed females. *Obstet. Gynecol.* 52:457–461, 1978.

Wilkinson, E., and Dufour, D.R. Pathogenesis of microglandular hyperplasia of the cervix uteri. *Obstet. Gynecol.* 47:189–195, 1976.

Williamson, H.O., and Satterfield, R.G. Diethylstilbestrol adenosis and dysfunctional uterine bleeding. *JAMA* 235:1687, 1976.

Wu, C.H. et al. Plasma hormones in DES-exposed females. *Obstet. Gynecol.* 55:157–162, 1980.

Yalom, I.D.; Green, R.; and Fisk, N. Prenatal exposure to female hormones, Effect on psychosexual development in boys. *Arch. Gen. Psychiatry* 28:554–561, 1973.

PERSPECTIVE:

DES Exposure in Utero: What Are the Effects?

Staffan R. B. Nordqvist

Diethylstilbestrol (DES) is a nonsteroidal estrogen which is structurally similar to steroidal estrogens and has the metabolic effects of an estrogen. Beginning in the 1940s, DES was commonly recommended as prophylactic therapy in situations of threatening and/or habitual abortion (Smith, Smith, and Hurwitz, 1946). Although the value of such therapy early was seriously questioned, the drug was continued to be used with these indications into the early 1970s. An estimated 1 to 4 million American women have received DES during pregnancy.

In 1971 the association was discovered between maternal ingestion of DES and subsequent development of clear cell adenocarcinoma of the cervix or vagina in female offspring (Herbst, Ulfelder, and Poskanzer 1971). A central registry for such cases was established (Herbst et al. 1972). In January 1979, 346 cases had been reported from all over the world although the vast majority were from the United States. Of 292 adequately analyzed cases, 182 had a history definitely positive for maternal ingestion of DES. Only 75 had a definitely negative history. In the remainder it was still uncertain (Herbst et al. 1979).

The incidence of clear cell adenocarcinoma in the female offspring has been estimated at 0.14 to 1.4 per thousand. Although the initial fear of an epidemic of clear cell adenocarcinoma never has materialized, it is evident that intrauterine exposure to DES increases the risk for the development of this neoplasm (Herbst et al. 1972, 1979; Nordqvist et al. 1976).

Screening examinations of large numbers of young DES progenies have led to a number of interesting observations. These suggest a teratogenic effect by DES when administered during the first 18 weeks of pregnancy resulting in an interference with the normal development of the female reproductive tract (Herbst, Kurman, and Scully 1972; Sherman et al. 1974; Fetherston 1975; Ng et al. 1975; Hart et al. 1975; Robboy et al. 1976; Burke and Antonioli 1976; Baggish, Robinson, and Passman 1976; Stafl 1974; Ng et al. 1975; Bibbo et al. 1977).

The vast majority of anomalies are benign and many are self-limited. Experimental work in animals done prior to any knowledge of DES-associated problems seems to offer explanations for many of the clinical, cytologic, and histopathologic observations reported.

The triggering mechanism for development of genital cancer in the DES offspring is largely unknown. Although attention was first directed to adenocarcinomas of the vagina and cervix, squamous cell neoplasia have also been described in these young women.

This paper will describe common observations as made by the author and as reported in the literature. Possible disease mechanisms will be discussed against the background of the embryology of the female genital tract in humans and in animals.

Benign Anomalies

The most common observation is that of an unusually large transformation zone (t-zone) involving the ectocervix and frequently also significant portions of the vagina. In the latter case the t-zone generally extends in a characteristic U or V shape in the anterior and posterior walls. Involvement of the lateral walls in general is much less pronounced. In our population of 106 young women, extension of the t-zone to the vagina was noted in 63.8% (Nordqvist, Medhat, and Ng, in press). Involvement beyond the upper third of the vagina was seen in 20.9%.

Squamous metaplasia, active or completed, was noted in all patients. In 54.7% surface-related adenosis was noted grossly or colposcopically in the vagina. In our opinion, the mere presence of a transformation zone in the vagina may not be equated with adenosis.

In the literature the prevalence of vaginal adenosis has been reported to vary from 35% to 40% by cytologic study (Ng et al. 1975; Hart et al. 1976; Robboy et al. 1976) to over 90% by histopathologic study (Sherman et al. 1974). The reasons for discrepancies are obvious since ctyology will only discover surface-related glandular epithelium. It is a recognized fact, however, that adenosis also may be present deep in the vaginal stroma (Nordqvist et al. 1976). Adenosis is particularly prominent in patients with vaginal hood, hypertrophic elongation of the anterior lip of the cervix (so-called cock's comb), and cervical pseudopolyps.

The mechanisms behind the formation of these latter anomalies are unknown. In our series vaginal hoods were seen in 16.0%, cock's combs in 17.9%, and cervical pseudopolyps in 3.8% (Nordqvist, Medhat, and Ng, in press). They are not known to have functional significance.

114

Adenosis in general is a self-limited condition which tends gradually to disappear in most patients by the process of squamous metaplasia (Ng et al. 1975, 1977). The end result is a mature stratified squamous epithelium indistinguishable histologically from native squamous epithelium. (fig. 4.5). The process occurs in both surface-related epithelium and deep in glandular crypts. It is accelerated by vaginal acidity, irritation, and cautery. Therapy may be directed to enhancement of vaginal acidity with local preparations but other measures are rarely indicated.

Adenocarcinoma

Ever since it was first described by Meyer in 1903 the histogenesis of mesonephric carcinoma has been much discussed and a variety of neoplasms have been included in this group (Fawcett, Dockerty, and Hunt 1966; Hameed 1968; Hart and Norris 1972; Nix and Wright 1967; Novak, Woodruff, and Novak 1954). Hameed's review demonstrated that, of these, clear cell carcinoma constitutes a separate biologic entity with respect to histology, age incidence, and prognosis. He concluded that the term mesonephric carcinoma should be abandoned. Herbst and Scully pointed out in 1970 that clear cell

Figure 4.5

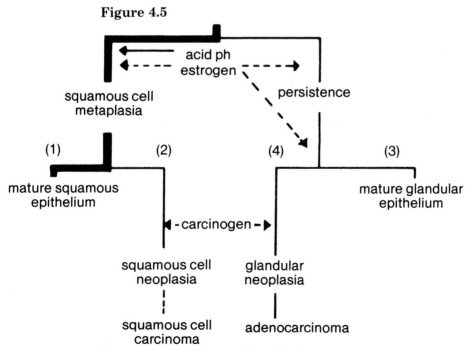

Proposed natural history of ectopic columnar epithelium in DES offspring.

carcinoma has never been demonstrated actually to arise from mesonephric remnants, and instead a Müllerian origin is currently favored by most investigators (Forsberg 1973; Herbst et al. 1974). Evidence supporting this concept includes factors such as the superficial and anterior location of most of the tumors; the association with vaginal adenosis and endocervical epithelium; the occurrence of clear cell carcinoma in the endometrium and similar Mullerian-related tumors in the ovaries (Herbst and Scully 1970; Scully and Barlow 1967); histochemical and ultastructural findings (Hameed 1968; Silverberg and DeGiorgi 1972).

The author's study in 1976 of 21 clear cell adenocarcinomas of the cervix and/or vagina lends further support to a Müllerian origin of these neoplasms. Nine were found to have coexisting vaginal adenosis. This included six of seven which were DES-related. In three, adenosis was demonstrated in the immediate vicinity of carcinoma, and although an origin from adenosis could not be proved, carcinoma was identified invading adenotic glands in two cases. In one, carcinoma was growing in continuity with benign endocervical glands, and in the other a focus of atypical ciliated endocervical cells was found in an area of tumor.

Embryologic Background

Johannes Müller in 1830 demonstrated the ducts which were named for him. He suggested that the fallopian tubes and uterine fundus developed from these ducts whereas the rest of the uterus and the vagina originated from the urogenital sinus. Although an overwhelming amount of work has since been published on the derivation and differentiation of the female reproductive tract, controversy still exists.

In 1963 Forsberg published a landmark study reviewing the world's literature on the subject and presenting his own data from the human, mouse, rat, hamster, rabbit, dog, and cow. He acknowledged the difficulty of determining by morphologic methods whether the vagina is derived from Müllerian, Wolffian, or sinus epithelium. Beginning during the first trimester, "the epithelium in the vaginal part of the Müllerian ducts undergoes a transformation from pseudostratified columnar epithelium into a stratified epithelium most closely resembling typical squamous epithelium. This stratified epithelium degenerates and is replaced by the cranially growing vaginal plate." The vaginal plate originates from the urogenital sinus, from Wolffian epithelium, or from both. Forsberg's histochemical studies seem to favor the Wolffian epithelium. Eventually the border between the epithelium of the vaginal plate and Müllerian endocervical epithelium marks the squamocolumnar junction.

Although differences exist among animals of various orders in the derivation of the vaginal epithelium, there are considerable similarities. With respect to study of the influence of steroid hormones on the developmental process, the mouse is particularly suitable. In this animal the process begins at the time of birth and concludes with puberty at the age of one month.

In 1969, by neonatal injections of 17β-estradiol, Forsberg had demonstrated interference with squamous transformation of the pseudostratified columnar epithelium of the cranial vagina and the cervix. The mechanisms of action appeared to be inhibition of a marked mitotic activity of the pseudostratified epithelium. As a result glandular epithelium persisted in the upper vagina as adenosis. This was particularly prominent at one month of age, a time at which mice enter puberty.

Later studies demonstrated DES to have a similar effect (Forsberg 1972), although cornification of the vaginal epithelium in DES-treated animals did not occur in those receiving 17β-estradiol. The development of adenocarcinoma has not been reported in these animals although a locally invasive pattern of adenosis was described (Forsberg, personal communication).

There is reason to assume that intrauterine exposure to DES in the human has a similar effect; that is, inhibition of the cephalad growth of the vaginal plate and/or interference with degeneration of the stratified Müllerian epithelium. Thus a more caudal position of the squamocolumnar junction will occur, and the persistence of glandular epithelium in the vagina is promoted. Further evidence was provided in 1972 by Herbst, Kurman, and Scully, who noted increasing frequency of adenosis the earlier during pregnancy DES medication was started.

No cytogenetic evidence has been produced suggesting adenosis as a precancerous condition. Lewis and associates (1973) found only diploid DNA contents in adenosis as opposed to clear cell adenocarcinoma, which invariably showed striking aneuploidy. If, however, the effect of DES is inhibition of cellular differentiation of the caudal Müllerian epithelium, persisting immature cells may be predisposed to malignant transformation under the influence of unknown endogenous or exogenous carcinogens. Since this cancer most often becomes evident shortly after puberty, one might also speculate on a partial hormone dependence of these neoplasms. Steroid hormone receptor studies could be of value in this respect.

The proposed natural history of persisting glandular epithelium is illustrated in figure 4.5.

Squamous Cell Neoplasia

In our study of women exposed to DES, colposcopic evidence of white epithelium was noted in 44 of 106 patients (41.9%). The degree of whiteness in general was most pronounced in patients found to have squamous cell neoplasia (that is, dysplasia or carcinoma in situ). It could, however, be significant also in cases of benign metaplasia.

Vascular patterns such as punctation and mosaic were noted in 38 patients (36.2%). The vessels were regular and of fine caliber in most instances,

117

with the exception of patients who were found to have squamous cell neoplasia, in whom the vessels were coarse and irregular. The total number of patients with any or all of the mentioned atypical patterns was 58 (55.2%).

Stafl and Mattingly (1974) reported abnormal colposcopic findings in 96% of women exposed to DES, while Fetherston (1975) found colposcopic abnormalities in 40 of 46 patients. In general we interpret white epithelium as being the result of the increased thickness of the immature metaplastic epithelium, which is a common occurrence in these patients. Thus the translucency of the epithelium is diminished. Another common observation and explanation for white epithelium is keratinization.

Stafl and Mattingly suggested that white epithelium is due to "arrested immature metaplasia," which in turn might place the DES progeny at increased risk for squamous cell neoplasia. A causal relationship in this regard is unknown in the human. Support for such a theory, however, can be found in the literature on experiments in animals.

Loeb and colleagues (1936) and Gardner and associates (1938) reported on cancer in the cervix and vagina of mice treated with estrogens. Dunn and Green (1963) administered DES to male and female mice on the day of birth. Autopsies were performed at 13 to 26 months, significantly later than in Forsberg's work. Female mice showed evidence of continuous estrogen stimulation (persistent estrous), as evidenced by vaginal cornification. Also, the endometrial mucosa showed epidermization. The ovaries contained no corpora lutea, but frequently there were follicular cysts and granulosa cell tumors. In male mice epididymal cysts were common, but sperm formation was frequently normal. It is interesting that epididymal cysts also have been reported in the human male DES offspring (Bibbo et al. 1977).

The most striking observation, however, was the presence of epidermoid hyperplasia with down-growth in the stroma and, in seven animals, epidermoid carcinoma. Two of these tumors were successfully transplanted. Epidermoid hyperplasia and preinvasive cancer were also noted under similar experimental conditions by Takasugi and Bern (1964) and by Kimura and Nandi (1967). To date there is no firm evidence to indicate that the human DES offspring is at increased risk for invasive squamous cell carcinoma of the cervix or vagina. If, however, the concept of arrested immature metaplasia (Stafl et al. 1974; Mattingly and Stafl 1976) is correct, this epithelium could conceivably retain over prolonged periods of time the apparent vulnerability to carcinogens attributed to physiologic squamous metaplasia during its dynamic phase (Coppleson, Reid, and Pixley 1967).

Prevalence rates of squamous cell neoplasia in the general female population between adolescence and 30 years of age range between 4% and 7% (Lindberg, Ahlgren, and Nordqvist 1977; Feldman 1976). The true rate in women exposed to DES is difficult to ascertain since most materials probably are strongly selective. Robboy and colleagues (1978) studied 1424 DES progenies in whom the prevalence of squamous cell neoplasia was 2.1%. Patients specifically referred with such a diagnosis, however, were excluded from the study. Bibbo and colleagues (1977) reported higher prevalence of dysplasia in women exposed to DES than in a control group. The highest rate, 18%, was reported by Mattingly and Stafl (1976). In their series the prevalence of carcinoma in situ was 1.4% which was five times higher than in a control group.

Our data indicate a prevalence of biopsy-proved squamous cell neoplasia in 11.3%. This is exceptionally high, but the material is too small and too selective to permit firm conclusions with regard to risk factors. In a previous study of a similar age group of women not exposed to DES the prevalence was 6.1% (Lindberg, Ahlgren, and Nordqvist 1977). It is interesting that only one patient in our series had vaginal extension of the neoplasia. More common involvement of the cervix has also been reported by others (Bibbo et al. 1977; Robboy et al. 1978).

Interpretation of the colposcopic picture in the DES progeny is significantly more difficult than in women not exposed to DES (Welch et al. 1978). As indicated by table 4.6, typical as well as atypical patterns are normally present. This places great demands on the skill and experience of the colposcopist. Much emphasis is placed on qualitative changes of the vascular pattern. Metaplasia is associated with fine-caliber regular vessels with short intercapillary distances. In the case of neoplasia, the vessels are of coarser caliber, and the intercapillary distance increases. Surface irregularities may also be seen; however, they are also common with hyperkeratosis.

Therapeutically the presence of squamous cell neoplasia presents a dilemma. It cannot be firmly stated at this point whether selective excision and/or destruction of the neoplastic epithelium is sufficient or if the entire transformation zone requires treatment. Future investigations should be directed to this question.

Conclusion

A great deal of controversy still exists regarding the teratogenicity and carcinogenicity of intrauterine DES exposure. Whether guided by great foresight, academic curiosity, or pure luck, our predecessors in medical science

Table 4.6
Colposcopy of the DES Progeny

Typical	Atypical
Distal OSC*	White epithelium
Ectopic columnar epithelium	Hyperkeratosis
Squamous metaplasia	Vascular pattern
Gland openings	Punctation
Nabothian-like cysts	Mosaicism

*OSC: original squamocolumnar junction.

have cast some light on these problems and set the stage for continued work. Dunn and Green in 1963 concluded that ". . . when clues to the etiology of cancer are sought in human populations, every effort should be made to obtain the prenatal and early postnatal history of patients with cancer." How right they were.

References

Baggish, M.S.; Robinson, D.; and Passman, B. Stilboestrol-induced Müllerian cervix: a colposcopic study. *Gynecol. Oncol.* 4:20–32, 1976.

Bibbo, M. et al. Follow-up study of male and female offspring of DES-exposed mothers. *Obstet. Gynecol.* 49:1–18, 1977.

Burke, L., and Antonioli, D. Vaginal adenosis. Factors influencing detection in colposcopic evaluation. *Obstet. Gynecol.* 48:413–421, 1976.

Coppleson, M.; Reid, B.; and Pixley, E. *Preclinical carcinoma of the cervix uteri.* Elmsford, N.Y.: Pergamon Press, Ltd., 1967.

Dunn, T.B., and Green, A.W. Cysts of the epididymis, cancer of the cervix, granular cell myoblastoma and other lesions after estrogen injection in newborn mice. *J. Natl. Cancer Inst.* 31:425–455, 1963.

Fawcett, R.J.; Dockerty, M.B.; and Hunt, A.B. Mesonephric carcinoma of the cervix uteri: a clinical and pathologic study. *Am. J. Obstet. Gynecol.* 95:1068–1079, 1966.

Feldman, J.M. et al. Abnormal cervical cytology in the teenager: a continuing problem. *Am. J. Obstet. Gynecol.* 126:418–422, 1976.

Fetherston, W.C. Squamous metaplasia of vagina related to DES syndrome. *Am. J. Obstet. Gynecol.* 122:176–181, 1975.

Forsberg, J.G. Derivation and differentiation of the vaginal epithelium. Lund, Sweden: H. Ohlssons Boktryckeri, 1963.

Forsberg, J.G. The development of atypical epithelium in the mouse uterine cervix and vaginal fornix after neonatal oestradiol treatment. *Br. J. Exp. Pathol.* 50:187–195, 1969.

Forsberg, J.G. Estrogen, vaginal cancer, and vaginal development. *Am. J. Obstet. Gynecol.* 113:83–87, 1972.

Forsberg, J.G. Cervicovaginal epithelium: its origin and development. *Am. J. Obstet. Gynecol.* 115:1025–1043, 1973.

Gardner, W.V. Carcinoma of the cervix of mice receiving estrogens. *JAMA* 110:1182–1183, 1938.

Hameed, K. Clear cell "mesonephric" carcinoma of uterine cervix. *Obstet. Gynecol.* 32:564–575, 1968.

Hart, W.R. et al. Cytologic findings in stilbestrol exposed females with emphasis on detection of vaginal adenosis. *Acta Cytol.* 30:7–14, 1976.

Hart, W.R., and Norris, H.J. Mesonephric adenocarcinomas of the cervix. *Cancer* 29:106–113, 1972.

Herbst, A.L. et al. Clear cell adenocarcinoma of the genital tract in young females. Registry report. *N. Engl. J. Med.* 287:1259–1264, 1972.

Herbst, A.L. et al. Clear cell adenocarcinoma of the vagina and cervix in girls: analysis of 170 Registry cases. *Am. J. Obstet. Gynecol.* 119:713–724, 1974.

Herbst, A.L. et al. An analysis of 346 cases of clear cell adenocarcinoma of the vagina and cervix with emphasis on recurrence and survival. *Gynecol. Oncol.* 7:111–122, 1979.

Herbst, A.L.; Kurman, R.J.; and Scully, R.E. Vaginal and cervical abnormalities after exposure to stilboestrol in utero. *Obstet. Gynecol.* 40:287–298, 1972.

Herbst, A.L., and Scully, R.E. Adenocarcinoma of the vagina in adolescence. A report of 7 cases including 6 clear cell carcinomas (so-called mesonephromas). *Cancer* 25:745–757, 1970.

Herbst, A.L.; Ulfelder, H.; and Poskanzer, D.C. Adenocarcinoma of the vagina: association of maternal stilboestrol therapy with tumor appearance in young women. *N. Engl. J. Med.* 284:878–881, 1971.

Kimura, T., and Nandi, S. Nature of induced persistent vaginal cornification in mice. IV. Changes in the vaginal epithelium of old mice treated neonatally with estradiol or testosterone. *J. Natl. Cancer Inst.* 39:75–93, 1967.

Lewis, J.L., Jr.; Nordqvist, S.R.B.; and Richart, R.M. Studies of nuclear DNA in vaginal adenosis and clear cell adenocarcinoma. *Am. J. Obstet. Gynecol.* 115:737–750, 1973.

Lindberg, L.G.; Ahlgren, M.; and Nordqvist, S.R.B. Cytologic screening and rescreening in detection and prevention of preclinical cervical cancer. *Gynecol. Oncol.* 5:121–133, 1977.

Loeb, L. Carcinoma-like proliferation in vagina, cervix, and uterus of mouse treated with estrogenic hormones. *Proc. Soc. Exp. Biol. Med.* 35:320–322, 1936.

Mattingly, R.F., and Stafl, A. Cancer risk in DES-exposed offspring. *Am. J. Obstet. Gynecol.* 126:534–548, 1976.

Meyer, R. Über adenom and karzinombildung an der ampulle des gartnerschen ganges. *Virchows Arch. (Pathol. Anat.)* 174:270–294, 1903.

Müller, J. Bildungsgeschichte der genitalien aus anatomischen untersuchungen an embryonen des menschen und der thiere. Düsseldorf: Arnz, u. Comp., 1830.

Ng, A.B.P. et al. Cellular detection of vaginal adenosis. *Obstet. Gynecol.* 46:323–328, 1975.

Ng, A.P.B. et al. Natural history of vaginal adenosis in women exposed to DES in utero. *J. Reprod. Med.* 18:1–13, 1977.

Nix, H.G., and Wright, H.L. Mesonephric adenocarcinoma of the vagina. *Am. J. Obstet. Gynecol.* 99:893–899, 1967.

Nordqvist, S.R.B. et al. Clear cell adenocarcinoma of the cervix and vagina. *Cancer* 37:858–871, 1976.

Nordqvist, S.R.B.; Medhat, I.; and Ng, A.B.P. Teratogenic effects of intrauterine exposure to DES in female offspring. *Compr. Ther.* In Press.

Novak, E.; Woodruff, J.D.; and Novak, E.R. Probable mesonephric origin of certain female genital tumors. *Am. J. Obstet. Gynecol.* 68:1222–1242, 1954.

Robboy, S.J. et al. Cytology of 575 young women with prenatal exposure to DES. *Obstet. Gynecol.* 48:511–515, 1976.

Robboy, S.J. et al. Squamous cell dysplasia and carcinoma in situ of the cervix and vagina after prenatal exposure to diethylstilboestrol. *Obstet. Gynecol.* 51:528–535, 1978.

Scully, R.E., and Barlow, J.F.: "Mesonephroma" of ovary. Tumor of Müllerian nature related to the endometrioid carcinoma. *Cancer* 20:1405–1417, 1967.

Sherman, A.I. et al. Cervical-vaginal adenosis after in utero exposure to synthetic estrogens. *Obstet. Gynecol.* 44:531–545, 1974.

Silverberg, S.G., and DeGiorgi, L.S. Clear cell carcinoma of the vagina. A clinical, pathologic and electron microscopic study. *Cancer* 29:1680–1690, 1972.

Smith, B.W.; Smith, G.V.S.; and Hurwitz, D. Increased excretion of pregnanediol in pregnancy from diethylstilbestrol with special reference to prevention of late pregnancy accidents. *Am. J. Obstet. Gynecol.* 51:411–415, 1946.

Stafl, A. et al. Clinical diagnosis of vaginal adenosis. *Obstet. Gynecol.* 43:118–128, 1974.

Stafl, A., and Mattingly, R.F. Vaginal adenosis. A precancerous lesion? *Am. J. Obstet. Gynecol.* 120:666–677, 1974.

Takasugi, N., and Bern, H.A. Tissue changes in mice with persistent vaginal cornification induced by early postnatal treatment with estrogens. *J. Natl. Cancer Inst.* 33:855–865, 1964.

Welch, W.R. et al. Comparison of histologic and colposcopic findings in DES-exposed females. *Obstet. Gynecol.* 52:457–461, 1978.

PART III

CARCINOMA OF THE CERVIX

Recent recommendations by the American Cancer Society regarding the cost effectiveness of routine annual cytologic smears of the cervix justify a detailed discussion of the management of patients with abnormal cervical cytology. Dr. Popkin emphasizes that cervical intraepithelial neoplasia are new diseases that produce no symptoms. He appropriately classifies cervical cytology as a screening rather than a diagnostic tool and suggests that it be used in the population at risk. As this includes all sexually active women, the "at risk" group is rapidly expanding as cultural values surrounding sexuality change. Both the techniques of obtaining the smear and the method of reporting results are discussed.

Dr. Ferenczy stresses the importance of early dysplasia and questions the reported tendency to spontaneous regression of mild and moderate dysplasia. He further suggests that the degree of dysplasia is irrelevant to the decision to institute treatment. Most important, he believes, is the exclusion of invasive cancer and the definition of the extent of the dysplastic process. His suggestion that mild dysplasia can progress directly to invasive carcinoma and that no mechanism exists to predict in which patients such progression will occur should provoke some anxiety in those of us who believe that focal mild dysplasia can be observed over time without treatment. Dr. Ferenczy describes those lesions necessitating cone biopsy and elaborates on the technique of cryotherapy.

Dr. Petrilli emphasizes the limitations of the cytologic smear in determining the degree of cervical abnormality and suggests that familiarity with the laboratory interpreting the smear will enhance the yield. He supports the guidelines of the American Cancer Society for the low-risk patient but notes that a pelvic examination has value on an annual basis independent of the cytologic smear. Special problems associated with the outpatient management of cervical intraepithelial neoplasia are discussed.

Perhaps the most controversial issue presented herein is that of the role of operative staging in the treatment of invasive carcinoma of the cervix. Dr. Berman, who has been closely involved in the design of new approaches to such procedures, describes his technique and discusses the advantages and limitations of the information obtained at operation. Dr. Jones expands the discussion to include patients with endometrial and ovarian carcinoma and stresses that the importance of the information gained is directly related to the ability to react to that information with treatment modifications carrying a reasonable rate of success.

Both operation and radiation fail to cure some patients with invasive carcinoma of the cervix. Since Brunschwig noted that approximately half such patients die with tumor confined to the pelvis, the operative removal of the bladder, uterus, vagina, anorectum, and supporting structures (total pelvic exenteration) has been advocated in the treatment of selected patients with recurrent disease. Although many patients initially were subjected to this procedure with purely palliative intent, it has now become mandatory to select patients for operation only with the intent to cure. It is thus necessary

124

to define those criteria on which curability is assessed prior to resection of the pelvic viscera. Dr. Morley details the preoperative assessment of candidates for pelvic exenteration and describes the investigations performed at the time of laparotomy to determine resectability. Drs. Weed and Creasman analyze a set of variables with respect to their ability to predict both resectability and outcome and suggest a potential scoring system for use in the evaluation of such patients.

Chapter 5

Management of the Patient with an Abnormal Pap Smear

PERSPECTIVE:

David R. Popkin

For many years cervical cancer has been the most common gynecologic malignancy and the cause of thousands of deaths among our female population. With the development of the cervicovaginal cytologic smear came the ability to detect preclinical cervical neoplasia. The majority of these preclinical lesions are confined to the cervical epithelium and have been called cervical intraepithelial neoplasia (CIN), a term proposed by Richart in 1967 to describe all dysplasias and carcinoma in situ. A significant proportion of CIN will, if left untreated, progress to invasive cervical cancer (Koss 1969; Kolstad and Klein 1976). It seems logical, therefore, to make every effort to detect cervical neoplasm in its preinvasive form and treat it before it becomes a lethal disease. The appropriate management of a patient with an abnormal Pap smear should result in a decrease in morbidity and mortality from cervical cancer.

Screening for Cervical Cancer

Diagnostic cytology for cancer of the cervix was introduced in 1943, when Papanicolaou and Trout published their now famous monograph on diagnosis of uterine cancer by the vaginal smear. It then took several years for the medical profession to appreciate the value of the technique and several more years to convince the public that a Pap test could detect cancer of the cervix in its earliest stage of development. As the Pap test became a routine examination by many doctors treating women, screening programs for the detection of cancer of the cervix developed.

127

Screening for cancer of the cervix has a particularly important advantage over screening for many other malignant conditions: the procedure is based on the detection of precursors of the truly invasive condition, and these precursors may be treated before the invasive malignant disease develops. Over the past 20 years, screening has revealed a large number of cases of preclinical disease that could only have been detected by cytologic means. Dysplasia of the cervix, carcinoma in situ, and microinvasive cancer of the cervix are all "new" diseases that do not give rise to symptoms. All are limited in extent and can be treated before invasive disease with its potential to metastasize develops.

The aim of a screening program is to detect disease at a stage when treatment is likely to be most effective. Current knowledge of cervical screening programs suggests that there are groups of women at different degrees of risk for carcinoma of the cervix. Tailoring the frequency of examination to the degree of risk rather than performing the annual Pap smear would result in the most efficient use of our resources. A Canadian report on cervical cancer screening programs suggests that cytologic screening programs are becoming effective in reducing mortality from carcinoma of the cervix (Walton et al. 1976). This report also suggests that a woman is considered at risk for the development of squamous carcinoma of the cervix as soon as she becomes sexually active. A high-risk subgroup is recognized consisting of those women who have had an early onset of sexual activity, especially with multiple partners. Women who have never been sexually active are in a low-risk group, as are those women over the age of 60 who have had repeated satisfactory smears without atypia. Although the accepted wisdom at present is to screen the female population with an annual Pap smear, it may be more efficient and less costly to change our approach to screening, concentrating on those women at highest risk for developing cervical cancer and reducing the frequency of Pap smears in the low-risk groups.

Cytology: The Papanicolaou-Trout Smear

The technique of cytologic sampling itself is important if one is to minimize the number of false negative results to an acceptable 5% or 10%. The cervix must be carefully inspected and the sample taken directly from the cervical epithelium and not from the posterior vaginal fornix. When the columnar epithelium is not everted onto the exocervix, an os aspiration using a glass pipette and a bulb syringe will increase the accuracy of the cytologic sampling. At our institution the cytopathologists do not use the Papanicolaou numerical classification for reporting cytology results, but they describe their findings in terms of the histology one would expect to find if a biopsy were performed on the cervical lesion. Since the correlation between this narrative cytology report and the actual histology is only 60% to 70%, one must investigate all abnormal Pap smears in the same manner whether the cytologist's prediction is a mild dysplasia or an invasive squamous cell cancer.

Abnormal and neoplastic cells will desquamate from areas of the female genital tract other than the cervix and also will be detected on cytologic examination. Endometrial cancer and fallopian tube and ovarian cancers have all been detected as a consequence of discovering neoplastic cells suggesting adenocarcinoma, thereby necessitating further investigation by way of fractional curettage, laparoscopy, or laparotomy. The Papanicolaou smear cannot be relied on, however, to detect genital neoplasia other than squamous cell lesions of the cervix, in which case it is 85% to 90% accurate (Hill 1966; Limburg 1958).

Investigation of Abnormal Squamous Cells on Pap Smear

Both the vulva and vagina as well as the cervix desquamate squamous cells so that, when investigating an abnormal Pap smear, a close inspection of the vulva and vagina is essential. The application of Lugol's solution (iodine) to the vagina and cervix will stain normal stratified squamous epithelium dark brown. Healthy squamous cells contain glycogen in large amounts, which accounts for the color reaction caused by the application of iodine. Neoplastic epithelial cells as well as cells which have been traumatized or are inflamed will not contain as much glycogen, will not stain dark brown, and should be biopsied. Since normal columnar epithelium does not stain brown, as does normal squamous epithelium, a distinct squamocolumnar junction can be seen on the cervix. Ninety to ninety-five percent of intraepithelium neoplastic lesions originate in the area of the squamocolumnar junction. Biopsies should be taken from the anterior and posterior lips of the cervix in nonstaining areas adjacent to the stained epithelium. If biopsies taken from nonstaining areas of the vagina or cervix reveal invasive cancer, the patient should be referred to a gynecologic oncologist for appropriate treatment. Patients whose biopsies reveal anything other than invasive cancer must be further investigated to determine the exact nature and extent of the abnormality. It should go without saying that any clinically suspicious lesion should be biopsied in the office or clinic. Although this is an extremely simple and relatively painless procedure requiring no more time than taking the Pap smear itself, this step, which could lead directly to the diagnosis of invasive disease, is often omitted. The finding of invasive cancer in a biopsy of the cervix eliminates the necessity of a cone biopsy. The only exception to this rule is when a diagnosis of microinvasion is made on the punch biopsy, in which case further investigation is necessary to rule out invasive cancer.

An essential part of the investigation of an abnormal Pap smear is the endocervical curettage (ECC), an outpatient procedure. This simple diagnostic test is performed with a Kevorkian curette. No analgesia is required, but there is often slightly more discomfort for the patient than experienced with the cervical punch biopsy. If the ECC is positive for CIN but does not show invasive cancer, a cone biopsy including the endocervical canal is necessary. If the endocervical curettage reveals no neoplastic cells, then further investigation of the cervix need only involve the ectocervix. The application of Lugol's solution will allow one to define the outer limits of the cone; thus the area of excision can be tailored for each individual patient. A cone biopsy has traditionally been performed in the hospital with the patient being confined for as long as eight or nine days. This procedure requires a general anesthetic and has an immediate morbidity of 10%. The risk of hemorrhage is greatest at the time of performing the cone and seven to eight days postoperatively. It was because of the risk of late hemorrhage that patients were hospitalized for such a long period of time.

During the past two years our experience at the Royal Victoria Hospital, McGill University, has indicated that cone biopsy can be just as safely done as a day care procedure with the patient being discharged four hours postoperatively if there is no immediate problem with hemostasis. No vaginal pack is used. The patient is advised to limit her activity for 10 days and to refrain from the use of tampons, douches, or sexual intercourse for 21 days.

If the cone biopsy removed all the abnormal epithelium and there is no invasive cancer, the patient has a 95% chance of being cured (Boyes, Worth, and Fidler 1970; Harris and Peterson 1955). Follow-up cytology every three months for one year and, if negative, yearly thereafter is important. The investigation of an abnormal Pap smear suggesting a neoplasia of squamous cell origin should involve the steps illustrated in figure 5.1.

Colposcopy

Cytology is undoubtedly the best method of detecting cervical neoplasia, but it is inadequate in the evaluation of this disease (Navratil et al. 1958). The diagnostic protocol using conization of the cervix has been proven over the years to be effective in diagnosing and treating preclinical cervical lesions (Bierra 1976; Boyes, Worth, and Fidler 1970; Kolstad and Klein 1976). Cone biopsy is not an innoxious procedure, and if a large portion of the endocervical canal is removed this could have detrimental effects on future fertility. This is an especially important consideration since CIN begins in the late teens and early twenties, when many women are deeply concerned about preserving their ability to conceive and bear children.

The colposcope was developed by Dr. H. Hinselman more than 50 years ago. It is essentially a low-power binocular microscope designed to view the cervix stereoscopically at 6- to 40-fold magnifications, using a strong light

Figure 5.1

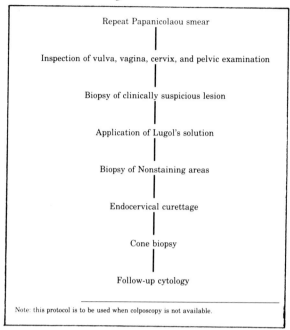

Repeat Papanicolaou smear

Inspection of vulva, vagina, cervix, and pelvic examination

Biopsy of clinically suspicious lesion

Application of Lugol's solution

Biopsy of Nonstaining areas

Endocervical curettage

Cone biopsy

Follow-up cytology

Note: this protocol is to be used when colposcopy is not available.

Diagnostic Protocol for Abnormal Pap Smear
Without Colposcopy

source. Colposcopy has recently been shown to be ideally suited for evaluating patients with an abnormal Pap smear and is without question an essential tool in the modern-day management of these patients. Several recent studies have demonstrated that diagnostic conization can be eliminated in over 90% of patients when colposcopy is used in experienced hands for investigation of abnormal Pap smears (Beller and Khatamee 1966; Donohue and Meriwether 1972; Hollyock and Chanen 1972; Krumholz and Knapp 1972; Stafl and Mattingly 1973; Ortiz, Newton, and Langlois 1969; Ostergard and Gondos 1973). The cone biopsy can be eliminated because the colposcope enables the colposcopist to assess the location, extent, and severity of the cervical lesion and to direct a biopsy to the appropriate areas. In this way the colposcopically directed biopsies can rule out invasive cancer. The addition of the colposcope to the evaluation scheme for the abnormal Pap smear allows a thorough assessment of the transformation zone, which is entirely visible in over 90% of patients. The transformation zone is that area of the cervix, once covered by columnar epithelium, which through a process of metaplasia has been transformed into stratified squamous epithelium. This is a physiological process, but occasionally, perhaps due to some external environmental factor such as a virus, the metaplastic epithelium becomes dysplastic. The

131

colposcopist recognizes the abnormal transformation zone because of its whiteness or because there are certain abnormal vascular patterns present. The entire transformation zone can be delineated in the majority of cases and directed biopsies taken from the most abnormal areas. An endocervical curettage should be a routine part of this colposcopic assessment even if the upper limits of the lesion are seen. If the entire extent of the lesion cannot be visualized using the colposcope, the examination should be reported as unsatisfactory and a cone biopsy performed. If on endocervical curettage neoplastic cells are found, a cone biopsy should also be performed. If the endocervical curettage is negative and the entire transformation zone is visualized and invasive cancer has been excluded by directed punch biopsy, a variety of treatments can be offered to the patient. The most valuable contributions that colposcopy makes to the evaluation of an abnormal Pap smear are in (1) localizing the abnormal area of the transformation zone so that a biopsy can be taken for histologic confirmation of the lesion and (2) delineating the extent of the abnormality. The latter is extremely important if local destructive therapy is to be the method of treatment. A diagnostic and therapeutic protocol using colposcopy in patients with abnormal Papanicolaou smears is shown in figure 5.2.

Treatment

As in most areas of medicine the effectiveness of the treatment is directly related to the accuracy of diagnosis. The diagnostic protocols in figures 5.1 and 5.2 are designed to rule out invasive cancer before conservative management is carried out. More radical therapy is of course necessary for invasive cancer. It is reasonable to attempt to minimize the use of the cone biopsy, provided other methods of diagnosis do not increase the likelihood of misdiagnosis and consequently result in inadequate treatment of invasive cancer.

Surgery

If the proper preoperative evaluation is carried out so that the extent of the lesion is accurately delineated and invasive cancer is ruled out, CIN I, II, and III can be treated equally well with conization or hysterectomy (Bjerra et al. 1976; Boyes, Worth, and Fidler 1970; Kolstad and Klein 1976). It must be emphasized that an experienced colposcopist must adequately assess the cervix prior to preceding directly to a simple hysterectomy. This assessment must include an endocervical curettage even if the entire squamocolumnar junction is visualized.

Special mention should be made of the pregnant cervix. The colposcope has been of invaluable assistance in the assessment of the pregnant patient with an abnormal Pap smear. Colposcopically directed biopsies can ade-

Figure 5.2

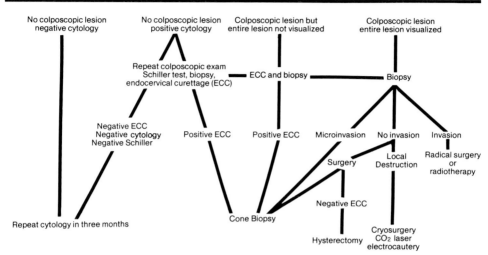

Diagnostic and Therapeutic Protocol Using Colposcopy for Patients with Abnormal Papanicolaou Smears.

quately assess the cervix in virtually all cases, and because of the eversion of columnar epithelium the entire transformation zone is almost always visible. An endocervical curettage should not be performed in pregnancy. Unless invasive carcinoma is diagnosed on colposcopically directed biopsy the patient is allowed to progress to term and is delivered vaginally. The cervix should be reevaluated three months postpartum. The use of the colposcope has virtually eliminated the need for a cone biopsy in pregnancy (De Petrillo et al. 1975).

Local Tissue Destruction

Cryosurgery

Numerous studies have appeared in the literature since 1970, indicating that cryosurgery is effective in treating cervical intraepithelial neoplasia if the cervix has been adequately assessed by an experienced colposcopist (Townsend and Ostergard 1971; Creasman et al. 1973; Kaufman et al. 1973; Popkin, Scali, and Ahmed 1978; Kaufman and Conner 1971; Crisp 1972; Crisp et al. 1970). Cure rates ranging from 85% to 96% have been reported. Prerequisites to the use of cryosurgery include (1) the exclusion of invasive cancer and (2) a nonpregnant patient. Under no circumstances should cryosurgery be used as treatment for CIN without a tissue diagnosis or colposcopic control, nor should it be used for the treatment of invasive cervical cancer including microinvasion.

Electrocautery

Electrocautery has been shown to be an effective method of local tissue destruction provided the same guidelines for patient selection and follow-up are used as with cryosurgery (Richart and Sciarra 1968; Connor and Kaufman 1970; Ortiz, Newton, and Tsai 1973).

CO_2 Laser Therapy

The CO_2 surgical laser is currently being used on an experimental basis for the treatment of selected patients with CIN. The radiant waves from the CO_2 laser destroy tissue by conversion of its energy to heat. In our experience this technique does not produce better cure rates for treatment of CIN than does cryosurgery. Patients seem to experience more local pain and bleeding than with cryosurgery, and one has to contend with the smoke produced as the tissue is destroyed. A continuous suction is very effective for this purpose. The healing of the treated area seems to occur more rapidly following laser therapy than cryotherapy. From preliminary data not yet published it would appear that the CO_2 laser will be as effective as cryosurgery in curing CIN but will not be competitive when ease of application and cost of equipment are considered.

References

Beller, F.K., and Khatamee, M. Evaluation of punch biopsy of the cervix under direct colposcopic observation. *Obstet. Gynecol.* 28:622–625, 1966.

Bjerra, B. et al. Conization as only treatment of carcinoma in situ of the uterine cervix. *Am. J. Obstet. Gynecol.* 125:143–152, 1976.

Boyes, D.A., Worth, A.J., and Fidler, H.K. The results of treatment of 4389 cases of preclinical cervical squamous carcinoma. *J. Obstet. Gynaecol. Br. Comm.* 77:769–780, 1970.

Conner, J.S., and Kaufman, R.H. Treatment of dysplasia of the cervix uteri by electrocauterization. *Surg. Gynecol. Obstet.* 131:726–728, 1970.

Creasman, W.T. et al. Efficacy of cryosurgical treatment of severe cervical intraepithelial neoplasia. *Obstet. Gynecol.* 41:501–506, 1973.

Crisp, W.E. Cryosurgical treatment of neoplasia of the uterine cervix. *Obstet. Gynecol.* 39:495–499, 1972.

Crisp, W.E. et al. Cryosurgical treatment of premalignant disease of the uterine cervix. *Am. J. Obstet. Gynecol.* 107:737–742, 1970.

DePetrillo, A.D. et al. Colposcopic evaluation of the abnormal Papanicolaou test in pregnancy. *Am. J. Obstet. Gynecol.* 121:441–445, 1975.

Donohue, L,. and Meriwether, D. Colposcopy as a diagnostic tool in the investigation of cervical neoplasias. *Am. J. Obstet. Gynecol.* 113:107–110, 1972.

135

Harris, J.H., and Peterson, P. Cold knife conization and residual preinvasive carcinoma of the cervix. *Am. J. Obstet. Gynecol.* 70:1092–1099, 1955.

Hill, E. Preclinical cervical carcinoma, colposcopy and the negative smear. *Am. J. Obstet. Gynecol.* 95:309–319, 1966.

Hollyock, V.E., and Chanen, W. The use of the colposcope in the selection of patients for cervical cone biopsy. *Am. J. Obstet. Gynecol.* 114:185–189, 1972.

Kaufman, R.H. et al. Cryosurgical treatment of cervical intraepithelial neoplasia. *Obstet. Gynecol.* 42:881–886, 1973.

Kaufman, R.H., and Conner, J.S. Cryosurgical treatment of cervical dysplasia. *Am. J. Obstet. Gynecol.* 109:1167–1174, 1971.

Kolstad, P., and Klein, V. Long term follow-up of 1121 cases of carcinoma in situ. *Am. J. Obstet. Gynecol.* 48:125, 1976.

Koss, L.G. Concept of genesis and development of carcinoma of the cervix in conference on early cervical neoplasia. *Obstet. Gynecol. Surv.* 24:850–860, 1969.

Krumholz, B.A., and Knapp, R.C. Colposcopic selection of biopsy sites. *Obstet. Gynecol.* 39:22–26, 1972.

Limburg, H. Comparison between cytology and colposcopy in the diagnosis of early cervical carcinoma. *Am. J. Obstet. Gynecol.* 75:1298–1301, 1958.

Navratil, E. et al. Simultaneous colposcopy and cytology used in screening for carcinoma of the cervix. *Am. J. Obstet. Gynecol.* 75:1292–1297, 1958.

Ortiz, R.; Newton, M.; and Langlois, P.L. Colposcopic biopsy in the diagnosis of carcinoma of the cervix. *Obstet. Gynecol.* 34:303–306, 1969.

Ortiz, R.; Newton, M.; and Tsai, A. Electrocautery treatment of cervical intraepithelial neoplasia. *Obstet. Gynecol.* 41:113–116, 1973.

Ostergard, D., and Gondos, B. Selection of patients with the use of colposcopy. *Am. J. Obstet. Gynecol.* 115:783–785, 1973.

Papanicolaou, G.N., and Trout, H.F. *Diagnosis of uterine cancer by the vaginal smear.* New York: The Commonwealth Fund, 1943.

Popkin, D.R.; Scali, V.; and Ahmed, M.N. Cryosurgery for the treatment of cervical intraepithelial neoplasia. *Am. J. Obstet Gynecol.* 130:551–554, 1978.

Richart, R.M. Natural history of cervical intraepithelial neoplasia. *Clin. Obstet. Gynecol.* 10:748–784, 1967.

Richart, R.M., and Sciarra, J.J. Treatment of cervical dysplasia by outpatient electrocauterization. *Am. J. Obstet. Gynecol.* 101:200–205, 1968.

Stafl, A., and Mattingly, R.F. Colposcopic diagnosis of cervical neoplasia. *Obstet. Gynecol.* 41:188, 1973.

Townsend, D.E., and Ostergard, D.R. Cryocauterization for preinvasive cervical neoplasia. *J. Reprod. Med.* 6:55–60, 1971.

Walton, R.J. et al. Cervical cancer screening program, epidemiology and natural history of cancer of the cervix. *Can. Med. Assoc. J.* 114:1003–1012, 1976.

PERSPECTIVE:

Management of the Patient with an Abnormal Pap Smear

Alex Ferenczy

Before discussing the rationale underlying the changing concepts in the diagnosis and management of preinvasive cervical carcinoma, it is useful to review the traditional terminology and therapy of cervical cancer precursors.

Lesions in which the full thickness of the epithelium is made of undifferentiated malignant cells are called carcinoma in situ (CIS). Lesions without full thickness dedifferentiation are referred to as dysplasias. These in turn are subdivided into very mild, mild, moderate, and severe forms according to the degree to which the epithelium is replaced by abnormal squamous cells.

The traditional management approach to women with noninvasive cervical disease is surgical for CIS and severe dysplasia. Lesser lesions are either followed with Pap tests or completely ignored. Women with severe dysplasia and CIS and those who no longer wish to conceive receive conization and simple hysterectomy, with or without vaginal cuff excision, respectively. Those who desire to preserve their reproductive functions are treated with conization, whereas those whose disease is detected during pregnancy are either followed by Pap tests or punch biopsies or receive conization and are subjected to transabdominal hysterectomy following delivery.

This two-disease (dysplasia-CIS) concept and management protocol are based on the following assumptions: (1) there is a high risk of developing invasive carcinoma from CIS compared to dysplasias; (2) very mild, mild, and moderate dysplasias have high spontaneous regression rates; (3) the cervix, endocervical canal, and vaginal fornix are often extensively involved by CIS and severe dysplasia; and (4) cervical cancer precursors have multifocal distribution. Although this surgical approach yields excellent cure rates, it is important to realize that the above assumptions derive from observations in treating women during the 1950s and 1960s. Indeed, these periods coincide with the early development of cervical cancer screening programs. As a result, many women were detected for the first time and thus were prevalence

137

cases; they had longstanding lesions. These tended to be high grade, large lesions with involvement of the endocervical canal, and on occasion the vaginal fornix. Also, in the light of today's knowledge, the high regression rates reported for early dysplasias are explained by the inaccurate morphologic ascertainment of cases studied and the poor design of prospective follow-up protocols and statistical analysis of cases (Richart 1967).

With current knowledge and understanding of the natural history of preinvasive cervical lesions and the improved techniques of evaluating their distribution and extent in the cervix by colposcopy, a trend toward a more conservative and highly individualized treatment of cervical cancer precursors has been developed in more recent years (Crisp et al. 1970; Conner and Kaufman 1970; Townsend et al. 1970; Kaufman and Conner 1971; Townsend and Ostergard 1971; Crisp 1972; Thompson et al. 1972; Tredway et al. 1972; Ostergard and Gondos 1973; Creasman et al. 1973; Kaufman et al. 1973; Stafl and Mattingly 1973; DiSaia, Townsend, and Morrow 1974; Chanen and Hollyock 1974; Creasman and Parker 1975; Underwood et al. 1976; Kohan et al. 1977; Kaufman 1978). In contrast to the traditional two-disease, dysplasia-CIS approach, the modern approach to patients with abnormal cytology is based on the concept that dysplasia and CIS are a part of a disease continuum, cervical intraepithelial neoplasia (CIN). Moreover, CIN, if untreated, may lead to invasive cancer of the cervix. The evidence favoring a unitarian concept of cervical cancer precursors and the underlying generic term CIN have been offered by Ralph Richart and associates. These investigators have conducted a series of carefully designed clinical and laboratory experiments of lesions believed to precede invasive squamous cell carcinoma of the cervix. Every objective test of these lesions reinforced the concept that they indeed form a continuum which begins as a well-differentiated lesion—very mild dysplasia—and ends with early stromal invasion (fig. 5.3).

With this concept of the disease, the question of whether a given lesion is mild, moderate, or severe dysplasia or CIS becomes irrelevant. (Richart 1967; Ferenczy 1977). It is important for the clinician as well as for the pathologist (1) to rule out invasive carcinoma; (2) if the lesion is noninvasive, to determine its size and distribution; and (3) to remove the lesion by using the easiest, fastest, most reliable, and least costly means possible, and if appropriate, to preserve the patient's reproductive functions. In the majority of cases with abnormal cytology, colposcopy can accurately determine the precise location and extent of the disease. Colposcopically directed punch biopsies coupled with thorough endocervical curettage can provide histologic confirmation of either CIN or invasive carcinoma (Ferenczy 1977). Using these outpatient diagnostic techniques, it is possible to eliminate the need for inpatient conization and its inherent high cost and complications in up to 95% of nonpregnant (Stafl and Mattingly 1973; DiSaia, Townsend, and Morrow 1974) and 99% (Stafl and Mattingly 1973; DePetrillo et al. 1975) of pregnant women. These rates are not only a reflection of our better understanding of the natural history of CIN but also of the extensive use of cervical cytology.

138

Figure 5.3

PRECURSORS TO INVASIVE CARCINOMA OF CERVIX

Cervical Intraepithelial Neoplasia

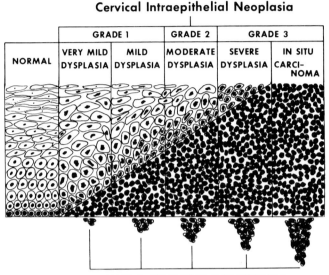

NORMAL	GRADE 1		GRADE 2	GRADE 3	
	VERY MILD DYSPLASIA	MILD DYSPLASIA	MODERATE DYSPLASIA	SEVERE DYSPLASIA	IN SITU CARCINOMA

MICRO INVASIVE CARCINOMA

*Schematic representation of cervical cancer
precursors. CIN grades 1, 2, and 3 correspond to
the traditional very mild to mild, moderate to
severe dysplasia and to CIS, respectively. They are
characterized by a progressive increase in the
number of undifferentiated, malignant cells and a
decrease in superficial cell differentiation
paralleling the increasing severity of CIN. Grading
CIN has no therapeutic implications, but it is
useful for epidemiologic and statistical
considerations. The schema also illustrates that
microinvasion, although more commonly associated
with a grade 3 lesion, may also develop directly
from any given stage of CIN. The risk of
developing microinvasion in different stages of
CIN, however, is not necessarily proportional to
that illustrated in the figure.*

Indeed, by rescreening women, we tend to discover incidence rather than prevalence cases, that is, newly established rather than longstanding CIN lesions. As a result, most of today's lesions are relatively small and located on the exposed portion of the cervix.

Treating "patient's disease" rather than "doctor's disease" requires not only a great deal of skill but also a thorough understanding of the natural history of the disease. Consequently, it is now appropriate to review briefly

139

the features of the CIN concept that are relevant to individualized patient care. Clinical studies designed to follow prospectively a large number of women with early CIN (dysplasia) using only cytology and colpomicroscopy as follow-up techniques are available. Unlike those studies that used biopsies for initial ascertainment of CIN and for follow-up (multiple biopsies actually remove many lesions and thus produce high spontaneous regression rates), in the Richart-Barron study (1973), most dysplasias either persisted or progressed to CIS. Only 6% of the earliest dysplasias regressed spontaneously. The study also showed a logarithmic increase in the progression transit times from very mild dysplasia, to mild, to moderate, and to severe dysplasia, ranging from a mean of 68 months in very mild dysplasia to 12 months in severe dysplasia. The calculated transit times correlated well with both the prevalence rates and the incidence of CIN observed in cytologic screening programs. Early dysplasias tending to last longer in the cervix are detected in a comparatively greater number than more severe forms of dysplasias or CIS lesions. The investigators, however, could not predict (nor could anybody else) (Koss 1978) the potential of regression, persistence, or progression of individual lesions to a more severe form of CIN or invasion. In fact, the data suggest that every CIN, regardless of degree of morphologic severity, has the same potential for invading the stroma at any given time in the individual patient. In other words, while microinvasion most commonly develops from CIN grade 3 lesion (CIS) in the aggregate, early stromal invasion may also develop directly from CIN grade 2 or 1 lesion in the individual patient (fig. 5.3). Since it is not possible to predict which patient will progress to invasion with a given CIN at a given time, a CIN lesion regardless of degree of morphologic severity, once detected, should be treated at once to prevent the occurrence of invasion (Richart 1967; Ferenczy 1977; Richart 1973; Koss 1978).

It has been shown that CIN originates in the squamous epithelium of the squamocolumnar junction of the transformation zone (t-zone), and its distribution coincides with that of the t-zone. CIN only rarely extends onto the native portio epithelium beyond the transformation zone, and expands by direct replacement (rather than transformation) of adjacent t-zone epithelium and of that lining the endocervical canal. Squamous metaplasia (SM) produces multiple islands of squamous epithelium in the t-zone, external os, and endocervical canal. SM is not involved, however, in the development of cervical squamous cell carcinoma. (Richart 1967; Ferenczy 1977; Richart 1973).

Ninety-five percent of CIN lesions develop in a single focus and have a single cell origin (Richart 1973). The field theory or multifocal carcinogenesis operating in predetermined fields of the cervical epithelium occurs in only 5% of CIN. This concept has important clinical implications since removal of a single CIN focus (large or small) should lead to a cure in about 95% of the cases. The overall treatment results strongly support the unifocal cervical carcinogenesis concept (Richart et al. 1979). Moreover, destruction of the t-zone epithelium (which is susceptible to carcinogenesis) at the same time explains the rarity of recurrences of new CIN in these patients. Furthermore, knowing that fields of SM are not at risk for carcinogenesis, the finding of isolated foci of SM in the endocervical canal does not present danger of malignancy in this region. Single and multiple lesions in the vaginal fornix and in the lower part of the vagina independent of the t-zone are either condylomata acuminata or primary vaginal intraepithelial or invasive neoplasias.

In summarizing the presently available data one can conclude the following: (1) CIN represents a continuum of epithelial alterations that precede invasive carcinoma of the cervix; (2) CIN originates at the squamocolumnar junction of the t-zone; (3) most CIN lesions are unifocal, have a single cell origin, and expand within the t-zone and into the endocervical canal; (4) at present, there are no objective means to predict the potential of progression to invasion of any CIN at a given time in the individual patient. Consequently, any and every CIN has the same unpredictable potential to invade the stroma in the individual patient at a given instant.

Acceptance and understanding of the natural history of CIN lead to the application of a triage approach to patients with abnormal Pap tests. This consists of distinguishing between normal epithelium and its variants (SM, atypia of inflammation, and so on) and CIN, and between CIN and invasive cancer. If CIN is found, its size and distribution are assessed, and the treatment is tailored according to the individual patient's need. The management flow chart is presented in figure 5.4.

Following an abnormal Pap test, the patient today is evaluated in most large medical centers by colposcopy. A colposcopist with good training (having first thoroughly examined a minimum of 10 patients a week for one year under supervision by an experienced colposcopist and then correlated colposcopy with histology) in most instances can accurately recognize the normal squamous epithelium and its variants as well as the abnormal transformation zone epithelium that may be associated with malignancy. The basic principles of good colposcopy imply attempts at visualizing the entire t-zone and its squamocolumnar junction as well as the lesional area. If this requires examination of the external os or endocervical canal, then an endocervical speculum should be used. By doing so, the entire limits of the abnormal epithelium can be visualized, and invasion can be excluded by colposcopy. It is of prime importance to remember that histologic sampling of the cervix provides the unequivocal diagnosis. As a result, all patients must receive a thorough, circumferential curettage of the endocervical canal and multiple punch biopsies. The latter should be applied to areas with greatest vascular abnormality and near the external os. Numerous new intraepithelial vessels with abnormal configuration and branching patterns growing parallel to the surface are the hallmarks of invasive carcinoma. Most invasive cancers are located near or within the anatomical external os. A biopsy should be performed in every case of hyperkeratosis to rule out keratinizing invasive cancer.

Patients with CIN lesions located on the exposed portion of the cervix who are reliable for long-term follow-up are best managed on an outpatient

Figure 5.4

ABNORMAL PAP SMEARS WITHOUT CLINICALLY VISIBLE CERVICAL CARCINOMA

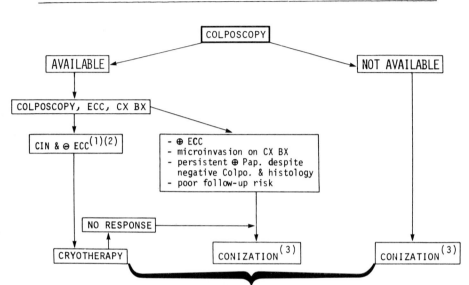

FOLLOW-UP WITH PAP TEST

Flow chart illustrating the diagnostic and therapeutic approach when colposcopic and cytopathologic expertise is available and not available.
ECC: *endocervical curettage;* CX BX: *cervical punch biopsies;* CIN: *cervical intraepithelial neoplasia. (1): if pregnant, delay treatment after delivery; (2): if sterilization desired, hysterectomy or cryotherapy and bilateral tubal ligation (BTL); (3): if sterilization desired, hysterectomy or BTL.*

basis using conservative techniques. Patients with abnormal findings other than the above will require inpatient diagnostic evaluation, and most commonly a cold-knife conization. These conditions include (1) lesions extending into the endocervical canal whose limit cannot be seen; (2) endocervical localization of lesion with normal portio (especially in older patients); (3) persistent positive cytology despite negative colposcopy or biopsy; (4) microinvasive carcinoma on biopsy (conization is performed to rule out stage I_b occult invasive carcinoma), and (5) patients unreliable for long-term follow-up.

Patients with CIN confined to the exposed portion of the cervix may be managed by electrocautery (Richart 1973), cryocauterization, and laser-beam therapy (Bellina 1974; Stafl et al. 1977; Carter 1978). Cryotherapy is now the most frequently used technique for exocervical CIN lesions, and its costs and complication rates are negligible compared to conization. Cryotherapy is preferred to electrocautery because it is less painful, faster to perform, and does not interfere with fertility (Weed et al. 1978). Carbon dioxide (CO_2) laser can be applied to treating CIN, but the results obtained so far are essentially identical with those of cryotherapy. The very high cost of the CO_2 laser, compared to that of cryotherapy, is its major disadvantage.

The treatment of patients with localized CIN and who wish to be sterilized is somewhat controversial. Some advocate simple hysterectomy for these patients, whereas others prefer cryotherapy and bilateral tubal ligation.

The best results of cryotherapy are obtained when the cervix, including the external os, is cleansed of excess mucus; a fine film of K-Y Jelly is applied to the cryoprobe tip (promotes cold transfer and even freezing); and freezing performed until the iceball extends circumferentially a minimum of 5 mm beyond the limits of the lesional tissue and that of the t-zone. For large lesions, the cryo-iceballs should be overlapped. Double freezing is generally not necessary, but may be carried out for postcryotherapy residual CIN. Large gas tanks (20 pounds or preferably 60 pounds) produce better freezing because of greater constancy and faster recovery of pressure. Nitrous oxide gas is preferred to CO_2 because the former is cleaner than the latter and keeps the pipes clean for a longer time.

One should wait three to four months before repeating cytology and colposcopy after cryotherapy to avoid false positive findings due to healing. Postcryotherapy follow-up protocol consists in reexamining the patient by means of cytology, colposcopy, and, if necessary, endocervical curettage and cervical biopsies every three months for the first year and by cytology once a year thereafter, for as long as the smears remain negative. Using colposcopy for long-term follow-up is not justified on a cost-benefit basis. A freeze cure is defined by obtaining three negative and satisfactory Pap smears beginning at three to four months within the first year postcryotherapy. In the author's colposcopy clinic, a thorough endocervical curettage is done in every patient during the third postcryotherapy visit to ascertain absence of disease in the canal. This overcaution is useful, since in many postcryo cervices, particularly those frozen more than once, the external os may be narrowed and the squamocolumnar junction located within the os. In these cases, colposcopic examination alone may be unsatisfactory.

A freeze failure is an abnormal smear or biopsy or endocervical curettage obtained during the first year of postcryotherapy. The freeze failure rate (residual or persistent disease) after one cryosurgical procedure in most large and recent series is approximately 12%. Refreezing residual CIN lesions may provide up to 95% overall therapeutic success rates (Richart et al. 1980). Further cryotherapy (third, fourth, and so on), however, tends to produce external os stenosis and is less effective in removing persistent disease. Therefore, compulsive cryotherapy for residual disease is not recommended, and these patients are best managed surgically by either conization or hysterectomy.

Most recently, important observations have been made regarding freeze-failure rates (Richart et al. 1980). It has been observed that failure rate is related to the size rather than the histologic grade of the CIN. In other words, when the results are analyzed according to lesional size and then correlated with histologic grades, the cure rate is independent of histology. Most small CIN lesions of grade 1, 2, or 3 have essentially similar freeze-failure rates: 9%, 8%, and 5%, respectively. Similarly, large CIN lesions, regardless of grades (1, 2, or 3), have a failure rate of 25% to 50%. These observations explain why one is less successful in treating a grade 3 as compared to a grade 1 CIN lesion, because in general CIN 3 tends to occupy larger areas than do its CIN 1 and 2 counterparts. Furthermore, since a grade 3 CIN develops in general from a grade 2, which in turn develops from a grade 1 CIN, it is unwise not to treat early CIN lesions, as they are likely to dedifferentiate, enlarge, and become more difficult to eradicate by conservative cryotherapy.

Another question often raised in related to the risks of developing a new CIN in patients who have received cryotherapy. The long-term recurrence rates of CIN in 2839 pooled cryotherapeutically treated patients followed for up to 15 years have recently been evaluated (Richart et al. 1980). According to life table analysis of pooled data from all CIN cases (amounting to 40,134 woman-years experience), 4 of 1000 women per year were observed to develop a new lesion following successful cryotherapy. This rate is essentially the same as the incidence of CIN: the occurrence of CIN in a previously CIN-free but sexually active population. In addition, all new cases were CIN 1 and were easily managed. The fact that no invasion occurred in this series of women negates the suggestion that after cryotherapy CIN may be buried within endocervical glands with normal surface epithelium, and that it can later become invasive carcinoma. The appearance of CIN in the treated compared to the untreated high-risk women is related to the cryotherapy itself. As has been suggested earlier, an adequate cryotherapy destroys not only the lesional area but also the entire t-zone. By doing so, the t-zone epithelium, which represents the susceptible area for subsequent carcinogenesis, is removed. This is the very reason why cryotherapy rather than excisional biopsy is recommended even for small lesions: the former also removes the t-zone, whereas the latter does not. The recurrence rates in postconization CIN patients, however, are reported to be comparatively higher than in patients treated with cryotherapy—up to 33% at 15 years—and include cases of invasive carcinoma (Richart et al. 1980).

A final issue of great concern to many physicians is the accuracy of colposcopy in distinguishing between CIN and invasive carcinoma. Indeed, an increasing number of women were recently observed with invasive carcinoma who were mismanaged by colposcopy and cryotherapy (Sevin et al. 1979). When these cases are carefully reviewed, however, it appears that a significant number of patients were examined poorly or not at all by cytology and/ or by colposcopy, and in most cases the mandatory endocervical curettage was ignored. If the endocervical curettage is eliminated from the triage approach, the risk of missing an invasive carcinoma is considerably increased

(Urcuyo, Romes, and Nelson 1977). It is the experience of most university medical centers that if colposcopy is coupled with endocervical curettage and cervical punch biopsies, invasive cancer is missed in 1 to 2 of 1000 patients with an abnormal smear (Richart et al. 1980). This error rate is closely similar to that for conization and hysterectomy. It should be reiterated that the outpatient colposcopic and cryotherapeutic approach must include in every case a thorough endocervical curettage followed by multiple punch biopsies sampling the most abnormal area of the t-zone, and that the procedures should be performed only by an experienced team of colposcopists and cytopathologists. Those clinicians who are in the process of learning colposcopy and cryotherapy or who do not have access to highly accurate cytology and pathology laboratories should either rely on conization as the major diagnostic and therapeutic modality or, if feasible, refer the patient for colposcopy consultation.

Among the many diagnostic and therapeutic modalities that have been advocated for CIN, colposcopy and cryotherapy appear highly effective in evaluating and treating CIN on an outpatient basis in the majority of cases. When all the steps of the procedures are carefully executed, treatment-failure and recurrence rates are negligible. Physicians with a clear understanding of the natural history of cervical cancer precursors who have access to cytopathologic expertise and to a relatively large number of patients with abnormal cytology are encouraged to become acquainted with the triage approach. The results obtained will be rewarding for both the patient and the clinician, and thus our contemporary medical care of women with abnormal Pap tests will improve significantly.

References

Bellina, J.H. Gynecology and the laser. *Contemp. Obstet. Gynecol.* 4:24–34, 1974.

Carter R. et al. Treatment of cervical intraepithelial neoplasia with the carbon dioxide laser beam. *Am. J. Obstet. Gynecol.* 131:831–836, 1978.

Chanen, W., and Hollyock, V.E. Colposcopy and the conservative management of cervical dysplasia and carcinoma in situ. *Obstet. Gynecol.* 43:527–534, 1974.

Conner, J.S., and Kaufman, R.H. Treatment of dysplasia of the cervix uteri by electrocauterization. *Surg. Gynecol. Obstet.* 131:726–732, 1970.

Creasman, W.T. et al. Efficacy of cryosurgical treatment of severe cervical intraepithelial neoplasia. *Obstet. Gynecol.* 41:501–506, 1973.

Creasman, W.T., and Parker, R.T. Management of early cervical neoplasia. *Clin. Obstet. Gynecol.* 18:233–245, 1975.

Crisp, W.E. Cryosurgical treatment of neoplasia of the uterine cervix. *Obstet. Gynecol.* 39:495–499, 1972.

Crisp, W.E. et al. Cryosurgical treatment of premalignant disease of the uterine cervix. *Am. J. Obstet. Gynecol.* 107:737–742, 1970.

DePetrillo, A.D. et. al. Colposcopic evaluation of the abnormal Papanicolaou test in pregnancy. *Am. J. Obstet. Gynecol.* 121:441–445, 1975.

DiSaia, P.J.; Townsend, D.E.; and Morrow, C.P. The rationale for less than radical treatment for gynecologic malignancy in early reproductive years. *Obstet. Gynecol. Surv.* 29:581–593, 1974.

Ferenczy, A. Cervical intraepithelial neoplasia. In *Pathology of the female genital tract,* ed. A. Blaustein. New York: Springer-Verlag, 1977.

Kaufman, R.H. et al. Cryosurgical treatment of cervical intraepithelial neoplasia. *Obstet. Gynecol.* 42:881–886, 1973.

Kaufman, R.H., and Conner, J.S. Cryosurgical treatment of cervical dysplasia. *Am. J. Obstet. Gynecol.* 109:1167–1174, 1971.

Kaufman, R.H., and Irwin, L.F. The cryosurgical therapy of cervical intraepithelial neoplasia. III. Continuing follow-up. *Am. J. Obstet. Gynecol.* 131:381–388, 1978.

Kohan, S. et al. Colposcopy and the management of cervical intraepithelial neoplasia. *Gynecol. Oncol.* 5:27–39, 1977.

Koss, L.G. Dysplasia. A real concept or a misnomer? *Obstet. Gynecol.* 51:374–379, 1978.

Ostergard, D.R., and Gondos, B. Outpatient therapy of preinvasive cervical neoplasia: selection of patients with the use of colposcopy. *Am. J. Obstet. Gynecol.* 115:783–785, 1973.

Richart, R.M. Natural history of cervical intraepithelial neoplasia. *Clin. Obstet Gynecol.* 10:748–784, 1967.

Richart, R.M. Cervical intraepithelial neoplasia: a review. In *Pathology annual 1973,* ed. S.C. Sommers. New York: Appleton-Century-Crofts, 1973.

Richart, R.M. et al. An analysis of long-term follow-up results in patients with cervical intraepithelial neoplasia treated by cryotherapy. *Am. J. Obstet. Gynecol.* 137:823–826, 1980.

Sevin, B.U. et al. Invasive cancer of the cervix after cryosurgery. *Obstet. Gynecol.* 52:465–468, 1979.

Stafl, A., and Mattingly, R.F. Colposcopic diagnosis of cervical neoplasia. *Obstet. Gynecol.* 41:168–176, 1973.

Stafl, A.; Wilkinson, E.J.; and Mattingly, R.F. Laser treatment of cervical and vaginal neoplasia. *Am. J. Obstet. Gynecol.* 128:128–136, 1977.

Thompson, B.H. et al. Cytopathology, histopathology, and colposcopy in the management of cervical neoplasia. *Am. J. Obstet. Gynecol.* 114:329–338, 1972.

Townsend, D.E. et al. Abnormal Papanicolaou smears: evaluation by colposcopy, biopsies and endocervical curettage. *Am. J. Obstet. Gynecol.* 108:429–434, 1970.

Townsend, D.E., and Ostergard, D.R. Cryocauterization for preinvasive cervical neoplasia. *J. Reprod. Med.* 6:55, 1971.

Tredway, D.R. et al. Colposcopy and cryosurgery in cervical intraepithelial neoplasia. *Am. J. Obstet. Gynecol.* 114:1020–1024, 1972.

Underwood, P.B.; Lutz, M.H.; and Fletcher, R.V., Jr. Cryosurgery. *Cancer* 38:546–552, 1976.

Urcuyo, R.; Rome, R.M.; and Nelson, J.H. Some observations on the value of endocervical curettage performed as an integral part of colposcopic examination of patients with abnormal cervical cytology. *Am. J. Obstet. Gynecol.* 128:787–792, 1977.

Weed, J.C. et al. Fertility after cryosurgery of the cervix. *Obstet. Gynecol.* 52:245–246, 1978.

147

PERSPECTIVE:

Management of the Patient with an Abnormal Pap Smear

Edmund Stephen Petrilli

Since cytologic screening for cervical neoplasia was introduced over 30 years ago, the primary responsibility of the physician in the management of the patient with an abnormal Pap smear has been to determine the presence or absence of invasive cervical carcinoma. Over the past decade the methods available to meet this obligation have expanded, due to the introduction of colposcopy. With appropriate skill in colposcopy, one can evaluate the patient who has abnormal cytology with an economy of cost, time, and morbidity. Colposcopy and directed biopsies can establish a diagnosis of invasive carcinoma or the grade and distribution of preinvasive disease that permits a selection of therapeutic options tailored to meet individual needs. This discussion considers the relationship of cervical neoplasia, cytologic screening, and colposcopic evaluation in the contemporary management of the patient with an abnormal Pap smear.

Cervical Neoplasia

Nonneoplastic and premalignant lesions of the cervix are responsible for most abnormal Pap smears. Even in a high-risk population, not more than 5% of patients with abnormal cytology have invasive carcinoma of the cervix (Townsend 1977). Richart (1967) introduced the term cervical intraepithelial neoplasia (CIN) to describe the precursors of invasive squamous carcinoma as a biologic continuum ranging from mild dysplasia (CIN 1) through severe dysplasia and carcinoma in situ (CIN 3). The progression from mild dysplasia to carcinoma in situ (CIS) occurs slowly in a patient population with a median transit time of 86 months, and all lesions do not advance to the next higher grade (Richart and Barron 1969). If untreated, 10% to 15% of CIN 1 and 2 lesions may eventually progress to invasive carcinoma (DiSaia, Morrow, and Townsend 1975). These concepts are supported by the fact that CIN 1 is the most common lesion and occurs in younger patients than CIN 3, which is least frequent and occurs later. In a review of cervical neoplasia, Briggs (1979) summarized the cytologic prevalence of dysplasia and CIS as ranging from 0.5% to 6.5% and 0.36% to 0.8% respectively. The incidence of new disease in patients previously screened as negative was 0.1% for dysplasia and 0.004% for CIS. Cytologic screening identifies those patients in the population who have cervical neoplasia.

Cytologic Screening

The accessibility of the uterine cervix to direct examination allowed a correlation of cytologic and histologic changes that formed the basis for Papanicolaou's classification system. Widespread cytologic screening became established in the United States over 30 years ago and is still the primary method by which cervical neoplasia are detected. Between 1955 and 1974, the rate of invasive squamous carcinoma of the cervix in British Columbia decreased from 28.5 to 8.6 per 100,000 women over the age of 20 and was directly related to the extent of screening during that period (Boyes et al. 1977). The Canadian Task Force on Cervical Cancer Screening Programs (1976) attributed the decreased mortality from cervical carcinoma over the past 20 years to cytologic screening. They suggest annual screening for high-risk patients who are defined as those having an early onset of sexual activity, multiple sexual partners, or previous CIN. They recommend cancer screening every three years for low-risk patients who have had three consecutive negative Pap smears, because this group is unlikely to develop cervical neoplasia. Alternatively, the annual examination also provides the health professoinal with an opportunity to search for systemic disease and early neoplasia of the breast, colon, and pelvic organs. It seems premature to abandon the annual examination in the low-risk group without further consideration of these benefits. An inordinate number of cases of invasive carcinoma occur in high-risk segments of the population who are not regularly screened. The degree to which this subgroup can be brought into screening programs will, to a large extent, determine further decreases in mortality from invasive cervical carcinoma.

Abnormal Cytology

According to Woodruff and Novak (1974), exfoliated surface cells show progressive changes as atypism in the cervical epithelium increases. These cellular features include nuclear hyperchromatism, increased chromatin gran-

149

ularity, increased nuclear to cytoplasmic ratios, and decreased cytoplasmic maturation. The ratio of mature to immature atypical cells indicates the degree of the underlying epithelial abnormality. No single feature characterizes a malignant cell, and the criteria for this diagnosis are not absolute. Features consistent with malignancy include nuclear irregularity, chromatin clumping, angularity of nucleoli, and extreme nuclear to cytoplasmic ratios. Degenerative or inflammatory processes may induce changes in cellular morphology that cause difficulty and confusion in cytologic interpretation. For accurate clinical correlation, evaluation, and management, it is essential that the clinician understand what information is being transmitted when an abnormal smear is reported because the interpretation and classification of abnormal cervical cytology may vary among different individuals and laboratories. To improve communication, recommendations have been made to include descriptive narrative statements and standardized terminology in addition to the numerical classification of abnormal Pap smears (Canadian Task Force 1976).

Limitations of Cervical Cytology

An effective screening test should have high sensitivity and low false negative error. False negative errors occur with cervical cytology and, although some are due to inherent limitations of the method or inaccurate interpretation, the most common cause is inadequate sampling. False negative results can be reduced to approximately 5% when both an exocervical scrape and an endocervical sample are taken (Wilbanks et al. 1968). Vaginal pool samples have a high incidence of false negative results and are not recommended. An excellent method for endocervical sampling is cervical os aspiration using a glass tube constricted at its distal portion and a 25 cc suction bulb (Richart 1973). Shingleton and co-workers (1975) compared two methods of endocervical sampling—os aspiration and cytology obtained with cotton-tipped applicators—and found similar results. Garite and Feldman (1978) reported a reduction in false negative smears when, in addition to an exocervical scrape, endocervical samples were obtained using a moistened cotton swab. One slide should be used for both specimens because it is more cost effective than separate slides, and the results are the same (Wilbanks et al. 1968).

The predictive value of an abnormal Pap smear to indicate the actual degree of histologic abnormality is limited. Ronk, Jimerson, and Merrill (1977) correlated cytologic and histologic diagnoses and found agreement within one degree of difference in only 67% of patients. The cytology was read as two degrees more severe than the tissue diagnosis in 20% of patients and less severe in 12%. In 11 patients with Pap smears indicating invasive carcinoma, two had invasion, six had CIS, one had severe dysplasia, and two had no pathologic change. Pap smears were interpreted as CIS in 13 patients; four had invasive carcinoma, eight had severe dysplasia or CIS, and one had no evidence of neoplasia. Moderate dysplasia by cytology occurred in 170 cases

150

of which three had invasive carcinoma, 37 were negative, and the remainder had CIN. Singleton and Rutledge (1968) reported that 21% of patients with a tissue diagnosis of CIS had Class I or II Pap smears. Twenty percent of their cases of stage I invasive carcinoma had Class I or II cytology, and only 63% had Pap smears consistent with overt malignancy. Richart (1964) reported a false negative cytology rate of 7% in patients with clinically obvious tumors. Visible cervical lesions require biopsy because Pap smear results may be misleading. These findings confirm the limitation of the Pap smear to a screening role for the identification of patients who require additional diagnostic procedures. In the past, the most common method to evaluate patients with abnormal Pap smears was the diagnostic cone biopsy. More recently, colposcopy has obviated the need for this procedure in a majority of patients.

Colposcopy

After abnormal cytology has identified a patient, further evaluation for cervical neoplasia should include repeat examination and Pap smear, colposcopy, directed punch biopsies, and endocervical curettage (ECC). Treatment of the cervix should never precede an accurate tissue diagnosis, and cone biopsy should be done after colposcopic evaluation when indicated. Although colposcopy was developed by Hinselman over 50 years ago, the difficult terminology and lack of a unifying theory made it initially unpopular in the United States. Colposcopy is an intervening link between abnormal cytology and tissue diagnosis and does not compete with the Pap smear as a screening method. The colposcope provides low-power magnification of genital tract tissues, and the application of 3% acetic acid is required to dissolve cervical mucus and enhance the appearance of abnormal epithelium. White epithelium, vascular punctuation, and mosaic patterns identify CIN lesions, and atypical vessels indicate invasive carcinoma (Coppleson, Pixley, and Reid 1971). Multiple directed punch biopsies are taken of the most advanced areas of epithelial abnormality. The identification of the transformation zone, the squamocolumnar junction, and the limits of a lesion are necessary for a satisfactory examination.

Except in pregnant patients, endocervical curettage (ECC) is an integral part of this evaluation and should accompany all colposcopic biopsies of the exocervix. A Kevorkian curette is used to scrape the entire circumference of the endocervical canal and is then rotated several times to pick up blood, mucus, and tissue fragments. The specimen is transferred to a small square of paper towel and submitted in fixative. Even if colposcopy is satisfactory, the ECC is necessary because it will provide objective tissue confirmation of this clinical impression, and it may also identify an occult adenocarcinoma of the endocervix. If the cervical biopsy or ECC reveals invasive carcinoma, cone biopsy is contraindicated, and primary therapy can be initiated promptly. When colposcopy is unsatisfactory or the ECC is positive, a cone biopsy is re-

151

quired. Invasive carcinoma has been reported in 11% to 18% of patients with a positive ECC (Shingleton, Gore, and Austin 1976; Townsend et al. 1970). Occult invasive carcinoma after a negative ECC is unusual; this occurred once in 500 cases treated at the USC-LAC Medical Center (Townsend 1977). Evaluation by a skilled colposcopist permits outpatient management in 85% of patients with abnormal Pap smears without the need for diagnostic cone biopsy (Stafl and Mattingly 1973). In older women the squamocolumnar junction is often located high in the endocervical canal. This frequently results in unsatisfactory colposcopy and the need for cone biopsy in this group (Tovell, Banogan, and Nash 1976).

Cytology and colposcopy are complementary. The abnormal Pap smear identifies patients with cervical neoplasia, and colposcopic-directed biopsies determine the degree and extent of disease with a precision that permits individualized outpatient therapy in most cases. As with any specialized technique, colposcopy requires training and skill to be effective, and if necessary, patients should be referred for evaluation.

Special Problems

Special problems often arise in regard to abnormal Pap smears. The patient with a Class II smear of the inflammatory process requires prompt diagnosis and treatment and repeat cytology after resolution of the condition. Persistent Class II smears may indicate continued inflammation or the presence of cervical neoplasia, requiring colposcopic evaluation. Nyirjesy (1972) found that 16% of patients with Class II smears had persistent cytologic abnormalities, and of those available for follow-up, 77% had preinvasive or invasive disease. Davis, Cooke, and Kirk (1972) reported that 31% of patients with persistent Class II smears had lesions of severe dysplasia or more.

If abnormal Pap smears persist after negative colposcopic evaluation, biopsies, and ECC, all material should be reviewed again with the pathologist for further information concerning the cytologic abnormality and tissue of origin. False positive smears can occur and are often due to interpretation errors (Feldman, Carrine, and Srebnik 1977). Iodine staining of the cervix and upper vagina with half-strength Lugol's solution should be used to identify any previously unrecognized epithelial abnormalities. Abnormal smears caused by tissue atrophy from hormonal deprivation can be corrected with topical estrogen cream. Such treatment may also enhance the clinical appearance of previously unrecognized epithelial lesions. If persistent abnormal Pap smears are unexplained, then cone biopsy, fractional curettage, and examination under anesthesia are required to search for occult disease located in the vagina, cervix, endometrium, fallopian tubes, and ovaries.

If abnormal Pap smears recur after cone biopsy or hysterectomy for CIN, repeat cytology and colposcopy are required. Kolstad and Klem (1976) found no difference in the rate of recurrence of CIS or invasive carcinoma (3.3%) in patients with CIS who were treated by cone biopsy and those treated by hysterectomy. Boyes, Worth, and Fidler (1970) reported persistent or new disease after cone biopsy for CIS in 12.7 of 1000 patient-years of follow-up as compared to 1.8 of 1000 for those treated by hysterectomy. The post-hysterectomy vaginal cuff requires careful inspection for apical, multifocal lesions; colpscopy, iodine staining, and directed biopsies can establish a diagnosis of vaginal intraepithelial neoplasia (Petrilli et al. 1980). If inflammatory or atrophic conditions are the cause of abnormal cytology, treatment should be followed with repeat smears.

One to 3% of pregnant patients with abnormal Pap smears require cone biopsy to exclude invasive carcinoma (DePetrillo et al. 1975; Benedet et al. 1977; Lurain and Gallup 1979). The hormonal and vascular changes of pregnancy enhance the colposcopic appearance of abnormal epithelium. Physiologic eversion of the cervix in the third trimester and the gentle use of ring forceps allow satisfactory evaluation of the endocervical canal in most patients. Although the ECC should not be done in pregnant patients, biopsies of suspicious cervical lesions are required even though this may result in active bleeding. The application of direct pressure, Monsel's solution, and, on occasion, a hemostatic suture will control this problem. Vaginal delivery is appropriate for CIN, but abdominal delivery is required if invasive carcinoma is present.

Summary

Patients with abnormal cytology should be evaluated by colposcopy, ECC, and directed biopsies. This will establish a precise diganosis in most cases without the need for diagnostic cone biopsy. Treatment alternatives for preinvasive disease include excisional punch biopsy for small focal lesions, cryotherapy, CO_2 laser therapy, cone biopsy, and hysterectomy. The most appropriate choice depends on the grade and distribution of the lesion, the reliability of the patient, and her interest in future fertility. Frequent follow-up with cervical cytology is necessary for all patients after therapy for cervical neoplasia.

References

Benedet, J.L. et al. Colposcopic evaluation of pregnant patients with abnormal cervical smears. *Br. J. Obstet. Gynaecol.* 84:517–521, 1977.

Boyes, D.A. et al. Recent results from the British Columbia screening program for cervical cancer. *Am. J. Obstet. Gynecol.* 128:692–693, 1977.

Boyes, D.A.; Worth, A.J.; and Fidler, H.K. The results of treatment of 4389 cases of preclinical cervical squamous carcinoma. *J. Obstet. Gynaecol. Br. Comm.* 77:769–780, 1970.

Briggs, R.M. Dysplasia and early neoplasia of the uterine cervix. A review. *Obstet. Gynecol. Surv.* 34:70–99, 1979.

Canadian Task Force. Cervical cancer screening programs. *Can. Med. Assoc. J.* 114:1003–1033, 1976.

Coppleson, M.; Pixley, E.; and Reid, B. *Colposcopy.* Springfield, Ill.: Charles C Thomas, 1971.

Davis, R.M.; Cooke, J.K.; and Kirk, R.F. Cervical conization—an experience with 400 patients. *Obstet. Gynecol.* 40:23–27, 1972.

DePetrillo, A.D. et al. Colposcopic evaluation of the abnormal Papanicolaou test in pregnancy. *Am. J. Obstet. Gynecol.* 121:441–445, 1975.

DiSaia, P.J.; Morrow, C.P.; and Townsend, D.E. *Synopsis of gynecologic oncology.* New York: J. Wiley & Sons, 1975.

Feldman, M.J.; Carrine, S.C.; and Srebnik, E. False positive cervical cytology: an important reason for colposcopy. *Am. J. Obstet. Gynecol.* 129:141–144, 1977.

Garite, T.J., and Feldman, M.J. An evaluation of cytologic sampling techniques—a comparative study. *Acta Cytol.* 22:83–84, 1978.

Kolstad P., and Klem, V. Long-term follow-up of 1121 cases of carcinoma in situ. *Obstet Gynecol.* 48:125–129, 1976.

Lurain, J.R., and Gallup, D.G. Management of abnormal Papanicolaou smears in pregnancy. *Obstet. Gynecol.* 53:484–488, 1979.

Nyirjesy, I. Atypical or suspicious cervical smears. *JAMA* 222:691–693, 1972.

Petrilli, E.S. et al. Vaginal intraepithelial neoplasia: biologic aspects and treatment with topical 5-fluorouacil and the carbon dioxide laser. *Am. J. Obstet. Gynecol.* 138:321–327, 1980.

Richart, R.M. Evaluation of the true false negative rate in cytology. *Am. J. Obstet. Gynecol.* 89:723–726, 1964.

Richart, R.M. Natural history of cervical intraepithelial neoplasia. *Clin. Obstet. Gynecol.* 10:748–784, 1967.

Richart, R.M. Cervical intraepithelial neoplasia. In *Pathology annual,* ed. S.C. Sommers. New York: Appleton-Century-Crofts, 1973.

Richart, R.M., and Barron, B.A. A follow-up study of patients with cervical dysplasia. *Am. J. Obstet. Gynecol.* 105:386–393, 1969.

Ronk, D.A.; Jimerson, G.K.; and Merrill, J.A. Evaluation of abnormal cervical cytology. *Obstet. Gynecol.* 49:581–586, 1977.

Shingleton, H.M. et al. The contribution of endocervical smears to cervical cancer detection. *Acta Cytol.* 19:261–264, 1975.

Shingleton, H.M.; Gore, H.; and Austin, J.M. Outpatient evaluation of patients with atypical Papanicolaou smears: contribution of endocervical curettage. *Am. J. Obstet. Gynecol.* 126:122–128, 1976.

Singleton, W.P., and Rutledge, F. To cone or not to cone—the cervix. *Obstet. Gynecol.* 31:430–436, 1968.

Stafl, A., and Mattingly, R.F. Colposcopic diagnosis of cervical neoplasia. *Obstet. Gynecol.* 41:168–176, 1973.

Tovell, H.M.; Banogan, P.; and Nash, A.D. Cytology and colposcopy in the diagnosis and management of preclinical carcinoma of the cervix uteri: a learning experience. *Am. J. Obstet. Gynecol.* 124:924–934, 1976.

Townsend, D.E. Detection and management of preinvasive cervical neoplasia. *Curr. Probl. Obstet. Gynecol.* 1:3–31, 1977.

Townsend, D.E. et al. Abnormal Papanicolaou smears. *Am. J. Obstet. Gynecol.* 108:429–434, 1970.

Wilbanks, G.D. et al. An evaluation of a one-slide cervical cytology method for the detection of cervical intraepithelial neoplasia. *Acta Cytol.* 12:157–158, 1968.

Woodruff, J.D., and Novak, E. *Gynecologic and obstetric pathology.* Philadelphia: W.B. Saunders, 1974.

Chapter 6

*The Value of Operative Staging
in the Treatment of
Invasive Carcinoma
of the Cervix*

PERSPECTIVE:

Michael L. Berman

Major advances in cervical cancer during the past 40 years have included prevention of the disease in many patients and improvements in therapy when invasive cancer is present. Preventive measures have included the widespread use of the Papanicolaou smear, often in conjunction with colposcopy. Noteworthy changes in the management of cervical cancer during this interval are the use of megavoltage radiation therapy, improved intraoperative and postoperative management of patients undergoing radical pelvic operations, and a better understanding of the biologic patterns of spread and risk factors associated with an increased likelihood of recurrence. The result of these changes has been a reduction in the number of new cases and increased survival in cervical cancer, which has fallen from the leading cause of cancer deaths in American women in the 1940s to the sixth leading cause in the 1970s. The overall five-year survival has increased from 47% to 56% during that interval while the death rate has fallen by more than 50% (National Cancer Institute 1972; U.S. Public Health Service 1953–1974).

While the central tumor, defined as that in the cervix, uterus, vagina, and parametria, can be controlled in most instances with radiation, surgery, or a combination of the two, the most frequent problem is recognition and eradication of lymph node metastases. Paunier, Delclos, and Fletcher (1967) reported the M. D. Anderson Hospital experience, where megavoltage therapy was performed upon 1705 patients with cervical cancer treated between 1954 and 1963. Only 7.7% of the patients did not achieve control of the central tumor, including 1.5% with stage I_b and II_a, 5% with stage II_b, 7.5% with stage III_a and 17% with stage III_b. On the other hand, 21% of the patients had recurrence with deep pelvic and regional lymphatic disease, and 15% had distant metastases. There is considerable overlap between these figures since patients who had recurrence in multiple sites are included for each location. Central disease, even when extensive, is usually controlled better than less bulky nodal disease because (1) higher doses of radiation can be delivered safely to the uterus and vagina using intracavitary therapy and (2) lymph node metastases usually are unrecognized when therapy is initiated and hence therapy is not modified to improve the likelihood of controlling the regional spread.

Staging

The accepted staging scheme for cervical cancer conforms to the recommendations of the International Federation of Gynaecology and Obstetrics (FIGO) based on clinical assessment and limited radiographic evaluation (American College of Obstetricians and Gynecologists, 1977). Evaluation consists of pelvic examination, cystoscopy, intravenous pyelography, sigmoidoscopy, barium enema, and chest roentgenogram. The inherent inaccuracies of clinical staging have been documented by numerous investigators who have attempted to correlate clinical evaluation with operative findings. Errors in comparative assessment of the clinical and surgical stage of tumor have been reported in excess of 30%, most frequently because of unrecognized lymph node metastases in the pelvic and periaortic regions (Berman 1977; Van Nagell, Roddick, and Lowin 1971; Averette, Dudan, and Ford 1972). Only when lymph node metastases are clinically apparent in the groin or supraclavicular areas can one document dissemination by the lymphatic route. Since metastases to these distant sites are uncommon while regional lymph node metastases occur frequently, most patients with lymph node metastases cannot be identified by clinical staging. An operative staging scheme using the tumor, nodes, metastases (TNM) system, as proposed by the International Union Against Cancer in 1964 and reported by Van Nagell, Roddick, and Lowin (1971) could be used to evaluate the status of regional lymph nodes and reduce the apparently inherent inaccuracies of clinical staging. The limitation of this approach is the risk of morbidity and mortality from a major operation to evaluate the lymph nodes and the uncertainty of benefits from the information gained. As a result, operative evaluation to date has been an experimental tool used only in an investigational setting.

Risk Factors for Lymph Node Metastases

The factor correlating most closely with risk of lymph node metastases is the stage of tumor. A review by Plentl and Friedman (1971) reported lymph node metastases in 15.4% of 3391 patients with stage I, 28.6% of 2952 women with stage II, and 47% of 217 women with stage III disease. When lymph node metastases are present, nodes in the pelvis generally are involved initially.

Metastases to the external iliac and obturator lymph nodes account for over 40% of metastases while hypogastric lymph nodes account for an additional 15% to 20%.

Metastases to the common iliac and periaortic lymph nodes occur secondarily to those in the pelvis. Data from the UCLA Medical Center (Berman et al. 1977) and from the M. D. Anderson Hospital (Wharton et al. 1977) reported that 44% of 82 patients with pelvic lymph node metastases found upon pelvic and periaortic lymphadenectomy had coexisting metastases involving the common iliac or periaortic lymph nodes. Rarely are metastases to these more distant areas found in the absence of pelvic lymph node spread. The importance of this finding is that some of the common iliac lymph nodes and all of the periaortic lymph nodes are outside the usual radiation portals. The overall prevalence of biopsy-documented periaortic lymph node metastases for each stage found upon lymphadenectomy is shown in table 6.1. As expected, the risk increases with more advanced stages.

A second important prognosticator for lymph node metastases is tumor volume. Although this factor frequently relates to the stage of disease, there is a wide range of tumor size and risk of regional spread within each stage. Piver and Chung (1975) found lymph node metastases in 21% of 132 patients undergoing radical hysterectomy and pelvic lymphadenectomy for stage I_b or II_a disease with tumors up to 3 cm in diameter. The prevalence doubled in 108 patients with bulkier tumors of similar stages. There was no significant difference in the risk of lymph node metastases between the two stages studied when corrected for tumor volume. Similarly, Burghardt and Pickel (1978) reported a progressive increase in the prevalence of lymph node metastases for tumors of greater size. Nodal metastases were found in none of 13 patients with tumors less than 1 cm in diameter, in 24% of 93 patients with

Table 6.1
Prevalence of Periaortic Lymph Node
Metastases in Cervical Cancer

Year	Reference	Stage				
		I_b	II_a	II_b	III_a	III_b
1977	Berman et al.	1/12	3/8	5/26	0/2	3/20
1977	Wharton et al.	0/21	0/10	10/47	11/34	—
1977	Delgado et al.	0/18	—	8/18	—	5/13
1977	Nelson et al.	—	2/16	7/47	—	15/39*
1974	Piver and Barlow	—	—	1/19	—	12/32
1975	Averette, Dudan, and Ford	7/145	2/20	3/20	0/3	4/16
1972	Buchsbaum,	0/4	0/1	1/11	—	7/20*
	Totals	8/200	7/55	35/188	11/39	46/140
	% of Totals	4	13	19	28	33

*Might include some patients with stage III_a.

tumors 1 to 3 cm in diameter, and in 52% of tumors greater than 3 cm in diameter.

Another prognostic factor which has been proposed to increase the risk of lymph node metastases is the histologic appearance of the tumor. Sedlacek and associates (1978) performed periaortic lymph node biopsies on 43 patients with stage I_b carcinoma of the cervix and found metastases in 5 of 25 patients with grade III tumors but none in 18 patients with grade I or II tumors. Similarly, in 1974 Piver and Barlow studied 56 patients with stage II_b or higher tumors and found an increased risk of periaortic lymph node metastases in patients with poorly differentiated tumors. Seven of 17 patients with poorly differentiated tumors and 8 of 31 patients with medium- or well-differentiated tumors had periaortic metastases. More data are necessary to interpret better the influence of histologic grade on the biological behavior of cervical cancers. A second microscopic feature that might influence the risk of lymph node metastases is the lymphocytic response to the tumor. In 1978, Van Nagell and associates found a significant increase in pelvic lymph node metastases and a decrease in survival of patients with stage I_b cervical cancer whose tumors showed mild lymphoplasmacytic infiltration as compared with those having a marked inflammatory response. The authors have interpreted a mild lymphoplasmocytic response to indicate a greater degree of immunologic impairment than a marked response, implying that immunocompetence might be a measure of risk of tumor dissemination and hence of curability in cervical cancer.

The location of the tumor within the cervix also might influence the risk of lymph node metastases. Plentl and Friedman (1971) reviewed the prevalence of lymph node metastases in over 1000 operated patients with cervical cancer by the site of origin. A total of 38.8% of patients with endocervical cancers had metastases, in contrast to only 24.6% with ectocervical tumors. This difference might reflect greater average tumor volume when diagnosed in the former group of patients since endocervical tumors often are asymptomatic even when extensive.

The importance of recognizing patients at increased risk for lymph node metastases is the inherently poorer prognosis when metastases are present. In a study of 118 patients with stage I_b cervical carcinoma who underwent radiation therapy in conjunction with pelvic lymphadenectomy at the City of Hope National Medical Center between 1956 and 1968, the five-year survival was 81.4%. Only 20% of the 20 patients with regional lymph nodes metastases survived, as compared with 93.6% of 98 patients with negative lymph nodes (Lagasse et al. 1974). Few series report cure rates in excess of 50% when regional lymphatic spread is documented, while many investigators report a five-year survival of 90% or greater in stage I_b when lymphadenectomy specimens are negative for metastatic tumor. Hence, information gained from lymphadenectomy in patients with cervical cancer is of prognostic importance. Similarly, this information permits the rational modification of therapy in patients with disease that is more extensive than can be found by clinical assessment alone. Whether survival is improved by identifying patients with lymph node metastases who therefore might benefit from modifying therapy to encompass the extent of recognizable tumor is not yet known.

Diagnosis of Lymph Node Metastases

Attempts to identify pelvic and periaortic lymph node metastases have included bipedal lymphangiography, selective lymph node biopsies, and lymphadenectomy. Although lymphangiography is of value in localizing primary malignancies including Hodgkin's disease and non-Hodgkin's lymphomas, characteristic changes in lymph nodes with metastatic cervical cancer frequently are not seen. This technique provides excellent visualization of the external iliac, common iliac, and periaortic lymph nodes, and, in instances where extensive replacement with tumor is present, unequivocal radiographic evidence of metastasis can be recognized. Unfortunately, negative and equivocal lymphangiograms correlate poorly with histologic findings following lymphadenectomy. In 1979, Lagasse and associates found agreement between lymphangiography and lymphadenectomy in 64 of 95 patients whose tumors were too extensive for primary operative treatment. Seventeen percent of patients had false positive or negative lymphangiograms in the common iliac or periaortic areas, and therefore would have been treated inappropriately based on lymphangiographic findings alone. If one elected to treat based on clinical assessment, 19% of those patients with metastases to the common iliac or periaortic lymph nodes who had tumor beyond the standard radiation ports would have been undertreated. Optimum therapy in this group of patients, therefore, could not be determined by clinical assessment, lymphangiography, or by combining the two means of evaluation. Lymphangiography can be used to identify lymph nodes that should be biopsied. When suspicious lymph nodes are seen, needle biopsy under fluoroscopic visualization can be of help in detecting metastases to pelvic and periaortic lymph nodes. This finding then could obviate operative evaluation and would permit modification of therapy based on the biopsy findings. If needle biopsy proved negative, operative intervention could be considered to assess the lymph nodes further.

Disappointment in lymphangiography as a useful diagnostic tool has led to the pretreatment operative evaluation, including pelvic and periaortic lymphadenectomy, of many patients identified at high risk for metastases (Berman et al. 1977; Averette, Dudan, and Ford 1972; Wharton et al. 1977; Delgado et al. 1977; Nelson et al. 1977; Piver and Barlow 1974; Averette et al. 1975; Buchsbaum 1972).

While this approach by the standard transperitoneal route has been useful in identifying patients with metastases and permitting modification of therapy tailored to the extent of disease, unacceptable morbidity and mortality from intestinal complications following postoperative radiation therapy have limited the applicability of this technique (table 6.2). Fourteen of 18

161

deaths reported by Berman and associates (1977) and Wharton and associates (1977) resulted from intestinal complications following lymphadenectomy and radiation therapy. Therapy in both series was modified according to the operative findings and some patients were treated with extended ports. Intestinal complications accounted for all of the reported serious morbidity in these two series. The excessive morbidity and mortality often resulted from segmental damage to loops of small intestine fixed to the posterior peritoneum by adhesions following transperitoneal lymphadenectomy (Berman et al. 1977). Doses of 5500 rad delivered to extended ports exceeded the tolerance of these immobilized loops of intestine.

To minimize adhesions, an extraperitoneal approach for performing pelvic and periaortic lymphadenectomies was devised (Berman et al. 1977). A J-shaped left lateral incision (fig. 6.1) is used to permit periaortic and bilateral pelvic lymph node dissections through an extraperitoneal approach. Since this approach eliminates an incision in the posterior peritoneum, loops of bowel are not at risk to adhere to this area. To evaluate the abdomen satisfactorily, the anterior peritoneum is opened and, when indicated, biopsies can be obtained from the liver, omentum, or other viscera. Thirty-nine patients so evaluated had no mortality and no morbidity requiring operative intervention. Radiation therapy to extended ports in eight patients with metastases to the common iliac or periaortic lymph nodes ranged from 4300 to 5100 rad.

When operative evaluation of the pelvic and periaortic nodes is performed, lymphadenectomy provides a better sampling than selective lymph node biopsies. Although massively enlarged fixed lymph nodes are easily identifiable as containing metastatic tumor, often clinically unsuspicious lymph nodes also contain metastases. When markedly enlarged nodes with metastatic tumor are found, an attempt at resection should be considered. Wharton and associates (1977) found that resecting nodes with metastatic cancer helped to control tumor within the treatment field and reported only one patient with failure on the pelvic sidewall alone. In the absence of

Table 6.2
Intestinal Complications of Lymphadenectomy Plus Irradiation: Transperitoneal Approach

Year	Source	Total Patients	Morbidity*	Mortality
1977	UCLA	33	10	2
1977	MDAH	116	32	16
	Totals (No./%)	149	42/28.2%	18/14.6%

*All patients required operative intervention.

162

grossly positive lymph nodes, there is no rational approach to selective biopsies; hence lymphadenectomy is preferred.

Treatment

When metastases to pelvic lymph nodes alone are found, radiation therapy should be modified by increasing the amount of external radiation administered to that pelvic sidewall and extending the radiation ports (Fletcher and Rutledge 1972). Patients with positive lymph· nodes in the external iliac chain should be treated with ports extended to the fourth lumbar vertebral body to encompass all the common iliac node-bearing tissue. Patients with metastases to the common iliac or periaortic lymph nodes should have radiation ports extended to the level of the 12th thoracic vertebral body. A dose of approximately 4500 to 5000 rad is delivered over five to six weeks to the extended ports. A dose of 5500 to 6000 rad has been associated with serious intestinal injury and mortality, as noted above (Wharton 1977; Piver and Bar-

Figure 6.1

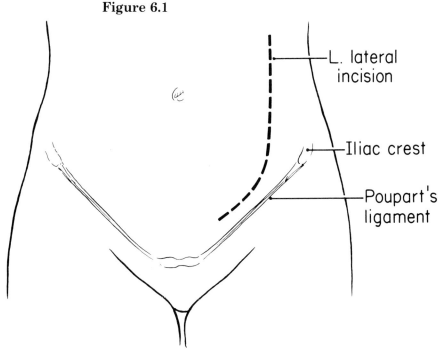

J-shaped left lateral incision for the performance of bilateral extraperitoneal pelvic and periaortic lymphadenectomy.

163

low 1977). The dose seems appropriate when the volume of metastatic tumor is small, since subclinical disease can be controlled with 5000 rad 90% of the time (Wharton et al. 1977).

Treatment Results

Patients with regional lymph node metastases in the pelvis often can be cured. Nodal spread can be eradicated employing either surgery or radiation therapy. Combined data from five institutions reporting to the Society of Gynecologic Oncologists in January 1979 found a five-year survival of 60% for 30 patients with confirmed pelvic lymph node metastases treated with radiation therapy, as compared with 59% for 144 such patients treated with operation only (Morrow 1979). All patients had stage I_b tumor on clinical assessment. In these combined series, recognition of regional disease often permitted control of tumor and apparent cures. Conversely, when the treatment plan does not encompass the full extent of regional spread, long-term survival is unlikely.

When metastases extend to second-echelon lymph nodes including the common iliac and periaortic chains, long-term survival is less frequent. Fletcher and Rutledge (1972) and Silberstein, Aron, and Alexander (1970) have shown that patients with periaortic lymph node metastases can be amenable to curative radiotherapy using extended ports. Although precise survival figures are difficult to find, in a preliminary report, 4 of 18 patients with periaortic lymph node metastases at the UCLA Medical Center were free of disease at five years (Ballon et al. 1980) Wharton and associates (1977) reported only 3 of 24 disease-free survivors at follow-up intervals of 13 to 38 months after extended field treatment with radiation therapy. Eight of 21 deaths resulted from complications of therapy. In 1977, Piver and Barlow reported 3 survivors of 21 patients with periaortic metastases at intervals of two to four years following completion of therapy. Four additional patients died from complications of therapy without evidence of recurrence. Many patients dying of cancer had distant metastases. Wharton reported that failure to control tumor in distant sites accounted for half of 50 reported deaths in his series of patients.

Analysis of survival by the presence and location of lymph node metastases is difficult on the basis of small numbers of patients evaluated and managed by different investigators. The data do demonstrate, however, that while regional failure can be reduced by lymphadenectomy and extended radiation therapy, satisfactory survival does not necessarily occur. Many deaths resulted from coexisting metastases in distant sites while others resulted from complications of the operative evaluation in conjunction with radiation therapy. It appears that deaths from complications can be minimized by the extraperitoneal operative approach; however, the problem of managing occult distant spread often present in patients with metastases to the common iliac and periaortic lymph nodes has not been solved. The failure of extended field therapy to cure more patients with lymph node metastases does not mitigate against further staging operations. Rather, it helps to identify a group of patients whose radiation therapy should be modified. Furthermore, it identifies a group of patients who are at great risk of suffering recurrence at distant sites and who would benefit from systemic chemotherapy or immunotherapy when active agents against cervical cancer become available.

References

American College of Obstetricians and Gynecologists. *Classification and staging of malignant tumors in the female pelvis. Technical bulletin number 47.* Chicago: American College of Obstetricians and Gynecologists, 1977.

American Joint Committee for Cancer Staging and End Results. *Clinical staging systems for carcinoma of the cervix.* Chicago: American Joint Committee for Cancer Staging, 1964.

Averette, H.E. et al. Staging of cervical cancer. *Clin. Obstet. Gynecol.* 18:215–232, 1975.

Averette, H.E., Dudan, R.C., and Ford, J.H. Exploratory celiotomy for surgical staging of cervical cancer. *Am. J. Obstet. Gynecol.* 113:1090–1096, 1972.

Ballon, S.C. et al. Lymph node metastases from carcinoma of the cervix. In *Lymphatic system metastasis,* eds. L. Weiss, H.A. Gilbert, and S.C. Ballon Boston: G.K. Hall, 1980.

Berman, M.L. et al. The operative evaluation of patients with cervical carcinoma by an extraperitoneal approach. *Obstet. Gynecol.* 50:658–664, 1977.

Buchsbaum, H.J. Para-aortic lymph node involvement in cervical carcinoma. *Am. J. Obstet. Gynecol.* 113:942–947, 1972.

Burghardt, E., and Pickel, H. Local spread and lymph node involvement in cervical cancer. *Obstet. Gynecol.* 52:138–145, 1978.

Delgado, G. et al. Paraaortic lymphadenectomy in gynecologic malignancies confined to the pelvis. *Obstet. Gynecol.* 50:418–423, 1977.

Fletcher, G.H., and Rutledge, F.N. Extended field technique in the management of the cancers of the uterine cervix. *Am. J. Roentgenol.* 114:116–122, 1972.

Koehler, P.R. Current status of lymphography in patients with cancer. *Cancer* 37:503–516, 1976.

Kolbenstvedt, A. Lymphography in the diagnosis of metastases from carcinoma of the uterine cervix stages I and II. *Acta Radiol. [Diagn.] (Stockh.)* 16:81–97, 1975.

Lagasse, L.D. et al. The effect of radiation therapy on pelvic lymph node involvement in stage I carcinoma of the cervix. *Am. J. Obstet. Gynecol.* 119:328–334, 1974.

Lagasse, L.D. et al. Pretreatment lymphangiography and operative evaluation in carcinoma of the cervix. *Am. J. Obstet. Gynecol.* 134:219–224, 1979.

Morrow, C.P. The postoperative management of stage I$_b$ carcinoma of the cervix with pelvic lymph node metastases. Presented at the Tenth Annual Meeting of the Society of Gynecologic Oncologists, Marco Island, January 1979.

National Cancer Institute. *End results in cancer, report no. 4.* DHEW Publication No. (NIH) 73–272. Washington, D.C. U.S. Government Printing Office, 1972.

National Center for Health Statistics, U.S. Public Health Service. *Vital statistics of United States, annual, 1950–1969.* Washington, D.C. U.S. Government Printing Office, 1953–1974.

Nelson, J.H. Jr. et al. The incidence and significance of para-aortic lymph node metastases in late invasive carcinoma of the cervix. *Am. J. Obstet. Gynecol.* 118:749–756, 1974.

Nelson, J.H., Jr. et al. Incidence, significance, and follow-up of para-aortic lymph node metastases in late invasive carcinoma of the cervix. *Am. J. Obstet. Gynecol.* 128:336–340, 1977.

Paunier, J.P; Delclos, L; and Fletcher, G.H. Causes, time of death and sites of failure in squamous cell carcinoma of the uterine cervix on intact uterus. *Radiology* 88:555–562, 1967.

Piver, M.S., and Barlow, J.J. Para-aortic lymphadenectomy is staging patients with advanced local cervical cancer. *Obstet. Gynecol.* 43:544–548, 1974.

Piver, S.M., and Barlow, J.J. High dose irradiation to biopsy confirmed aortic node metastases from carcinoma of the uterine cervix. *Cancer* 39:1243–1246, 1977.

Piver, M.S., and Chung, W.S. Prognostic significance of cervical lesion size and pelvic node metastases in cervical carcinoma. *Obstet. Gynecol.* 46:507–510, 1975.

Plentl, A.A., and Friedman, E.A. Clinical significance of cervical lymphatics. In *Lymphatic system of the female genitalia.* Philadelphia: W.B. Saunders, 1971.

Sedlacek, T.V., et al. Exploratory celiotomy for cervical carcinoma: the role of histologic grading. *Gynecol. Oncol.* 6:138–144, 1978.

Silberstein, A.B.; Aron, B.S.; and Alexander, L.L. Para-aortic lymph node irradiation in cervical carcinoma. *Radiology* 95:181–184, 1970.

Van Nagell, J.R., Jr. et al. The significance of vascular invasion and lymphocytic infiltration in invasive cervical cancer. *Cancer* 41:228–234, 1978.

Van Nagell, J.R., Jr.; Roddick, J.W.; and Lowin, D.M. The staging of cervical cancer: inevitable discrepancies between clinical staging and pathologic findings. *Am. J. Obstet. Gynecol.* 110:973–978, 1971.

Wharton, J.T., et al. Pre-irradiation celiotomy and extended field irradiation for invasive carcinoma of the cervix. *Obstet. Gynecol.* 49:333–338, 1977.

PERSPECTIVE:

The Value of Operative Staging in the Treatment of Invasive Carcinoma of the Cervix

Howard W. Jones III

A precise knowledge of the extent of disease is an important prerequisite in planning the treatment of any malignancy. This is generally referred to as staging the cancer, and for most gynecologic malignancies this means using clinical techniques with only the most simple diagnostic surgical procedures such as biopsy or curettage. Since many patients with cervical and endometrial cancer are treated by radiation therapy alone, no abdominal surgical procedure is part of their treatment, and thus the status of the pelvic organs and retroperitoneal lymph nodes is never investigated. Nevertheless, a clinical staging system was adopted for these malignancies so that patients treated with either operation or radiation could be uniformly staged, enabling institutions with different treatment policies to compare results and complications. Clinical staging techniques, however, are not sufficiently sensitive to demonstrate pelvic or aortic lymph node metastases in many cases or even the extent of the primary cancer in some patients. In cervical carcinoma, for instance, Van Nagell, Roddick, and Lowin (1971) compared patients' clinical stages with the actual stages as found by surgery and demonstrated a 25% error in patients with clinical stage I disease and a 62% error in women who were felt to have clinical stage II$_b$ cervical cancer.

Because radiation therapy has become more effective at controlling metastatic cancer in regional lymph nodes, and clinical staging techniques are often inadequate to demonstrate its presence, several investigators in the last 10 years have studied this problem by using pretreatment staging laparotomy to document the precise spread of the disease before beginning radiation therapy so that all the areas of cancer, including regional lymphatic metastases, could be adequately treated.

It should also be noted that this approach provides an opportunity for a combined form of therapy—surgical excision of the tumor bulk with radiation to "clean up" subclinical foci of persistent cancer.

Cervical Cancer

As discussed above, the clinical staging techniques for evaluation of cervical cancer are inadequate for diagnosing the presence of retroperitoneal lymph node metastases. Even lymphangiography has not provided consistent diagnostic accuracy, especially in small nodes with minimal involvement. Improvement in radiation therapy techniques has led to improved control of pelvic lymph node metastases, but it has become apparent that some patients are not cured because of metastatic cancer in the aortic lymph nodes, not covered by the standard treatment fields. In a series of surgically explored and biopsied patients with stage III cervical cancer, Rutledge and Fletcher (1958) reported aortic or high common iliac lymph node metastasis in 17%. With improvements in the ability of radiation therapy to control pelvic disease and several reports of long-term survival following successful aortic radiation in patients with aortic lymph node metastasis, it was felt that if these patients with aortic nodal metastases could be identified, some could perhaps be cured by extended field irradiation.

The results of several studies shown in table 6.3 indicate that the overall incidence of aortic lymph node metastasis is about 25% for the group of patients with clinical stage II_b and greater cervical cancer. In all these investigations, patients with advanced cervical cancer underwent exploratory laparotomy with lymph node biopsies prior to any therapy and then were treated with full radiation postoperatively with the size of the field determined by the surgical findings. As might be predicted, the incidence of extrapelvic lymph node metastases increases with advancing clinical stage (table 6.4).

In addition to lymph node metastasis, Buchsbaum (1979) reported that pretreatment exploratory laparotomy detected 16 patients (10.7%) with intraperitoneal sites of metastatic cancer such as small bowel, rectosigmoid, bladder peritoneum, and liver.

These studies clearly demonstrate that the incidence of metastatic cancer outside the standard pelvic radiation field is appreciable, and they have improved our knowledge of the pathologic behavior of the disease, but have we been able to use this newfound knowledge to improve the cure rate of patients with advanced cervical cancer?

The complications of transperitoneal lymph node biopsies followed by high-dose radiation therapy have been considerable. In a series of 120 patients, Wharton and associates (1977) reported 16 deaths among 32 serious complications usually involving bowel injury. In a recent report Lagasse and associates (1979) have advocated an extraperitoneal approach which has reduced the incidence of intestinal complications from 30% in their first 30 patients to less than 5% in their last 60 cases. Thrombophlebitis and pulmonary

Table 6.3
Incidence of Positive Aortic Nodes in Patients
with Stages II$_b$ to IV Cervical Cancer

Year	Author	Total Number of Patients	Aortic Node Metastasis (No./%)
1972	Averette	21	5/23.8
1979	Buchsbaum	129	39/30.2
1979	Lagasse et al.	57	10/17.5
1974	Nelson et al.	61	18/29.5
1973	Piver and Barlow	56	15/26.8
1972	Ucmakli and Bonney	23	5/21.8
1977	Wharton et al.	89	24/26.9
	Totals	436	116/26.6

embolus have also been common problems, and lymphocysts with leg edema have occurred in patients who had pelvic lymph node sampling followed by irradiation.

It has been suggested that lymphangiography might be an accurate way to identify lymph node metastases without subjecting the patient to the risks of surgery. Despite a previous report by Piver and colleagues (1971), however, who found 97% accuracy when positive nodes were diagnosed by lymphangiogram, both Buchsbaum and Lagasse and associates found only about a 51% accuracy (table 6.5). There was better agreement when the nodes were thought to be uninvolved on the basis of lymphangiogram. Piver and Barlow (1973) reported positive nodes on biopsy in 19.6% of patients who were said to have negative nodes by lymphangiogram while the recent studies of

Table 6.4
Incidence of Common Iliac and Aortic Lymph
Node Metastases in Cervical Cancer

Clinical Stage	Patients	Positive Common Iliac and Aortic Nodes (No./%)
I$_b$	21	0
II$_a$	10	0
II$_b$	47	10/21.2%
III$_a$	34	11/32.3%
III$_b$ and IV	8	3/37.5%
Totals	120	24/20.0%

SOURCE: *Modified from Wharton 1977.*

Table 6.5
Correlation of Lymphangiography with
Actual Lymph Node Biopsy

| | Node Biopsy | | |
Lymphangiogram	Positive	Negative	Total
Positive	14	15/51.7%	29
Negative	10/11.5%	77	87
Total	24	97	

SOURCE: Buchsbaum 1979; Lagasse et al. 1979.

Buchsbaum and Lagasse missed 11.5% of the patients with biopsy-proven nodal metastases.

Newer techniques such as computerized tomography and thin-needle biopsy of retroperitoneal nodes have been reported, but it remains to be seen if
such procedures will be helpful in identifying those patients with a relatively
small volume of metastatic disease who stand the best chance for cure by external irradiation.

The complication rate of such extended field radiation therapy itself is
not negligible. In a series of 36 patients, only 5 of whom had prior surgical
exploration, Lepanto and associates (1975) reported a 19.5% incidence of complications with 5.5% mortality when the aortic area was treated to approximately 5000 rad. Only 5 of 15 patients followed three years or longer were
still alive.

The published reports concerning survival for patients with aortic node
metastasis have been somewhat limited due to the short follow-up period, but
table 6.6 lists some of the results for patients who have been surgically
staged. It is apparent that while the survival is not high, patients with aortic
lymph node metastases can be cured in a few cases. Both Buchsbaum and
Hughes (1978) have patients who have shown no evidence of disease for more
than five years. If we assume, however, that approximately 30% to 40% of all
patients with stage III cervical cancer have positive aortic nodes and that
15% of these may be long-term survivors, we are only talking about 5% overall improvement in the stage III cure rate. The morbidity and occasional mortality, not to mention the cost, must be balanced against the overall improvement in survival, since all patients would require surgical staging to identify
those with aortic nodal metastasis, and others who were destined to fail in
the pelvis or distantly would also be treated with aortic radiation.

Chism, Park, and Keys have published an excellent analysis of the overall situation (1975). They made several assumptions: (1) patients who were
cured by standard radiation therapy techniques would not need or benefit
from extended field radiation; (2) patients who had persistent or recurrent
disease in the pelvis would not benefit because the central disease was not
controlled anyway; (3) patients who developed distant metastases within 12

Table 6.6
Survival and Node Status in Patients with
Cervical Cancer

Year	Reference	Clinical Stage	Overall Living Patients (No./%)	Positive Aortic Nodes Living Patients (No./%)
1979	Buchsbaum	Stage I_b–II_b	19 of 28/67.8%	2 of 5/40%
		Stage III_a–IV	30 of 94/31.9%	4 of 27/14.8%
1979	Wharton	All stages	45 of 120/37.5%	3 of 24/12.5%
1978	Hughes	All stages		3 of 31/9.3%

months would not benefit, since these lesions were probably already present prior to therapy; and (4) only those patients with distant metastases alone, which occur more than 12 months after radiation therapy, might benefit. Using these assumptions to analyze the patients treated at Walter Reed, they calculated that, overall, 20 of some 530 patients (3.7%) might benefit from aortic nodal irradiation. This benefit could be achieved only if 100% of the eligible patients were cured by extended field irradiation—an unlikely assumption. The greatest potential improvement in survival occurred among patients with stage II_b lesions where 17 of 227 women (7.4%) might benefit from extended field irradiation. A similar result is obtained when the survival and site of recurrence data are analyzed from the M. D. Anderson Hospital (table 6.7).

Although many patients with advanced cervical cancer suffer recurrence in the pelvis within the treatment field, in many cases positive aortic nodes are merely an indicator of widespread metastatic cancer. For example, Buchsbaum found that 34.8% of patients with aortic lymph node metastasis also had tumor that had spread to the scalene nodes.

Attempts are now underway to add chemotherapy or immunotherapy to radiation, to improve radiation techniques, and to refine the surgical approach so that the surgical staging of cervical cancer will be not only accurate, but associated with minimal morbidity and a significantly improved survival. Pretreatment staging laparotomy in cervical cancer is useful in determining the extent of the disease, but we do not yet know how to turn this information into improved results, and, if the analysis by Chism and his associates is correct, until we improve central control and/or learn how to handle distant metastases, staging laparotomy should be used only in an investigational setting.

Table 6.7
Theoretical Analysis of the Possible Benefits
of Aortic Radiation

Stage	Walter Reed		M. D. Anderson	
	Number of Patients	Possible Benefit (No./%)	Number of Patients	Possible Benefit (No./%)
I	200	0	407	10/2.4%
II_a	34	0	327	13/3.9%
II_b	227	17/7.4%	291	20/6.8%
III	44	2/4.5%	599	38/6.3%
IV	15	0	81	4/4.9%
Totals	520	19/3.6%	1705	85/5.0%

NOTE: *Patients who might benefit are those who are not cured but do not develop pelvic recurrence and distant metastatic disease within 12 months of treatment (modified from Chism et al. 1975).*

Endometrial Cancer

Following the lead of the cervical cancer investigations, Creasman, Boronow, DiSaia, and Morrow (1976) have started an investigation into the operative staging of endometrial cancer. This differs somewhat from the studies of cervical cancer where the surgery is purely diagnostic, for in the case of endometrial cancer a hysterectomy as part of the therapy is done in addition to the diagnostic lymph node sampling. This group has now investigated over 200 patients with stage I carcinoma of endometrium. Masubuchi and associates (1979) have also reported the results of a similar study, although they did not study the incidence of aortic node metastasis.

A preliminary report of the lymph node findings of Creasman and associates is presented in table 6.8. More recent reports from this study indicate an overall 7.5% incidence of aortic lymph node metastasis in patients with stage I endometrial cancer. These investigators have also reconfirmed the prognostic significance of histologic grade, endocervical involvement, and depth of myometrial invasion. They have also introduced the importance of peritoneal cytology in this disease, since Creasman has reported that 16.5% of patients with stage I endometrial cancer have positive washings and that in this group there is a 35.7% recurrence rate.

In the case of endometrial cancer, it appears that this type of surgical staging and treatment approach will be beneficial since the complication rate is low, surgery for a hysterectomy is usually done, and the results of the surgery provide specific indications for postoperative radiation therapy. In many cases it appears that routine radiation therapy can be eliminated, and in cases involving positive aortic nodes or washings additional therapy is indicated. It seems that treatment of these patients may prove more successful

Table 6.8
Incidence of Pelvic and Aortic Lymph Node Metastases in Stage I Adenocarcinoma of the Endometrium

	% Positive Pelvic		% Positive Aortic	
I_a, G1	2.6 ⎫		2.6 ⎫	
G2	6.9 ⎬ 6.2		3.5 ⎬ 3.8	
G3	16.7 ⎭		8.3 ⎭	
I_b, G1	3.9 ⎫		0 ⎫	
G2	14.3 ⎬ 18.0		4.8 ⎬ 11.7	
G3	54.0 ⎭		46.0 ⎭	

SOURCE: Creasman et al. 1976.

173

than in cervical cancer since the possibility of central pelvic persistence or recurrence has been virtually eliminated by hysterectomy.

Ovarian Cancer

Since ovarian cancer is a surgically staged disease already, one may wonder why it is discussed in this section. It is included because several developments in recent years have raised the question as to how well this disease was actually being staged at the time of initial surgery.

Piver and associates (1976) reviewed the operative reports of 100 consecutive patients with ovarian cancer who initially underwent surgery elsewhere and were referred to the Roswell Park Memorial Institute for postoperative treatment. Only 24% of these reports included a detailed description of the upper abdomen including the diaphragm, liver, and aortic nodes.

In 1973, Bagley and his colleagues from the National Cancer Institute reported finding metastatic ovarian cancer implants on the undersurface of the diaphragm in several patients referred to them for chemotherapy after being described as having stage I or II disease at recent laparotomy. In subsequent reports, using the laparoscope to restage patients previously operated upon, they noted 7 of 16 women with alleged stage I or II ovarian cancer who had biopsy-proved metastatic cancer on the diaphragm.

Other reports have noted the incidence of aortic lymph node metastases and positive peritoneal cytology and stressed the importance of evaluating these aspects at the time of surgery. Piver, Barlow, and Lele (1978) have recently reviewed the incidence of such subclinical metastases in early ovarian cancer.

With increasing awareness of these findings it is hoped that gynecologists are attempting to be more thorough and precise in the intraoperative staging of ovarian cancer. This is of vital importance if we hope to be able to evaluate the effect of various treatment regimens in this malignancy.

Summary

A review of the studies reported indicates that exploratory laparotomy for staging purposes prior to any therapy provides a significantly improved evaluation of the extent and location of gynecologic cancers. In the case of endometrial cancer this staging procedure may be done as part of a therapeutic hysterectomy and postoperative therapy selected or omitted as surgical pathologic findings dictate. This may result in an improved survival but will also almost certainly result in fewer stage I patients being treated with radiation therapy, therefore reducing morbidity, time, and expense.

In cervical cancer, however, the staging laparotomy increases the morbidity, time, and expense and most often results in the discovery of more advanced cancer which we do not yet know how to manage successfully. Continued studies on improved local control and treatment of systemic disease need to be carried out as part of a pretreatment surgical staging protocol. Therefore, this technique cannot yet be recommended in the routine evaluation and treatment of patients with cervical cancer.

References

Averette, H.E., Dudan, R.C., and Ford, J.H., Jr. Exploratory celiotomy for surgical staging of cervical cancer. *Am. J. Obstet. Gynecol.* 113:1090–1096, 1972.

Bagley, C.M. et al. Ovarian carcinoma metastatic to the diaphragm frequently undiagnosed at laparotomy. *Am. J. Obstet. Gynecol.* 116:397–400, 1973.

Buchsbaum, H.J. Extrapelvic lymph node metastases in cervical carcinoma. *Am. J. Obstet. Gynecol.* 133:814–824, 1979.

Chism, S.E.; Park, R.C.; and Keys, H.M. Prospects for para-aortic irradiation in treatment of cancer of the cervix. *Cancer* 35:1505–1509, 1975.

Creasman, W.T. et al. Adenocarcinoma of the endometrium: its metastatic lymph node potential. *Gynecol. Oncol.* 4:239–243, 1976.

Lagasse, L.D. et al. Pretreatment lymphangiography and operative evaluation in carcinoma of the cervix. *Am. J. Obstet. Gynecol.* 134:219–224, 1979.

Lepanto, P. et al. Treatment of para-aortic nodes in carcinoma of the cervix. *Cancer* 35:1510–1513, 1975.

Masubuchi, S.; Fujimoto, I.; and Masubuchi, K. Lymph node metastasis and prognosis of endometrial carcinoma. *Gynecol. Oncol.* 7:36–46, 1979.

Nelson, J.H., Jr. et al. The incidence and significance of para-aortic lymph node metastases in late invasive carcinoma of the cervix. *Am. J. Obstet. Gynecol.* 118:749–756, 1974.

Piver, M.S., and Barlow, J.J. Para-aortic lymphadenectomy, aortic node biopsy, and aortic lymphangiography in staging patients with advanced cervical cancer. *Cancer* 32:367–370, 1973.

Piver, M.S.; Barlow, J.J.; and Lele, S.B. Incidence of subclinical metastasis in stage I and II ovarian carcinoma. *Obstet. Gynecol.* 52:100–104, 1978.

Piver, M.S.; Lele, S.; and Barlow, J.J. Pre-operative and intraoperative evaluation in ovarian malignancy. *Obstet. Gynecol.* 48:312–315, 1976.

Piver, M.S.; Wallace, S.; and Castro, J.R. The accuracy of lymphangiography in carcinoma of the uterine cervix. *Am. J. Roentgenol.* 111:278–283, 1971.

Rosenoff, S.H. et al. Peritoncoscopy in the staging and follow-up of ovarian cancer. *Semin. Oncol.* 2:223–228, 1975.

Rutledge, F.N., and Fletcher, G.H. Transperitoneal pelvic lymphadenectomy following supervoltage irradiation for squamous cell carcinoma of the cervix. *Am. J. Obstet. Gynecol.* 76:321–334, 1958.

Ucmakli, A., and Bonney, W.A., Jr. Exploratory laparotomy as routine pretreatment investigation in cancer of the cervix. *Radiology* 104:371–378, 1972.

Van Nagell, J.; Roddick, J.W.; and Lowin, D.M. The staging of cervical cancer: inevitable discrepancies between clinical staging and pathologic findings. *Am. J. Obstet. Gynecol.* 110:973–978, 1971.

Wharton, J.T. et al. Preirradiation celiotomy and extended field irradiation for invasive carcinoma of the cervix. *Obstet. Gynecol.* 49:333–338, 1977.

Chapter 7

Pelvic Exenteration: Who is a Candidate?

PERSPECTIVE:

George W. Morley

Ever since 1948, when Brunschwig described the principles and method of pelvic exenteration as a therapeutic approach to certain forms of pelvic malignancy, several technical changes have been advanced and many guidelines have been established in the overall care of these patients. This has resulted in a significant improvement in survival. To maintain this excellence in overall survival, the established criteria must be adhered to when considering patients as candidates for pelvic exenterative therapy.

During the most recent 15-year period, over 80 patients have been treated with some type of pelvic exenteration at the University of Michigan Medical Center. Forty of 66 patients treated in this institution were alive and free of disease at five years—a 60% five-year survival. The postoperative mortality in this series was 2.5%. It must be remembered that the primary goal of every surgeon performing this procedure should be the control and cure of the existing disease, with palliation seldom an indication.

Of the patients treated with this form of radical pelvic surgery, over 75% were treated with total pelvic exenteration (Morley, Lindenauer, and Cerney 1971). The remainder were treated with either resection of the bladder anteriorly or excision of the bowel posteriorly, depending on the origin and location of the tumor. One must not be too conservative, however, in selecting the type of pelvic exenteration to be performed while trying to avoid more than one diversionary procedure. Such conservatism may not only lead to fistulous complication but may unfavorably affect survival, since microscopically extended disease cannot be seen by the naked eye or palpated by the examining finger.

The primary diagnosis was recurrent carcinoma of the cervix in more than two-thirds of the cases. In the order of decreasing frequency, the remaining cases involved the vulva, vagina, uterus, and urethra. One patient had a well-differentiated carcinoma of the ovary but her survival was limited to only one year.

In selecting the patients for pelvic exenterative therapy, several criteria should be met. These include (1) the constitutional factors, (2) the type of disease, and (3) the extent of disease.

Constitutional Factors

Whereas age itself is not an absolute contraindication, the patients' lack of acceptance and compromised medical status will decrease significantly the frequency with which this procedure is performed after 70 years of age. If, however, after all other criteria are met and the patient has been acquainted with the details of the procedure, then age itself should not be an eliminating factor. The patient's medical status and her physical and emotional condition must be thoroughly evaluated before one embarks on this type of radical pelvic surgery. Given a healthy, normal woman, then, one should not be too conservative in choosing radical surgery as treatment of this potentially fatal disease.

Type of Disease

The lesions most suitable for pelvic exenterative surgery are those of the squamous cell variety since spread of this type of tumor beyond the primary organ often occurs in continuity and in contiguity during the earlier stages of recurrence. For this reason, then, patients with recurrent squamous cell carcinoma of the cervix are the most ideal candidates for this treatment. A patient with primary squamous cell carcinoma of the vulva may very well be a candidate for either an anterior or posterior pelvic exenteration since the location of the primary lesion may be perilously close to the bladder anteriorly or to the bowel posteriorly. If, however, the lesion is so advanced that a total pelvic exenteration would be required to control the disease, then the chance of cure decreases significantly. Patients with carcinoma of the ovary are not to be considered candidates for this type of radical pelvic surgery since the pattern of recurrent growth in this disease is one of disorganized abdominal dissemination. Carcinoma of the endometrium, on the other hand, is a more favorable lesion than is carcinoma of the ovary; however, its pattern of growth is also unpredictable. Some patients with sarcomas or melanomas of the vagina or vulva who form a very limited group have benefited from this surgical approach.

Extent of Disease

"Why should you take the ureters out of the bed of neoplasm, only for the patient to die in some other way?" This often-heard question reminds us that the extent of the disease is obviously of paramount importance. This type of radical pelvic surgery, therefore, is indicated only when there is central pelvic recurrence.

There are many diagnostic tests available today that can be used to determine quite accurately the extent of the disease without subjecting the patient to exploratory surgery. Whereas most patients can tolerate a surgical exploration reasonably well, the emotional impact of being declared inoperable can be overwhelming. Therefore the physician must make every effort to determine the operability of the lesion before subjecting the patient to surgical exploration. In fact, the more thorough the preoperative investment, the more likelihood the exenteration will be performed at the time of exploration. One gynecologic oncologist stated that he explored six patients for every pelvic exenteration he performed. In our institution, approximately two-thirds of all patients explored for this purpose are treated with pelvic exenterative surgery as planned.

Diagnostic Studies

The preoperative evaluation of a patient not only includes a routine physical examination and thorough pelvic evaluation but also basic laboratory and roentgenologic studies, confirmatory biopsies, and specialized diagnostic tests. The basic laboratory and roentgenologic studies should include a complete blood count, urinalysis, renal and liver function assays, chest x-ray, intravenous pyelogram, and barium enema examination. Should the chest x-ray examination be suspicious, a tomographic study of this area can be most helpful. The confirmatory biopsy of the tumor is carried out under direct visualization or by needle aspiration of the pelvic mass whenever possible. On occasion, the presence of recurrence cannot be detected in this manner, and surgical exploration is required.

The specialized studies include radioisotopic scanning, computerized axial tomography, lymphangiography, and transcutaneous needle aspiration of regional lymph nodes under fluoroscopic control. Unfortunately, the lymphangiography is considered unreliable in many institutions; however, with improved techniques and better interpretation this diagnostic evaluation can be of immeasureable assistance. When accurate lymphangiography is available and the report suggests the presence of abnormal regional lymph nodes, then a confirmatory biopsy can be performed utilizing the transcutaneous needle aspiration technique. To date, over 45 transcutaneous needle aspirations have been performed at the University of Michigan Hospital with approximately 75% accuracy on first aspiration. More recently, a second aspiration has been performed if the first aspirate was reported negative for metastasis, and approximately 50% of these specimens have confirmed the suspicous abnormality of the lymphangiogram. On one occasion, the pathology report of a third aspirate finally correlated with the positive lymphangiogram. Parenthetically, if the lymphangiogram is reported negative, no attempt is made at randomized sampling of lymph nodes by this technique. These patients are surgically explored.

Whereas electromyography is included in our diagnostic armamentarium, its indications are limited and its findings are only suggestive rather than diagnostic. Given, however, a patient with radiation of pain down one of her lower extremities, probably secondary to regional lymph node involvement, this test can be most complementary in the overall evaluation of the patient.

It has been suggested by others that a routine biopsy of the scalene lymph node or fat pad in the left supraclavicular area be included in the preoperative investigation of these patients. Whereas we have not used this diagnostic aid routinely in our institution, it certainly cannot be criticized.

Whereas (1) an abnormal pyelogram, (2) lower extremity edema, and (3) sciatic distribution of pain have often been referred to as the "triad of trouble," they cannot always determine the candidacy of a patient for pelvic exenterative therapy. They, suggest, however, that the recurrent lesion is inoperable. The presence of any one of these abnormalities suggests that there is pelvic lymph node or lateral pelvic wall involvement with tumor extending from the primary site. This, coupled with a clinical suspicion that the lesion extends out to the lateral pelvic wall, makes surgical exploration highly unsuccessful. If all three of the triad or if two of the three abnormalities are present, then exploration is usually contraindicated. If only one of the triad is present, however, then exploration is justified. Again, whenever one is in doubt as to the resectability of the lesion and the curability of the disease, then exploratory laparotomy is indicated irrespective of the results of the preoperative investigation. Remember, the court of last resort is not in the conference room, but in the operating room.

The gynecologic oncologist has still another and final opportunity to analyze the extent and involvement of the disease at the time of the exploratory laparotomy when pelvic exenteration is anticipated. A careful and thorough inspection of the intraabdominal contents and the regional lymph nodes must be carried out before one commits the patient to such radical surgical therapy. At the time of this intraoperative investigation the peritoneal surfaces, the liver, the omentum, the small and large intestine as well as the paraaortic and pelvic lymph nodes must be accurately assessed for the presence or absence of metastatic disease. Frozen section examination should be utilized liberally in the evaluation of all suspicious masses encountered during this exploration. It is the consensus among gynecologic oncologists doing pelvic exenterative therapy that, given a patient with positive pelvic lymph nodes, this probably should be a contraindication to pelvic exenterative therapy. It is estimated that the five-year survival of a patient undergoing pelvic exenteration is approximately 2% to 3% if regional lymph nodes are positive. In our own series, all 10 patients with positive pelvic lymph nodes on whom pelvic exenterative surgery was performed were dead or dying of their disease within one year.

Finally, and again before one commits the patient to radical pelvic surgery, the resectability of the primary lesion must be proved. This can be carried out very easily by opening up the broad ligament on both sides of the pelvis and by dissecting down into the pelvis laterally as well as anteriorly and posteriorly to determine if the lesion can be resected without leaving behind malignant tissue in the pelvis. If one is in doubt at this point, a sample of the tissue lateral to the dissected cleavage plane can be sent to pathology for frozen section examination. One also should thoroughly palpate the paraureteral and presacral areas since on occasion metastatic disease is detected in these locations.

To confirm our suspicions that this preoperative and intraoperative investigative program has been a most satisfactory one, we recently reviewed the cases of patients on whom an exploratory laparotomy only was performed, since all the criteria for proceeding with the pelvic exenteration were not met. There were 28 patients investigated. Twenty-one of these patients (75%) were dead at one year; 26 of them (93%) were dead at two years following only exploratory laparotomy.

It is realized that rehabilitation is not within the scope of this discussion, but the author suggests that one of the contraindications to the primary surgery is the inability of the surgeon to see the need and accept the responsibility for long-term rehabilitation of these patients postoperatively (Morley, Lindenauer, and Youngs 1973). Sexual and social readjustments are extremely important in the aftercare of these patients, since the tolerance of the diversionary devices and the loss of normal sexual function may be the unfortunate sacrifices made in the attempt to control advanced cancer of the pelvic organs. We must all be cognizant of the patient's pride in her own femininity.

Summary

Over the past 30 years, pelvic exenterative therapy has become increasingly successful in the control of pelvic gynecologic malignancy when the lesion was centrally located in the female genital tract. It is believed that when all of the criteria are met, the overall five-year survival of patients so treated should approximate 60%. The criteria, as described, deal primarily with the type and extent of disease. The more sophisticated diagnostic tools now available can be most helpful in the complete evaluation of these patients before surgery. When any doubt as to resectability and curability of a lesion exists, then exploratory laparotomy must be performed. It is at this time that still further diagnostic procedures can be carried out before one is committed to performing the radical surgical procedure described above. The prolonged hospitalization, the potential complications, and the protracted period of rehabilitation certainly do not benefit the patient should we not be successful in controlling the disease in this way.

References

Brunschwig, A. Complete excision of pelvic viscera for advanced carcinoma. *Cancer* 1:177–183, 1948.

Morley, G.W.; Lindenauer, S.M.; and Cerney, J.C. Pelvic exenterative therapy in recurrent pelvic carcinoma. *Am. J. Obstet. Gynecol.* 109:1175–1186, 1971.

Morley, G.W.; Lindenauer, S.M.; and Youngs, D. Vaginal reconstruction following pelvic exenteration: surgical and psychological considerations. *Am. J. Obstet. Gynecol.* 116:996–1002, 1973.

PERSPECTIVE:

Pelvic Exenteration: Who is a Candidate?

John C. Weed, Jr. and
William T. Creasman

Pelvic exenterative surgery is a form of potentially curative therapy for patients with advanced, persistent, or recurrent pelvic malignancy. Approximately 75% of exenterative surgery is performed for patients with recurrence of cervical or vaginal carcinoma after irradiation therapy (Rutledge et al. 1977; Symmonds, Pratt, and Webb 1975). Primary neoplasms of the vulva, urethra, bladder, uterus, or colon may be treated with extensive surgery and account for the remainder of exenterative operations. Primary exenterative surgery for advanced cervical cancers was performed on only 5 of 37 patients reported by Symmonds and colleagues. Some authors have suggested that primary exenterative surgery should be performed if the bladder is involved in patients with cervical cancer; however, Million and associates (1972) reported 28% survival of patients with bladder invasion managed only by radiation therapy. This survival was equivalent to survival after exenteration, and no fistulae developed in these patients. On the basis of this study, these authors preferred radiation therapy to primary exenteration in patients with advanced cervical carcinoma involving the bladder.

Neoplasms of the vulva, urethra, and vagina are more frequently considered suitable for primary exenteration. Vulvovaginal lesions requiring inguinal, pelvic, and perineal dissections are treated frequently with primary exenteration as these areas are intolerant to radiation therapy. Unusual lesions such as melanomas, sarcomas, and, more recently, adenocarcinomas, seem to respond more favorably to primary surgery.

All patients with persistent or recurrent pelvic cancer should be considered candidates for exenterative surgery because it is the only remaining treatment offering the chance of long-term survival. Histologic documentation should be required, but occasionally it may not be possible in some heavily irradiated patients. Unfortunately, only 8% to 14% (Ketcham et al. 1970; Morley and Lindenauer 1976) of patients considered for exenterative surgery will be operable.

Evaluation of the patient involves three progressive levels. First, an historical review is made of the general medical background, psychosocial environment, previous therapy, and general physical status. Second, a careful assessment is made of the extent of disease by physical examination and laboratory diagnostic studies. Finally, surgical exploration for operative determination of the extent of disease and resectability is performed. The evaluation may be stopped at any point where findings preclude surgery; however, the only absolute contraindication to exenteration is the demonstration of disease outside the bounds of resectability.

Historical Data

Age

The patient's age at diagnosis is an important but highly variable factor. Rutledge (1974) notes that patients over 70 years of age generally have serious physical impediments to exenterative surgery; however, Symmonds reported 23% of 198 exenteration patients were greater than 60 years of age and 5% were over 70 years. Just as older candidates should not be excluded by age alone, younger patients may have poor prognosis factors downgraded in the hope that they will be found resectable at exploration.

General Medical Status

Thorough evaluation of the exenteration candidate for systemic medical illness and nutritional status is required. The ability to tolerate an operative procedure lasting six hours or longer with blood loss approaching 3000 cc and a 33% rate of serious complications must be considered carefully. Evaluation of the general physical status of the patient is important during the initial appraisal. Individuals who have a history of recent marked weight loss, anemia, and hypoproteinemia often will be found to have advanced, generalized disease which is not amenable to exenteration. Pain, particularly hip pain with radiation down the posterior thigh, is a poor prognostic sign usually indicating an unresectable extension of tumor into lumbosacral nerves.

Obvious disease outside the treatment field should be sought carefully. Metastases to supraclavicular lymph nodes may be palpable, and confirmation by biopsy should be obtained prior to any intensive preoperative evaluation. An early chest x-ray will detect pulmonary metastases and should preclude further extensive studies.

The technical disadvantages of obesity relative to blood loss and stoma function are considerable. Renal reserve must be evaluated in the light of an

11% rate of postoperative urinary tract complications (Rutledge et al. 1977). The presence of preoperative renal compromise demonstrated chemically or by changes in the intravenous pyelogram is indicative of poor outlook for the patient. Urinary diversion required for exenterative surgery predisposes compromised renal units to retrograde flow and the serious effects of chronic renal infection. The vascular system must have sufficient reserve to tolerate the hypotension, blood replacement, and electrolyte fluctuations which are associated with an 11% rate of early cardiovascular complications (Rutledge et al. 1977). Coronary artery disease and chronic hypertensive cardiovascular disease may seriously deplete myocardial reserve. Obesity, extensive pelvic dissection, inflammation, prolonged convalescence, and the hypercoagulability associated with malignant disease may predispose to venous thromboses and embolic phenomena. Serious medical illnesses such as the collagen diseases may result in poor healing of the surgical incisions and intestinal anastomoses. Diabetes mellitus, in addition to its known deleterious effects on the vasculature in the form of coronary artery disease and renal vascular disease, may predispose to complications of infection. All of these factors must be carefully weighed in the preoperative evaluation of patients considered for exenterative surgery.

History of Primary Therapy

The history of primary therapy is important. Postsurgical recurrence of radiosensitive tumors may be treated by radiation therapy. Surgery is reserved for postirradiation recurrence. Some authors (Creasman and Rutledge 1972; Rutledge et al. 1977) feel that patients who have received 6000 rad or more to the whole pelvis are not candidates for exenterative surgery, inasmuch as the complications in this group of patients are tremendous.

Psychosocial Aspects

The successful exenterative operation returns the patient to a productive life. A prolonged convalescence is the rule even after an extensive hospitalization during which the basic skills of stoma management are taught. Considerable expertise is gained only through the personal experience of stoma management. The impact of major surgery on the family situation requires careful evaluation because of the total patient dependence upon the family for emotional and physical support. Any failure of the family to understand or accept the patient and her postsurgical changes will be devastating. Social ostracism will lead to the patient's physical demise. Recent studies by Lamont and associates (1978) have shown that the support of the spouse and his reassurance are key factors in the sexual rehabilitation of exenterative patients. Without an accepting and supporting spouse, reconstructive procedures for restoration of vaginal function are for naught. The rehabilitation of postoperative exenteration patients requires a contribution from physicians, paramedical personnel, social service agencies, and, most importantly, the family. Without the availability of coordinated team effort, the successful outcome may be jeopardized.

Metastatic Survey

The second major level of preoperative evaluation consists of a thorough documentation of the extent of disease. Complete hematologic profiles, including careful assessment of anemia or coagulation defects, are performed. Renal and liver function studies are reviewed, with particular attention given to pyelographic abnormalities and evidence of hepatic metastasis. Bone scans have been helpful in overall evaluation of these patients. Bipedal lymphangiography is performed to evaluate iliac and paraaortic adenopathy. Abnormal lymph nodes may be sampled via fine needle aspiration to confirm tumor involvement which precludes exenterative surgery. Other studies such as barium enema, lung scan, and brain scan may be useful.

Creasman and Rutledge (1972) have reviewed their experience with exenterative surgery from the standpoint of preoperative evaluation. Five factors were found to be useful predictors of resectability, survival, and complications. One is symptoms of disease. These include pelvic, back, or hip pain; bladder symptoms; and vaginal discharge or bleeding. Those patients without symptoms had a greater chance of resectability and survival than did those with symptoms. The percentages of resectable patients were 64 (symptomatic) and 70 (symptom-free) (table 7.1).

The second factor is the elapsed time from primary treatment to recurrence. The longer the latent period before recurrence, the better was the two-year survival (table 7.2).

The third factor is the status of the urinary system as demonstrated by pyelography (table 7.3). Poor survival is associated with any pyelographic abnormality, regardless of degree.

The remaining factors are location of recurrence and the surgeon's estimate of resectability. Clearly, a small central lesion that the surgeon feels is

Table 7.1
Clinical Symptoms and Resectability

	Exploratory Operation	Resection Performed (No./%)	Survived Resection 2 Years (No./%)	Overall 2-Year Survival of Patients with Exploratory Operation (No./%)
No symptoms	41	29/70	21/72	21 of 41/51
Any symptoms	219	141/64	66/47	66 of 219/30

Table 7.2
Time from Primary Treatment to Recurrence

Time from First Treatment to Recurrence (yr)	Exploratory Operation	Resection Carried Out (No./%)	Survived Resection 2 Years (No./%)	Overall 2-Year Survival of Patients with Exploratory Operation (No./%)
0–2	178	104/58	48/46	48 of 178/27
2–5	44	33/75	19/58	39 of 82/47
>5	38	33/87	20/61	

resectable has a greater chance of extirpation as well as survival than larger lesions (tables 7.4 and 7.5).

Table 7.6 presents the resectability and survival with the multiple factors summarized. A positive finding in any factor is given a score of one and a negative finding is given a score of zero. The summation of this score is correlated with exploration, resection, and two-year survival.

Abdominal Exploration

The ultimate evaluation for exenteration is made at celiotomy. Various authors report that 23% to 66% of patients explored actually underwent exenteration (Ketcham et al. 1970; Lamont, DePetrillo, and Sargeant 1978;

Table 7.3
IVP and Resectability of Tumor

	Exploratory Operation	Resection Performed (No./%)	Survived Resection 2 Years (No./%)	Overall 2-Year Survival of Patients with Exploratory Operation (No./%)
Normal IVP	144	117/81	69/59	69 of 144/48
Abnormal IVP				
Unilateral deviation	17	10/59		
Unilateral hydronephrosis	55	21/38		
			17/34	17 of 114/15
Bilateral hydronephrosis	12	5/42		
Unilateral nonfunction	30	14/47		

189

Table 7.4
Location of Pelvic Recurrence and
Resectability

	Explored	Resection Performed (No./%)	Survived Resection 2 Years (No./%)	Overall 2-Year Survival of Patients with Exploratory Operation (No./%)
Central lesion	112	92/82	57/62	57 of 112/51
Large central lesion not fixed	24	18/75		
Fixed unilateral	67	26/39		
Fixed bilateral	28	14/50 } 78/53	30/38	30 of 148/20
Lower 1/3 vagina involved	10	7/70		
Multiple combinations	19	13/68		

Rutledge et al. 1977; Symmonds, Pratt, and Webb 1975). The determination of disease outside the bounds of resectability may only be possible at operation. Subclinical liver metastases and spread of disease into the peritoneal cavity are considered contraindications to exenteration. We employ immediate peritoneal washings for cytologic screening upon entering the abdomen. Positive washings for malignant cells are grounds to abandon the procedure. Symmonds feels that peritoneal penetration in the cul-de-sac of Douglas may not absolutely contraindicate exenteration, although Rutledge disagrees.

Table 7.5
Estimate of Clinical Resectability Compared
with Surgical Resection

	Exploratory Operation	Resection Performed (No./%)	Survived Resection 2 Years (No./%)	Overall 2-Year Survival of Patients with Exploratory Operation (No./%)
Thought clinically to be resectable	176	132/75	75/57	75 of 176/43
Thought clinically to be unresectable	63	27/43	10/37	10 of 63/16

Table 7.6
Resectability and Survival with Multiple
Variables

Score	Exploratory Operation (number of patients)	Resection Performed (No./%)	Survived Resection 2 Years (No./%)	Overall 2-Year Survival of Patients with Exploratory Operation (No./%)
0	7	7/100	7/100	7 of 7/100
1	41	36/88	28/78	28 of 41/68
2	63	52/83	26/50	26 of 63/41
3	52	32/62	12/38	12 of 52/23
4	36	18/50	7/39	7 of 36/20
5	37	11/30	4/36	4 of 37/11

Paraaortic lymph node metastases preclude exenteration; however, the significance of pelvic lymphadenopathy is under discussion. Creasman and Rutledge, reviewing the subject in 1974, pointed out that 25% of patients with positive pelvic nodes survived five years compared with 36% of patients with negative nodes in a series of 170 patients. The point was made that not all patients undergoing exenteration had a lymphadenectomy performed, and some of these patients may have harbored positive nodes. Morley reported that all resected patients with positive pelvic nodes had recurrence or died with disease within two years of operation. In his 1977 review, Rutledge states that small pelvic lymph nodal disease may not be a contraindication, but his results show that only 2 of 30 such patients were long-term survivors. Symmonds and associates report 39% five-year survival in patients without lymph node metastasis in the internal iliac or obturator groups as opposed to 13% survival if these nodes contain cancer.

A few patients may fall into the category of nonresectability because of extreme fixation of heavily irradiated tissues to the pelvic wall and pelvic vessels. These patients generally tend to be younger, and they have usually received high doses of megavoltage roentgen therapy for bulky disease. They are explored as a last hope for cure in young patients with recurrent disease.

All patients with postirradiation recurrence of cervical cancer should be considered candidates for pelvic exenterative surgery as long as there is no proven disease outside the area of resection. This absolute contraindication may be obvious or more subtle. The task involves deciding the point at which the sum of relative contraindications equals an absolute contraindication. This judgment requires the compassion, skill, and experience of well-trained gynecologic oncologic surgeons.

References

Creasman, W.T., and Rutledge, F. Preoperative evaluation of patients with recurrent carcinoma of the cervix. *Gynecol. Oncol.* 1:111–118, 1972.

Creasman, W.T., and Rutledge, F. Is positive pelvic lymphadenopathy a contraindication to radical surgery in recurrent cervical carcinoma? *Gynecol. Oncol.* 2:482–485, 1974.

Ketcham, A.S. et al. Pelvic exenteration for carcinoma of the uterine cervix: a 15-year experience. *Cancer* 26:513–521, 1970.

Lamont, J.A.; DePetrillo, A.D.; and Sargeant, E.J. Psychosexual rehabilitation of exenterative surgery. *Gynecol. Oncol.* 6:236–242, 1978.

Million, R.R.; Rutledge, F.; and Fletcher, G.H. Stage IV carcinoma of the cervix with bladder invasion. *Am. J. Obstet. Gynecol.* 113:239–246, 1972.

Morley, F.W., and Lindenauer, S.M. Pelvic exenterative therapy for gynecologic malignancy: an analysis of 70 cases. *Cancer* 38:581–586, 1976.

Rutledge, F.N. Pelvic exenteration. In *Gynecologic surgery: errors, safeguards, and salvage.* ed. J.H. Ridley. Baltimore: Williams and Wilkins, 1974.

Rutledge, F.N. et al. Pelvic exenteration: an analysis of 296 patients. *Am. J. Obstet. Gynecol.* 129:881–892, 1977.

Rutledge, F.N., and Burns, B.C., Jr. Pelvic exenteration. *Am. J. Obstet. Gynecol.* 91:692–708, 1965.

Symmonds, R.E.; Pratt, J.H.; and Webb, M.J. Exenterative operations: experience with 198 patients. *Am. J. Obstet. Gynecol.* 121:907–918, 1975.

PART IV

CARCINOMA OF THE ENDOMETRIUM

Adenocarcinoma of the endometrium has become the most commonly diagnosed invasive tumor of the female reproductive tract. Although stage for stage this disease is as lethal as carcinoma of the cervix, the overall survival of women with endometrial cancer remains high because most cases are diagnosed when the tumor is confined to the uterine fundus (stage I). The treatment of stage I endometrial carcinoma is thus of enormous practical importance. Drs. Johnson and Berman use those prognostic criteria of importance in patients with stage I disease and arrive at different conclusions. The reader is encouraged to critically evaluate the literature in the light of the information provided by Dr. Lamb on the statistical analysis of clinical trials in cancer.

High rates of detection of early endometrial carcinoma are achieved because of an increasing awareness on the part of the patient and her physician of the implications of abnormal uterine bleeding in the perimenopausal and postmenopausal years; however, a real increase in the incidence of this tumor has been reported by several investigators. It is well documented that postmenopausal estrogen users have an increased risk to develop adenocarcinoma of the endometrium. Dr. Cohen discusses the implications of this information with respect to the relative morbidity and mortality rates of osteoporosis and endometrial cancer and suggests an appropriate use of replacement estrogens in the postmenopausal years in an attempt to maximize benefits while reducing the risks.

Chapter 8

Osteoporosis versus Endometrial Carcinoma: Are Estrogens the Cure or the Cause of Lethal Disease?

PERSPECTIVE:

Carmel J. Cohen

Life expectancy in the United States is increasing along with the population itself. The average age for menopause in North America is 51 years, and, in the United States, there are approximately 30 million women who have achieved this age. This group may expect to live more than 20 years in the postmenopausal state, and during this time they will face an increasing cumulative risk of the occurrence of several metabolic and neoplastic disorders. One of these, osteoporosis, is a condition of loss of bone substance which seems to increase dramatically in postmenopausal women, imposes complications as a direct function of age from time of menopause, and occurs as a function of estrogen deprivation. This latter observation has stimulated a variety of investigators to prescribe estrogens, either prophylactically or therapeutically, in an attempt to prevent or reverse the demineralization process in the bones of postmenopausal women (Avioli 1978; Gordan 1977, 1978; Lindsay et al. 1976, 1978; Meema et al. 1975, 1976).

This attempt is worthy and rational because, though men and women both lose bone mass progressively with age, the rate of loss in women increases dramatically after age 50 and can result in the loss of 50% of the total bone mass in aged women, whereas in men at the age of 80 only 20% to 25% of bone mass is lost as determined by photodensitometry studies (Meema et al. 1973). During this postmenopausal state, women experience 50 to 70 fractures per 1000 women per year, and the rate of fracture is at least eight times greater than in men of comparable age. Gordan estimates that of the 1600 participating hospitals during 1972–73 which reported on the incidence of hip fractures, there were 10,000 deaths associated with 135,000 fractures. This group of hospitals represents only one-third of the short-term-care hospitals in the United States. Women accounted for approximately 80%, or

8000, of these deaths. This statistic obviously omits consideration of suffering and disability from fracture in the aged and economic burden to the immediate family, insuring agencies, and governmental resources.

Another of the diseases prevalent in postmenopausal women is endometrial cancer. Ninety-five percent of endometrial neoplasms are adenocarcinomas, and at least 80% of these occur in the postmenopausal state. The incidence of this cancer is rising in the United States, and a significant number of these cancers appear to be hormone-dependent. More recently, evidence has accumulated that the administration of exogenous estrogen might be associated with the development of this disease. (Gray, Christopherson, and Hoover 1977; Greenwald, Caputo, and Wolfgang 1977; Hoogerland, Buchler, and Crowley 1978; Mack et al. 1976; McDonald et al. 1977; Smith et al. 1975; Studd 1976; Ziel and Finkle 1975, 1976).

In this brief discussion, we shall attempt to clarify the role of postmenopausal osteoporosis in producing morbidity in aged women, the role of estrogens in preventing or reversing this event, the evidence for production or development of endometrial cancer as a function of estrogen activity, and the ultimate quest for controlling both osteoporosis and endometrial cancer.

Hormone Dependence of Endometrial Cancer

The evidence for hormone dependence of endometrial cancer has been summarized in some detail by Gusberg (1978) from the experience in our own institution as well as from the reports of other investigators. Experimental work employing animal models has demonstrated the production of endometrial hyperplasia and endometrial carcinoma in rabbits that became infertile and anovulatory as a result of liver damage, in rabbits exposed to unopposed long-term estrogen administration, and in rabbits rendered diabetic. Griffiths and associates (1963) demonstrated the protective effect of progesterone in resisting estrogen stimulation in this same animal model.

In the human, one may observe the frequent association of endometrial cancer precursors as well as invasive endometrial cancer in the uteri of patients with granulosa-theca cell tumors of the ovary. This relationship is even stronger as patients age, so that with length of exposure to unopposed estrogen elaboration, the risk of endometrial cancer increases. In the young patient, endometrial cancer is usually found in the anovulatory model. Infertility and lack of ovulation in the cystic ovary syndrome are the predominant concomitance of endometrial cancer when it exists in the premenopausal patient. The coincidence of obesity with attendant peripheral conversion of estrogen precursors by aromatization and the development of endometrial cancer has been noted by many investigators. The development of endometrial cancer precursors, such as adenomatous hyperplasia, in association with prolonged estrogenic stimulation, has been noted not only by Gusberg but by others who have studied the histologic progression of these precursors. Finally, the increasing number of case control studies suggesting an increase in risk of endometrial cancer for women receiving long-term estrogen therapy is notable. Such studies, to be sure, have many critics, for their design is variable, there are few prospective studies, and the selection of controls differs among the various studies. One might note in favor of the validity of the studies, however, that there is a definite relationship between dose and risk. There is also a relationship among dose, length of exposure, and risk. The range of risk of all of the studies (4 to 14 times, depending on subgroups and stratifications) is remarkably similar despite the disparate geographic distribution and populations from which the studies were reported.

The final consideration among the body of evidence for hormone dependence of endometrial cancer is the response of this cancer to hormone therapy. Since the report of Kelly and Baker (1961), there have been numerous publications documenting the response of one-third of these cancers to treatment with gestagens (Kohorn 1976). More recently, with the identification of estrogen and progesterone receptors in normal endometrium and in endometrial cancers, the mechanisms of action of each of these hormones in the metabolism of the endometrium are better understood. The role of estrogen in cell replication emerges with increasing clarity, and the capacity of the gestagen to alter the number of estrogen receptors as well as to elaborate enzymes which lead to conversion of estrodiol to estrone, thus producing a weaker estrogen, support the clinical observations noted since the work of Kelly and Baker. Finally, the observation that cancers with greater differentiation have a larger number of progesterone receptors and also respond best to progestational treatment clearly underlines the hormone dependence of many endometrial cancers. The latest work suggesting that tamoxifen, an "antiestrogen," is active against endometrial cancers which have failed to respond to conventional therapy, including progestational therapy, is further support for this thesis.

Osteoporosis

An understanding of osteoporosis requires some consideration of normal bone structure (Wheeler 1976). In the human, bone is formed in a succession of layers or lamellae by osteoblasts. Some of these forming cells are trapped within the bone and are transformed into osteocytes that remain the metabolically active cells of "resting" bone. The living cells entrapped in the resting bone have access to the blood supply and are subject to the stimuli provided through blood transport. Each isolated metabolic unit within the bony structure communicates through a weblike system of filaments. During the process of new bone formation, the first product is matrix or osteoid. This is composed mainly of collagen which provides the template on which minerals are deposited. Collagen is a unique protein substance in that it contains the amino acids hydroxyproline and hydroxylysine in high concentrations. Once the collagen is deposited, mineralization occurs: calcium is deposited, resulting in the rigidity of bone. Mineralization is not a passive process, as suggested by the observation that not all collagen calcifies. It is known that osteocytes play an active role in mineralization, but the inhibition of mineralization of collagen in certain locations is not well understood. Once bone is mature, it is renewed by a process called remodeling. In this process, osteocytes are transformed into osteoclasts, which are multinucleated cells responsible for causing bone resorption. When the calcium is thus absorbed from the bone structure, the osteoclast converts once more into the osteoblast, and bone formation proceeds. During the process of remodeling, collagen is cleaved, and the resulting hydroxyproline is released with a concomitant elevation in urine levels. Thus the urinary ratio of hydroxyproline to creatinine reflects the extent of bone resorption.

Osteoporosis is the condition in which the composition, the shape, and the essential morphology of bone are normal, but the total skeletal mass is decreased. There are numerous disorders that result in diminished bone density. In the context of our discussion, we shall refer to osteoporosis in women as a normal process of diminished bone density, occurring spontaneously in adult women with marked acceleration in the face of hypoestrogenic or postmenopausal states. This implies the absence of other disease processes that might be considered in the differential diagnosis. This list includes subtle forms of thyrotoxicosis, multiple myeloma, metastatic carcinoma, bilateral corticoadrenal nodular hyperplasia without the classical signs of Cushing's syndrome, and adult forms of osteogenesis imperfecta tarda. In addition, primary hyperparathyroidism, megadose vitamin A therapy, diabetes mellitus, chronic alcoholic abuse, and hereditary bone absorption disorders may all mimic osteoporosis (Avioli 1978).

In normal bone metabolism in the adult woman, remodeling occurs constantly and is an ongoing process in which osteoclastic activity (bone resorption) and osteoblastic activity (new bone formation) are in constant evidence. Factors that influence this process include many hormones as well as a significant list of dietary, constitutional, and environmental factors. Parathormone is associated with both osteoblastic and osteoclastic activity; however, its major effect is with the latter process. Estrogen, on the other hand, seems to block bone resorption by a mechanism that is still unclear. Progesterone maintains bone density in the face of increased bone resorption, suggesting that it stimulates active bone formation at a rate exceeding that of bone resorption, resulting in maintenance of bone density by a mode complementing rather than exaggerating the effect of estrogen. Vitamin D, prostaglandins, phosphorus, calcitonin, smoking, and alcohol ingestion all affect the ratio of resorption to new bone formation, presenting a very complex pattern of variables at work in bone metabolism.

Management of Postmenopausal Osteoporosis

In 1941, Albright and his co-workers recognized the importance of meno-pause in the occurrence of osteoporosis in women. This observation has been confirmed by many authors, and Gordan's review (1977) documents their con-tribution. One of the difficulties in studying osteoporosis is the absence of clear diagnostic criteria, so that a comparison of data from different series is difficult. Radiologic diagnosis alone is inaccurate because variation in radi-ographic technique or in positioning of the patient will compel different interpretations. Moreover, random repeat readings of the radiograph by the same group of diagnosticians will result in wide variations of reporting. Cal-cium balance studies are good reflections of bone metabolism but require measurement of urinary and fecal calcium levels, and these are notoriously poor parameters in terms of reproducibility. Bone biopsy is diagnostic but is obviously impractical for serial study. The technique of photon absorption densitometry, which can measure bone density, usually in peripheral bones, has a high degree of reproducibility. Several studies have correlated bone density in the distal phalanges with the occurrence of vertebral fractures. Thus by combining clinical evaluation, the presence or absence of bony frac-tures, serial measurement of bone density, and a measurement of the ratio between urinary excretion of hydroxyproline and creatinine, one can develop diagnostic parameters. Certainly, these can be applied in following single pa-tients serially.

By measuring the bony density of the radius in 82 postmenopausal women who had been entered into a program of estrogen treatment, Meema and Meema demonstrated in 1976 that at the time of menopause or castra-tion, if patients were treated with equine-conjugated estrogens in cylic fash-ion, their bone deposition increased, whereas those patients who were untreated sustained a marked diminution in bone density. Lindsay and his co-workers (1976), in a prospective randomized study, found that treatment with estrogen for five years prevented the reduction in bone mineral content observed in women treated during the same time with a placebo. If the pa-tient received no therapy for three to six years after oophorectomy and then was treated with estrogen, there was a highly significant increase in the bone mineral content during the first three years of treatment. Following that, there was no further increase in bone mineral. During this time, the placebo-treated groups continued to lose bone annually.

In another study by Lindsay's group, in 1978, a group of 43 patients in whom oophorectomy had been performed and who were randomized to treat-ment by estrogen or treatment by placebo were investigated. Patients receiv-ing estrogen for eight years showed no significant amount of bone loss during these eight years. Patients in the placebo-treated control group initially lost bone at the rate of 2.6% per annum and later averaged a loss of 0.75% per annum. Of special importance is the group of patients who were treated with estrogen for four years and who then were treated with placebo for the second four years. This group lost no bone during the four years of treatment with estrogen, but when they were then given placebo for four years, their bone density was indistinguishable from that of the patients who had received placebo for eight years. This suggests that estrogen therapy must be ongoing if its prophylactic effects are to be maintained.

In addition to the preventive role of estrogen in the patient with hypoestrogenism, there is increasing evidence that postmenopausal bone loss may be reversed to some degree by the administration of estrogen (Gordan and Jemand 1978) and that patients with fractures can experience arrest of further demineralization by the administration of estrogen.

Nonestrogenic treatment includes the daily administration of calcium carbonate or low-dose calcitonin (one Medical Research Counsel unit intramuscularly three times a week). These regimens will decrease bone resorption and will increase bone accretion but may lead to problems from hypercalcemia in some women. Ingestion of elemental calcium (1 gm/day), elimination of smoking, provision for daily sustained exercise programs, and administration of androgens in some patients to stimulate an androgen-dependent calcitonin action may all be helpful in lieu of estrogen therapy.

Resolution of the Dilemma

The results of two important investigations bearing on this problem have recently been published; the first, a retrospective case control study of the metabolic and neoplastic effects of long-term estrogen replacement therapy (Hammond et al. 1979a, 1979b), and the second, a 10-year prospective study of the effects of estrogen replacement on osteoporosis, carcinoma, and cardiovascular and metabolic problems (Nachtigall et al. 1979a, 1979b). In the retrospective study, Hammond and his co-workers studied equal numbers of postmenopausal or postoophorectomy patients who had been treated with or without estrogen. He found that the estrogen-treated group experienced lower rates of new cardiovascular disease, hypertension, osteoporosis, and fractures. There was a fourfold increase, however, in the risk of endometrial adenocarcinoma over the patients who did not receive estrogen. Of interest is the fact that no patient receiving a synthetic progestin in addition to the estrogen treatment developed endometrial cancer. This observation was statistically significant in Hammond's series.

In the prospective randomized 10-year, double-blind study by Nachtigall and co-workers, the estrogen treatment arm included conjugated estrogen tablets at a dose of 2.5 mg daily with medroxyprogesterone acetate tablets at a dose of 10 mg daily for seven days of each month. This study concluded that when estrogens were administered within three years of the menopause, osteoporosis was prevented or reversed. When the program was initiated longer than three years after the menopause, replacement therapy halted the osteoporotic process, with no new osteoporosis developing during the 10 years of treatment. There were no differences between the treatment group and the placebo group in the incidence of thrombophlebitis, myocardial infarction, or uterine cancer. There was an increase in cholelithiasis in the group receiving estrogen therapy. It is apparent, however, that by the addition of the progestational agent, the 84 patients studied over a 10-year period did not sustain an increase in their risk for endometrial cancer.

From the studies which have been published, the following information is thus available: (1) osteoporosis in women is a normal function of aging and is accelerated by hypoestrogenic states; (2) this process can be arrested, possibly reversed, and might be prevented by alteration of the hormone milieu in women, including the prescription of estrogen; (3) the minimal dose of estrogen required to achieve this end is unknown; (4) the minimal length of time required to secure prophylaxis is unknown, but cessation after short-term therapy results in rapid progression of osteoporosis; (5) the administration of unopposed estrogen to adult women increases the risk of developing endometrial cancer by 4 to 14 times; (6) in preliminary studies, the administration of a progestational agent in addition to conjugated estrogen prevented osteoporosis and did not increase the risk for endometrial cancer; (7) although the incidence of endometrial cancer is rising in this country, the morbidity and mortality arising indirectly from osteoporosis is probably increasing at a faster rate.

Since numerous studies have demonstrated the capacity to detect endometrial cancer in its precursor or noninvasive states by simple outpatient screening techniques, it would seem reasonable to assign all patients entering a hypoestrogenic state at a young age to a program of prophylactic administration of estrogen with a gestagen. Such people must be monitored by routine periodic sampling of the endometrial cavity and routine measurement of bone density, parameters of cardiovascular functions, measurement of circulating lipoproteins, screening for breast cancer, and other careful observations of potential complications from such open-ended therapy.

For those women spontaneously entering menopause at the normal age, a prospective randomized collaborative study should be mounted by the various regional or specialty-oriented collaborative groups in this country. Such a program could confirm the findings of the previously cited smaller studies, could establish optimum dose schedules and drug regimens, and could educate patients in how to diminish their own risk factors through improvement of metabolic function leading ultimately to a heightened sense of well-being.

References

Albright, F.; Smith, P.H.; and Richardson, A.M. Postmenopausal osteoporosis: its clinical features. *JAMA* 116:2465, 1941.

Avioli, L.V. What to do with "postmenopausal osteoporosis"? *Am. J. Med.* 65:881–884, 1978.

Gordan, G.S. Postmenopausal osteoporosis: cause, prevention, and treatment. *Clin. Obstet. Gynecol.* 4:169, 1977.

Gordan, G.S., and Jemand, H.K. Postmenopausal osteoporosis: is it a preventable disease? *Contemp. Obstet. Gynecol.* 11:47–59, 1978.

Gray, L.A., Sr.; Christopherson, W.M.; and Hoover, R.N. Estrogens in endometrial carcinoma. *Obstet. Gynecol.* 49:385–389, 1977.

Greenwald, T.; Caputo, T.A.; and Wolfgang, P.E. Endometrial cancer after menopausal use of estrogen. *Obstet. Gynecol.* 50:239–243, 1977.

Griffiths, C.T. et al. Effects of progestins, estrogens, and castration on induced endometrial cancer in rabbits. *Surg. Forum* 14:399–401, 1963.

Gusberg, S.B. Cancer of the endometrium: diagnosis and histogenesis. In *Corscaden's gynecologic cancer,* fifth ed. Baltimore: Williams and Wilkins, 1978.

Hammond, C.B. et al. Effects of long-term estrogen replacement therapy: I) metabolic effects. *Am. J. Obstet. Gynecol.* 133:525–536, 1979a.

Hammond, C.B. et al. Effects of long-term estrogen replacement therapy: II) neoplasia. *Am. J. Obstet. Gynecol.* 133:537–547, 1979b.

Hoogerland, D.L.; Buchler, D.A.; and Crowley, J.J. Estrogen use: risk of endometrial carcinoma. *Gynecol. Oncol.* 6:451–458, 1978.

Kelly, R.N., and Baker, W.H. Progestational agents in the treatment of carcinoma of the endometrium. *N. Engl. J. Med.* 264:216–222, 1961.

Kohorn, E.I. Gestagens in endometrial carcinoma. *Gynecol. Oncol.* 4:398–411, 1976.

Lindsay, R. et al. Long-term prevention of postmenopausal osteoporosis by oestrogen. *Lancet* 5:1038–1040, 1976.

Lindsay, R. et al. Bone responses to termination of oestrogen treatment. *Lancet* 6:1325–1327, 1978

Mack, T.M. et al. Estrogens in endometrial cancer in a retirement community. *N. Engl. J. Med.* 294:1262–1267, 1976.

McDonald, T.W. et al. Exogenous estrogen in endometrial carcinoma: case control and incidence study. *Am. J. Obstet. Gynecol.* 127:572–580, 1977.

Meema, S.; Bunker, M.L.; and Meema, N.E. Preventive effect of estrogen on postmenopausal bone loss. *Arch. Intern. Med.* 135:1436–1440, 1975.

Meema, S., and Meema, H.E. Menopausal bone loss and estrogen replacement. *Isr. J. Med. Sci.* 12:601–606, 1976.

Nachtigall, L.E. et al. Estrogen replacement therapy: I) a 10-year prospective study in the relationship to osteoporosis. *Obstet. Gynecol.* 53:277–281, 1979a.

Nachtigall, L.E. et al. Estrogen replacement therapy: II) a prospective study in the relationship to carcinoma and cardiovascular and metabolic problems. *Obstet. Gynecol.* 54:74–79, 1979b.

Smith, D.C. et al. Association of exogenous estrogen and endometrial carcinoma. *N. Engl. J. Med.* 293:1164–1167, 1975.

Studd, J. Estrogens as a cause of endometrial carcinoma. *Br. Med. J.* 1:1144–1145, 1976.

Wheeler, M. Osteoporosis. *Med. Clin. North Am.* 60:1213–1224, 1976.

Ziel, H.K., and Finkle, W.D. Increased risk of endometrial carcinoma among users of conjugated estrogens. *N. Engl. J. Med.* 293:1167–1170, 1975.

Ziel, H.K., and Finkle, W.D. Association of estrone with the development of endometrial carcinoma. *Am. J. Obstet. Gynecol.* 124:735–740, 1976.

Chapter 9

The Treatment of Stage I Carcinoma of the Endometrium

PERSPECTIVE:

Gary H. Johnson

Endometrial cancer has now become the most common invasive gynecologic malignancy. Data from the American Cancer Society reveal that 27,000 new cases of endometrial cancer occurred in 1975 and during that year accounted for approximately 3500 deaths among American women (table 9.1).

Unfortunately, some physicians have developed a complacent attitude in their approach to patients with endometrial cancer. They believe that five-year survival is optimal; therefore there would be little benefit from improved treatment techniques. In reality, large contemporary studies indicate that five-year survival is similar, stage for stage, to cancer of the cervix. Four thousand one hundred ninety-seven cases collected by Kottmeier and a collected series of 2432 cases from Morrow form the basis for the data presented in table 9.2. Gynecologists commonly believe that treatment results are superior in patients with endometrial cancer when compared to results for patients with cancer of the cervix, but their impressions are biased simply because we see many more patients with early stage I endometrial cancer (75% of cases) than with early stage I cervical cancer (Boronow 1976). The increasing number of patients with endometrial cancer, as well as the five-year survival data reflecting a need for improved treatment modalities, have renewed interest in defining the optimal therapy of endometrial cancer. This discussion is limited to the therapeutic modalities and treatment schemes related to stage I endometrial cancer, both because of the increased number of patients presenting with early disease and the continued controversy related to the treatment of early endometrial cancer.

Table 9.1

Cancer Incidence and Death in U.S. Women

Site	Incidence		Deaths	
	Number	Percent Total	Number	Percent Total
Breast	88,000	27	32,600	20
Colorectum	51,000	15	25,400	15
Corpus uteri	27,000	8	3,300	2
Lung	19,000	6	17,600	11
Cervix	19,000	6	7,800	5
Ovary	17,000	5	10,800	6

SOURCE: *Morrow, DiSaia, and Townsend 1976.*

The Development of Methods Used to Treat Early Endometrial Cancer

Despite 30 years of accumulated experience in the treatment of endometrial carcinoma, we are still searching for the ideal method of therapy. This on-going search continues primarily because no clearly superior method has emerged which is soundly based on adequate clinical investigation (Lewis, Mortel, and Slack 1977).

As early as 1878, hysterectomy became the therapy of choice in the treatment of endometrial cancer and still prevails as the cornerstone of therapy. With the advent of radiotherapy, Heyman, in 1927, challenged the supremacy of surgery as the only method of treatment. His data demonstrated equal five-year survival using radiation alone in patients deemed to be op-

Table 9.2

Endometrial Cancer Five-Year Survival by Clinical Stage

Stage	Kottmeier Annual Report 1973		Morrow Collected Data 1973	
	Five-Year Survival	Number of Patients	Five-Year Survival	Number of Patients
I	70.0	3025	76.0	1860
II	47.0	595	51.0	205
III	28.0	428	26.0	256
IV	4.7	149	8.8	113
All stages	60.0	4197	68.0	2432

SOURCE: *Boronow 1976.*

erative candidates (Gusberg 1976). Further evaluation through large group studies has failed to substantiate radiation alone as an effective treatment modality in early endometrial cancer. Those centers initially enthusiastic in the use of only radiation therapy now employ hysterectomy in the treatment plan of most patients whenever possible (Jones 1975). The importance of the role of hysterectomy can be appreciated from the data in table 9.3 (Morrow, DiSaia, and Townsend 1976).

With the knowledge that either surgery or radiation was therapeutically effective in controlling endometrial cancer, the trial of a combination of both treatments naturally developed. By 1934 reports appeared in the literature indicating that increased survival was possible by using surgery and some form of radiation therapy. The number of patients in each reported series has been small and holds no statistical significance. Reports as recently as 1976 state:

> In many quarters the superiority of combination therapy is accepted as established dogma and re-examination of treatment policies viewed as heretical. Despite the confident air of this position, a life sparing effect specifically attributable to the radiotherapeutic component of combination regimens has not been proven (Morrow, DiSaia, and Townsend 1976).

Nevertheless, the demonstrated radiosensitivity of endometrial cancer underlies our continued attempt to combine surgery and radiation as an ideal treatment method, and it has become the most common form of therapy in the United States today.

With statistical validity, one fact has emerged from our studies of combination therapy. The rate of vaginal recurrence is significantly lower when combination therapy is used, as opposed to surgery alone (Goodman and Hellman 1974) (table 9.4). Some would question the risk of vaginal recurrence when stage I endometrial cancer is treated by surgery alone, but this query may be answered by a report from Price, Hah, and Rominger (1965). Information from 196 patients with stage I carcinoma of the endometrium treated

Table 9.3
Corrected Five-Year Survival in Stage I
Endometrial Carcinoma

| Reference | Surgery with or without Radiation | | Radiation Only | | P |
	Number	Percent Five-Year Survival	Number	Percent Five-Year Survival	
Bickenbach	137	87	136	69	< 0.005
Joelsson	517	90	197	71	< 0.0005

SOURCE: Morrow, DiSaia, and Townsend 1976.

Table 9.4

Incidence of Vaginal Recurrences

Reference	Surgery Only (No./%)	Intracavitary Radium		Preoperative External Beam (No./%)
		Preoperative (No./%)	Postoperative (No./%)	
Shah, Green	37/16	46/4.0	34/6.0	—
Graham	33/12	59/3.0	31/0.0	—
Dobbie	64/11	——	84/2.4	—
Price et al.	41/14	110/3.6	16/0.0	—
Lampe	——	——	——	121/0.8
Sala, del Regado	——	——	——	126/0.0

SOURCE: Goodman and Hellman 1974.

by surgery alone revealed a vault recurrence rate of 4.4% with well-differentiated histology, 5.7% with intermediate histology, and 13.6% with anaplastic histology. With no invasion of the myometrium, the vault recurrence rate was 3.7%, with superficial invasion, 4.7%, and with deep invasion, 15.1%. Also of interest was the fact that the extent of surgery did not seem to be related to the incidence of vault recurrence. Twenty-six patients had 2 cm or more of vaginal cuff removed at surgery and had a 7.6% vault recurrence. In 143 patients with minimal or no cuff removed, there was a 6.9% recurrence.

The development of treatment programs using chemotherapy in early endometrial cancer has been limited. Progestins have been shown to be active in the therapy of endometrial carcinoma, but to date, their benefit in the treatment of primary stage I disease has not been identified (Lewis et al. 1974).

Virulence Factors

Gusberg and others (1976) have identified a number of characteristics associated with stage I endometrial cancer affecting the outcome of therapy. Histologic differentiation of the tumor was reported as early as 1923 to be one significant factor. In that year, Mahle reported 136 patients with four grades of cancer. He reported all patients with grade I cancers, 71% of grade II, and 38% of grade III as living, and no survivors with grade IV disease. The prognostic value of this grading system has been substantiated by others and has subsequently been shown to be associated with increased depth of myometrial invasion and increased frequency of lymph node metastasis with dedifferentiation of the tumor.

Myometrial invasion is a second valuable prognostic factor independent of the histologic grade of the tumor. Numerous reports in the literature now attest to the fact that survival is inversely proportional to the depth of myometrial invasion.

Cervical involvement also decreases survival, as reflected by the outcome in stage II as compared to stage I malignancies (table 9.1). These patients are of concern in this discussion because sometimes patients with clinical stage I disease have occult cervix involvement detected at hysterectomy.

Although increased uterine size has traditionally been associated with a poor prognosis, the evidence for this is meager. In a study by Javert and Douglas (1956) 100 hysterectomy specimens were examined from patients with stage I endometrial cancer. The uterus was enlarged in 54%, but in only eight cases was this due to tumor. Morrow, DiSaia, and Townsend (1973) and Lewis, Mortel, and Slack (1977) feel that neither uterine size, cavity measurement, nor uterine weight has proved to be of material value in assessing the extent of disease or affecting the ultimate clinical outcome.

Selection of a Treatment Method for Early Endometrial Cancer

The management of stage I endometrial carcinoma remains controversial. Treatment programs advocated vary from surgery alone to combinations of radiation before and after hysterectomy. Variations among study groups and a lack of prospective randomized trials make it difficult to attain comparisons between one treatment method and another. Because of the relatively high survival in early endometrial cancer, large numbers of patients are necessary to acquire statistically significant figures. For example, Jones points out that if the only advantage of combined therapy were a 5% increase in five-year survival (from 85% to 90%) over surgery alone that it would take 300 to 400 patients in each group to attain a P value of less than 0.05. I know of no randomized, prospective study with nearly that number of evaluable patients.

Another factor making evaluation of treatment in stage I disease difficult is the general lack of acceptance of a staging system. Staging on a clinical basis is necessary to evaluate patients treated totally with radiation who will never undergo surgical exploration. But since the number of patients who do not undergo surgical exploration in this country are few in reality, it appears that a surgical pathologic staging system might be advantageous. This would permit more precise evaluation of each of the factors known to influence survival and would allow more individualized treatment. Until the results of well-planned clinical trials become available, it behooves those treating endometrial cancer to study carefully all regimens and to utilize that treatment program which is efficacious in the greatest number of patients.

At the University of Utah in 1971 we adopted a prospective, nonrandomized protocol for the evaluation and treatment of newly diagnosed clinical stage I endometrial cancers (Ohlsen et al.). This protocol consisted of preoperative intrauterine and vaginal cesium followed within 72 hours by total abdominal hysterectomy and bilateral salpingo-oophorectomy. Those patients with poorly differentiated tumors, deep myometrial invasion, occult cervical involvement, or pelvic metastasis were then considered for external beam radiotherapy to the whole pelvis because of increased risk of involvement of pelvic nodes or other pelvic structures. To date, 99 patients with endometrial cancer clinically confined to the uterus have been treated by this protocol. Only 1 of 16 patients at high risk for recurrence, treated with external radiation, has failed with recurrence in the pelvis, and no vaginal recurrences have been identified. The overall Berkson-Gage actuarial survival at three years, uncorrected for death from intercurrent disease, is 85.8% (fig. 9.1 and table 9.5). The operative morbidity associated with hysterectomy immediately following intracavitary irradiation was low and did not affect the outcome.

Other literature also reports that using similar treatment techniques has achieved excellent results (Underwood et al. 1977; Boronow 1969). Since 1977, at the University of Utah we have included sampling the pelvic and paraaortic nodes in an attempt to define further the extent of disease and

Figure 9.1

BERKSON–GAGE ACTUARIAL SURVIVAL–UNCORRECTED

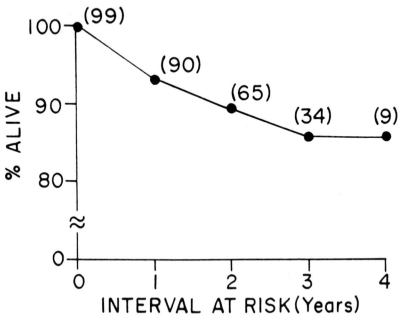

Actuarial survival curve for patients included in the preoperative intracavitary irradiation protocol, calculated by Berkson-Gage method.

Table 9.5
Survival of Patients at Risk for Various
Intervals

Years at Risk	Number of Patients	Alive without Evidence of Disease	Lost to Follow-up	Dead of Cancer	Dead of Other Causes	Alive with Disease
> 1	99	83	3	7	5	1
> 2	75	60	3	6	5	1
> 3	45	32	3	5	4	1
> 4	12	9	1	0	2	0

modify therapy. Those patients with positive pelvic nodes will have external radiation, with extended fields if the paraaortic nodes are positive. The curative value of paraaortic and pelvic irradiation is not established, but improvement in our institution in custom shaped, multiple field, external beam radiation techniques has rendered the morbidity sufficiently low to warrant the curative attempt.

Rationale for Selection of Preoperative Radium Followed Immediately by Hysterectomy

As previously discussed, surgery alone subjects a significant number of patients to the risk of vaginal vault recurrence. The actual risk varies depending on the virulence factors previously presented. It has been well documented that enough patients with even stage I_a, grade I neoplasm develop vault recurrence (Price, Hah and Rominger 1965; Boronow 1973) that it appears beneficial to give adjunctive treatment to all stage I tumors, regardless of grade. In addition, reports of grade I neoplasm with deep myometrial invasion in 21% of patients would persuade one to use adjunctive radiotherapy in this group (Morrow 1973). Because of the low morbidity associated with intracavitary preoperative radiation and the untested theoretical benefits described above, we will continue to use adjunctive, preoperative radiation for all stage I endometrial cancers regardless of grade.

We have elected to use preoperative intrauterine and vaginal brachytherapy followed immediately by hysterectomy because:

1. To reduce vault recurrence, we theoretically feel that the vaginal and paracervical lymphatic network, and not just the vaginal epithelium alone, needs to be treated by adjunctive therapy. We think this can best be done by a radium syste, with contributions from the uterine and cervical tandem rather than from vaginal sources alone (Lewis et al. 1975).

2. Adjunctive radium is beneficial in that it may prevent the surgeon's having to remove the upper one-third of the vagina to prevent vault recurrences—a procedure which, according to Price, is not beneficial, with vault recurrences having no relationship to the amount of vaginal epithelium removed at the time of hysterectomy (Price, Hah, and Rominger 1965).

3. It would theoretically be advantageous to use radiation at a time when

215

tissue oxygenation was optimal, rather than after hysterectomy and alteration of the paravaginal vasculature.

4. If vault recurrences are associated with implantation at the time of surgery or with tumor cells displaced into the paravaginal lymphatics and venous system at the time of surgical manipulation, the preoperative irradiation would prevent such recurrences.

5. Suit and Gallagher (1964) have shown that increasing doses of radiation decrease the transplantability of normal tumor cells.

6. Occult cervical involvement in stage I endometrial carcinoma is estimated to occur in 10% of patients (Lewis et al. 1975). A higher and more uniform parametrial dose can be achieved with the preoperative system previously described as opposed to a vaginal system administered postoperatively or by external therapy.

7. The described system could potentially treat microscopic disease peripheral to the surgical field encompassed by a simple hysterectomy.

8. A radium system accompanied by immediate hysterectomy avoids the delay of surgery necessitated by external radiation.

9. Potentially, the complications from a radium system would be less than with whole pelvic irradiation.

10. The treatment can be accomplished during one hospitalization.

11. A radium system with immediate hysterectomy provides a surgical specimen for histopathologic evaluation without changes that might be induced with whole pelvic irradiation and irradiation of the lesion prior to surgical pathologic staging.

12. Individualized treatment can be afforded on the basis of the surgical staging and histopathologic features of the surgical specimen.

13. Preoperative radiation could potentially decrease bowel exposure. Postoperative therapy might increase segmental radiation of the gastrointestinal tract if adhesions are present following removal of the uterus.

14. Because uterine size does not appear to be related to survival and is frequently associated with causes other than neoplasm, we have elected not to use intrauterine packing techniques with Heyman's capsules but to use the system described and tailor postoperative whole pelvis therapy to the patient as needed.

Conclusion

Preoperative intracavitary irradiation followed promptly by hysterectomy appears to have numerous theoretical advantages in the therapy of stage I endometrial cancer. It appears to be associated with a favorable survival and low treatment morbidity. Until such time that needed preoperative, clinical trials randomizing various treatment modalities are completed, we shall continue to use this combination therapy in our early endometrial cancers.

References

American Cancer Society. *Cancer facts and figures.* New York, 1975.

Boronow, R. Carcinoma of the corpus—treatment at M. D. Anderson Hospital. In *Cancer of the uterus and ovary.* Chicago: Year Book Medical Publishers, 1969.

Boronow, R. A fresh look at corpus cancer management. *Obstet. Gynecol.* 42:448–451, 1973.

Boronow, R.C. Endometrial cancer, not a benign disease. *Obstet. Gynecol.* 47:630–634, 1976.

Goodman, R., and Hellman, S. The role of postoperative irradiation in carcinoma of the endometrium. *Gynecol. Oncol.* 2:354–361, 1974.

Gusberg, S.B. The evolution of modern treatment of corpus cancer. *Cancer* 38:603–609, 1976.

Javert, C., and Douglas, R. Treatment of endometrial adenocarcinoma. *Am. J. Roentgenol.* 75:580, 1956.

Jones, H.W. III. Treatment of adenocarcinoma of the endometrium. *Obstet. Gynecol. Surv.* 39:147–169, 1975.

Lewis, G.C. et al. Adjuvant progestogen therapy in the primary definitive treatment of endometrial cancer. *Gynecol. Oncol.* 2:368–376, 1974.

Lewis, G.C., Jr.; Mortel, R.; and Slack, N.H. Endometrial cancer—therapeutic decision and staging process in "easy disease." *Cancer* 39:959–966, 1977.

Lewis, J.L. et al. Managing endometrial cancer. *Contemp. Obstet. Gynecol.* 6:106–148, 1975.

Mahle, A. The morphological histology of adenocarcinoma of the body of the uterus in relation to longevity. *Surg. Gynecol. Obstet.* 36:385, 1923.

Morrow, C.P.; DiSaia, P.J.; and Townsend, D.E. Current management of endometrial carcinoma. *Obstet. Gynecol.* 42:399–406, 1973.

Morrow, C.P.; DiSaia, P.J.; Townsend, D.E. The role of postoperative irradiation in the management of stage I adenocarcinoma of the endometrium. *Am. J. Roentgenol.* 127:325–329, 1976.

Ohlsen, J.D. et al. Combined therapy for endometrial carcinoma: preoperative intracavitary irradiation followed promptly by hysterectomy. *Cancer* 39:659–664, 1977.

Price, J.; Hah, G.; and Rominger, C. Vaginal involvement in endometrial cancer. *Am. J. Obstet. Gynecol.* 91:1060–1065, 1965.

Suit, H., and Gallagher, H. Intact tumor cells in irradiated tissue. *Arch. Pathol.* 78:648–651, 1964.

Underwood, P.B. et al. Carcinoma of the endometrium: radiation followed immediately by operation. *Am. J. Obstet. Gynecol.* 128:86–98, 1977.

PERSPECTIVE:

The Treatment of Stage I Carcinoma of the Endometrium

Michael L. Berman

Optimal management of stage I endometrial cancer has not yet been determined. Two commonly used approaches include initial preoperative radiation therapy followed by abdominal hysterectomy with bilateral salpingo-oophorectomy (Wade, Kohorn, and Morris 1967) and initial operation followed by radiation therapy when indicated by operative findings (Morrow, DiSaia, and Townsend 1976). There have been advocates of more extended operations (Lees 1969), but no data suggest improved survival in patients so treated (Rutledge 1974; DeMuelenaere 1973); obesity and advanced age commonly encountered provide relative contraindications to this approach. When preoperative radiation is used, often it is administered by the Heyman packing technique or with Suit-Fletcher afterloading devices (Fletcher 1973). Some investigators prefer using external beam therapy preoperatively, especially with more poorly differentiated tumors. Postoperative radiation can be administered either to the whole pelvis or to the vaginal vault alone (Morrow, DiSaia, and Townsend 1976). Despite the multiplicity of treatment regimens currently advocated, no data support a clear superiority of one approach over another.

The dilemma of choosing the best treatment for early endometrial cancer without data identifying such a program is disquieting. Although radiation therapy alone can cure patients with endometrial cancer and reduce vaginal vault recurrences, it is unclear whether its use with surgery improves survival, and the optimal method, timing, and dosage of administration is unknown. The most compelling explanation for these unanswered questions is the inability to compare data between and within studies reported in the literature. Bias in patient selection and failure to control within treatment groups for factors that influence prognosis prevent meaningful comparison of treatment modalities. By necessity, therefore, a rational approach to the selection of a treatment regimen must be based both on an understanding of the biological patterns of spread of endometrial cancer and an assessment of those risk factors that influence prognosis.

Biological Patterns of Spread

The biology of endometrial cancers must be understood to treat areas at greatest risk for occult spread and hence subsequent recurrence. The commonest areas of recurrence are the vagina and regional lymph nodes. Treatment, therefore, often must include both the primary tumor within the uterus and possible vaginal and lymphatic metastases.

Most frequently vaginal recurrences result from dissemination via paravaginal lymphatics as inferred from data of Truskett and Constable (1968). The belief commonly held that vaginal metastases result from tumor implantation at the time of hysterectomy was contradicted by their demonstration that the incidence of vaginal metastases was independent of the presence or absence of residual tumor in the uterus at the time of hysterectomy. These data imply that intraoperative manipulation of the uterus has little influence on the risk of vaginal recurrences and that there is no theoretical advantage of preoperative over postoperative radiation in the prevention of vaginal recurrences.

Pelvic and periaortic lymph node metastases result from lymphatic dissemination which can follow the dual blood supply of the uterus. Metastases can involve the uterine, hypogastric, external, and common iliac nodes accompanying their respective vessels, or can go directly to the periaortic nodes along the lymphatic chains that follow the ovarian vessels. Creasman and associates (1979) performed pelvic and periaortic lymphadenectomies on 228 patients with stage I endometrial cancer and found that 17 of 23 patients with pelvic lymph node metastases also had periaortic metastases. They did not report periaortic metastases in the absence of pelvic metastases. These data suggest that in most instances periaortic nodes are involved secondarily after pelvic lymph node metastases occur and that the prevalence of coexisting pelvic and periaortic nodal metastases is high. The therapeutic implications include the importance of identifying patients at high risk for lymph node metastases and the necessity to evaluate by biopsy and consider treatment of the periaortic lymph nodes when the pelvic lymph nodes have metastatic tumor.

Seen less frequently are distant spread by the hematogenous route and intraperitoneal dissemination. In general, protocols for the management of stage I endometrial cancer have not been directed toward treatment of occult spread to these more distant sites. The risk of such dissemination has not been quantified but seems to be low, and the potential to eradicate it by chemotherapy or immunotherapy cannot be assessed.

Risk Factors

Many studies have helped to identify factors associated with an increased likelihood of subsequent recurrences and reduced survival. These risk factors include depth of myometrial invasion, histologic grade, uterine size, and patient age (Lewis, Stallworthy, and Cowdell 1970; Frick et al. 1973; Jones 1975; Sall, Sonneblick, and Stone 1970). Of these factors, myometrial invasion appears to be the most important, correlating most closely both with lymph node metastases and vaginal recurrences. Because well-differentiated tumors tend to be superficial while poorly differentiated tumors most frequently are deeply invasive, histologic grade also is an important risk factor. Nevertheless, approximately 12% of well-differentiated tumors are deeply invasive (Cheon 1969) and appear to have a risk of lymph node metastases similar to deeply invasive, poorly differentiated tumors (Boronow 1976). On the other hand, poorly differentiated superficial tumors are less likely to metastasize than deeply invasive tumors of any grade. Uterine enlargement also correlates with a poorer overall prognosis; however, when corrected for the grade of tumor, it does not appear to influence survival (Malkasian 1978). Advanced age is associated with more anaplastic tumors and advanced stage (Jones 1975; Homesley, Boronow, and Lewis 1976), but when corrected for these risk factors and when deaths from intercurrent disease are excluded, age per se has not been shown to affect survival.

These risk factors have been evaluated primarily for vaginal and lymph node metastases. Accordingly, an estimate of the risk of local and regional recurrence can be used to determine if specific therapy including operation and/or radiation should be directed to these areas.

Vaginal Recurrences

The risk of vaginal recurrences in stage I endometrial cancer increases with more deeply invasive and more anaplastic tumors. The Mayo Clinic reported recurrences in 1% of 196 patients without myometrial penetration, 4% of 179 patients with tumors invading up to 5 mm, and 8% of 171 patients whose tumors were more deeply invasive (Brown et al. 1968). Stander (1956) and Price, Hahn, and Rominger (1965) found a similar association between tumor grade and vaginal recurrences with 5 of 196 recurrences (2.5%) with well-differentiated tumors and 8 of 72 with poorly differentiated tumors (11.1%). It has not been shown whether the risk of vaginal recurrences with more anaplastic tumors is independent of the depth of myometrial penetration. Ng and Reagan (1970) have demonstrated that anaplastic tumors confined to the endometrium have a worse prognosis than superficial tumors of lower grade; therefore, even superficial anaplastic tumors must be viewed as capable of early dissemination, and when high-grade tumors are present the vagina should be considered at risk for recurrence. The increased risk of vaginal recurrences with myometrial invasion or anaplastic tumors can be diminished with adjuvant vaginal radiation.

Lymph Node Metastases

As with vaginal recurrences the risk of lymph node metastases increases with deeper myometrial invasion and tumor dedifferentiation. Of these two factors the depth of myometrial penetration provides a more accurate measure of risk since superficial tumors, independent of histologic grade, rarely metastasize to pelvic or periaortic lymph nodes. Data compiled from Creasman and associates (1979), Lewis, Stallworthy, and Cowdell (1970), Carmichael and Bean (1967), and Javert (1952) help to quantify the risk of lymph node metastases according to the depth of penetration. These authors found lymph node metastases in 10 of 339 patients (3%) with tumors either confined to the endometrium or superficially invasive, in 6 of 43 with moderate invasion (14%), and in 31 of 75 with deep invasion (41%). Therefore, patients with deeply invasive tumors of any histologic grade should either undergo pelvic lymphadenectomy and periaortic lymph node biopsies, or in the case of an unsuitable candidate for extensive retroperitoneal dissection, adjuvant radiation therapy to the whole pelvis. Such radiation would include the upper vagina, also at high risk for recurrence.

The importance of assessing or treating the pelvic lymph nodes relates to the potential to cure many such patients. In five collected series of 34 patients with stage I endometrial cancer metastatic to the pelvic lymph nodes, 41.2% were cured with aggressive therapy (Lewis, Stallworthy, and Cowdell 1970; Homesley, Boronow, and Lewis 1976; Graham 1971; Hulbert 1969; Dobbie, Taylor, and Waterhouse 1965). Those patients not cured frequently have concomitant metastases elsewhere, including periaortic lymph nodes, peritoneal cavity, lungs, and other sites (Homesley, Boronow, and Lewis 1977). In the absence of demonstrable metastases to these other sites, more than half of the patients with lymph node metastases can be cured.

Treatment

Radiation versus Surgery

Surgery should be an integral part of the management of the patient with stage I endometrial cancer. Only patients with severe medical conditions such as a recent myocardial infarction or severe pulmonary insufficiency should be treated with radiation therapy alone. Obesity and advanced age should not preclude operation in the absence of more absolute contraindications. Although radiation therapy alone often can cure early endometrial cancer, five-year survival figures are significantly poorer than for operation with or without radiation. Bickenbach and associates (1967) studied 137 pairs of patients matched for age, intercurrent disease, and uterine size from the University Hospitals in Munich and Hannover, West Germany. The two treatment groups studied were radiation therapy alone and operation with or without radiation therapy. The 5- and 10-year survival for the operated group were 87% and 76% while comparable figures for the radiated group were 69% and 52%, respectively. Because some patients in the operated group had adjuvant radiation, it is not possible to compare radiation with surgery alone from this study. Nevertheless, the group of patients treated with radiation alone did substantially worse than the operated group.

When radiation therapy alone is employed in patients with severe medical problems that preclude operation, treatment can include both intrauterine and external beam therapy. Because patients with well-differentiated tumors and uteri with a depth of 8 cm or less are at low risk to have lymph node metastases, intracavitary therapy often is curative. Landren and associates (1976) recommended intrauterine packing with Heyman capsules, delivering a total of 6000 mg hours of radium in two applications separated by two weeks. Vaginal radiation can be delivered simultaneously using protruding tandem sources or colpostats to deliver 7000 to 8000 rad surface dose to the upper half of the vagina. When the uterus is large or the cavity irregular, three packings, each separated by two weeks, can deliver up to 8000 mg hours of radium. Multiple applications are important to provide tumoricidal doses of radiation distributed homogeneously when variation in the shape of the uterine cavity and geographic location of the tumor mass might otherwise preclude optimal therapy. When poorly differentiated stage I tumors are treated only with radiation therapy, the vagina and pelvic lymph nodes must be treated in addition to the uterine fundus. Initial treatment consists of 4000 to 5000 rad to the whole pelvis, including the upper half of the vagina, over four to five weeks. A rest period of two weeks is provided to permit reduction in the tumor volume and uterine size, after which 3000 to 4000 mg hours of intracavitary therapy and 3000 to 4000 rad surface dose to the vaginal mucosa are administered in one or two applications. When a small uterine cavity does not permit application of multiple Heyman capsules, suitable doses of radiation can be administered using a tandem loaded 20–15–10 mg of radium.

Radical versus Nonradical Surgery

Although most investigators recommend total abdominal hysterectomy and bilateral salpingo-oophorectomy in stage I endometrial cancer, others have advocated radical hysterectomy, bilateral salpingo-oophorectomy, and pelvic lymphadenectomy. Those advocating more extensive operations have pointed out that for each stage of endometrial cancer the survival is no better than for cervical cancer (table 9.6) and that biological patterns of spread to the vagina, parametria, and pelvic lymph nodes are similar. The frequency of

Table 9.6
Comparison of Survival between Cervical
Cancer and Endometrial Cancer

Stage	Cervical Cancer		Endometrial Cancer	
	Number of Cases	5-Year Survival	Number of Cases	5-Year Survival
I	17,833	14,348/80.5%	12,655	9,670/76.4%
II	21,845	12,916/59.1%	2,185	1,089/49.8%
III	16,959	5,565/32.8%	1,596	480/30.1%
V	2,866	202/7.0%	585	54/9.2%
Totals	59,503	33,031/55.5%	17,021	11,293/66.3%

*SOURCES: cervical cancer: Kottmeier 1976;
endometrial cancer: Lewis, Stallworthy, and
Cowdell 1970; Kottmeier 1976.*

lymph node metastases as high as 28% in some series supports this approach
(Javert 1952). Because endometrial cancer rarely spreads to the parametria
without cervical extension, their removal in patients with stage I disease is
not justified, and because vaginal recurrences have not been reduced by more
radical operations, subtotal vaginectomy also is not warranted (Shah and
Green 1972). In addition, the increased morbidity and mortality in elderly
patients, who often are obese and have intercurrent medical illnesses, preclude extensive pelvic dissection and prolonged operative procedures.

Whether removal of the pelvic lymph nodes should be carried out in patients at risk for occult metastases who are suitable operative candidates has
not been evaluated fully. When complete lymphadenectomy is carried out,
the need for adjuvant whole pelvis radiation is eliminated in the absence of
metastases. When metastases are present, knowledge of their location helps
to direct the radiation therapy. The hazards of lengthy operations and technical difficulties encountered in performing retroperitoneal dissections in
these patients, however, have not been shown to be offset by improved survival. Furthermore, some patients who undergo lymphadenectomy also
might require adjuvant radiation, and the risk of intestinal injuries with this
approach could be prohibitive. These risks are greatest when extended ports
are used or when more than 5000 rad are delivered to operative site (Wharton et al. 1977; Piver, Vongtoma, and Barlow 1975). While limitation of
whole pelvis radiation following lymphadenectomy to no more than 5000 rad
might reduce the risk of complications, data are not yet available to assess
either risk or potential benefit from this approach.

Adjuvant Radiation Therapy

Since most patients with stage I endometrial cancer do not undergo lymphadenectomy, the most frequent use of radiation is the prophylactic treatment

of patients at high risk for occult metastases. Therapy usually is administered in conjunction with a total abdominal hysterectomy and bilateral salpingo-oophorectomy.

Advocates of preoperative radiation often use intracavitary therapy, external beam therapy, or both according to the uterine size and tumor grade. Theoretical advantages offered for preoperative radiation include prevention of tumor implantation at operation by reducing the tumor volume, sealing lymphatic channels, and injuring viable tumor cells, whereby attachment to the vaginal cuff and peritoneal cavity are prevented. These proposed advantages are contradicted by the data of Truskett and Constable cited above and by the absence of any data suggesting that recurrences are prevented more effectively by radiation administered preoperatively as compared with postoperatively. Data compiled by Jones (1975) show a reduction of vaginal recurrences from greater than 10% in patients treated with hysterectomy alone to approximately 5% in patients treated with adjuvant radium therapy. There was no difference in the recurrence rate reported in patients treated postoperatively as compared with those treated preoperatively. Furthermore, no data show improved survival in patients treated with preoperative radiation as compared with those treated after surgery.

Another proposed advantage of preoperative radiation might be a reduction in the incidence of radiation-induced complications. Advocates of preoperative radiation have suggested that initial operation might cause loops of intestine to adhere to the operative site, subjecting the bowel to excessive doses of radiation administered following operation. Reported bowel complications are infrequent, however, with either preoperative or postoperative radiation. In fact, the only group of patients treated with a combination of simple hysterectomy and radiation reported to be at increased risk for radiation-induced complications are those treated with both preoperative intracavitary and postoperative whole pelvis therapy. In 63 patients so treated, Joelsson, Sandri, and Kottmeier (1973) reported a 16% incidence of radiation injuries to the bowel or urinary tract as compared with 2% in 113 patients who received whole pelvis therapy only following abdominal hysterectomy. These data, therefore, suggest a potential increase in complications for those patients managed with preoperative intrauterine radiation, since it is impossible to predict accurately those patients who might also require whole pelvis radiation. For example, when patients treated with intracavitary radiation followed by operation are found to have lymph node metastases, ovarian spread, deep myometrial penetration, or occult cervical extension, whole pelvis radiation should be administered. While this combination of preoperative and postoperative radiation can be avoided by treating with preoperative radiation to the whole pelvis, unnecessary morbidity and delays in definitive therapy can be avoided by assessing instead the need for radiation following hysterectomy.

Another disadvantage of preoperative intracavitary radiation is that risk factors for occult lymphatic and vaginal spread that include deep myometrial penetration and extension to the uterine isthmus and cervix can be obscured. Hence, patients with a high likelihood of lymph node metastases are not identified and lymphadenectomy and/or pelvic radiation might be withheld inappropriately. This problem can be minimized if operation is carried out within a week following radiation, before tumor in the uterus is eradicated by therapy, but is avoided altogether by withholding preoperative radiation.

Initial operation is preferable to preoperative radiation because it (1) provides a rational approach to adjuvant therapy by permitting assessment of the surgical and pathologic features that influence prognosis and biological patterns of spread, (2) often reduces treatment time and cost, and (3) can reduce the number of treatment complications. When disseminated tumor is found at operation, radiation therapy is reserved for palliation only, and the expense and risks of a combined surgery and radiation approach can be avoided. The absence of deep myometrial penetration even in the presence of a grade 3 tumor would eliminate the need for whole pelvis radiation since lymph node metastases rarely are seen with superficial tumors. On the other hand, deep myometrial penetration associated with 10% to 12% of well-differentiated tumors is not obscured by this approach, and such patients should have treatment directed to the pelvic lymph nodes because of the high risk of metastases. If lymphadenectomy or lymph node biopsies are carried out, the identification of metastases permits administration of appropriate radiation therapy and consideration of adjuvant chemotherapy if periaortic metastases are found. This approach, therefore, reduces the number of patients requiring radiation therapy and eliminates patients treated both with preoperative and postoperative radiation therapy, thereby minimizing the risk of radiation complications. It provides a logical approach to the administration of radiation when indicated and does so without compromising survival. It also permits objective assessment of the biological patterns of spread of early endometrial cancer, which still have not been elucidated completely. Finally, operation prior to radiation prevents unnecessary delays in the treatment of some radioresistant tumors.

Treatment Summary

Patients with stage I endometrial cancer able to withstand a general anesthetic and an abdominal operation should undergo total abdominal hysterectomy and bilateral salpingo-oophorectomy. When well-differentiated tumors in the uterine fundus are confined to the endometrium or invade less than one-third of the myometrial wall, operation alone will cure more than 90% of patients, and radiation therapy is unnecessary. When tumors involve the uterine isthmus, extend to the cervix, are higher grade, or are more deeply invasive, radiation should be administered postoperatively. If lymphadenectomy is carried out at the time of hysterectomy in this high-risk group of patients, the absence of lymph node metastases permits therapy to be administered to the vaginal vault only, delivering 7000 to 8000 rad to the vaginal mucosa using colpostats or a vaginal mold. If lymph node metastases are found at lymphadenectomy, it is unclear whether adjuvant radiation adds to the survival; however, because of the poorer prognosis in this group of patients, I favor administration of 5000 rad to the whole pelvis, with ports extended one node chain above the level of the highest involved lymph node. If periaortic lymph node metastases exist, the ports should be extended to the level of the twelfth thoracic vertebral body. The upper half of the vagina should be included in the ports. When lymphadenectomy is not carried out, administration of radiation is determined by the grade of tumor, the depth of penetration, and the location of the tumor within the uterus. When these tumors invade more than one-third of the myometrial thickness or are located in the uterine isthmus or cervix, radiation should be delivered to the whole pelvis, administering 5000 rad over a period of five weeks because of the high risk of pelvic lymph node metastases. When grade 2 and 3 tumors are superficially invasive only, the risk of lymph node metastases is small while the risk of recurrence in the vagina is increased. Accordingly, vaginal vault radiation should be administered as outlined above. Because of the great importance placed on depth of myometrial penetration and geographic location of the tumor in managing these patients, it is essential that the entire uterus be processed to determine the greatest depth of invasion and the location of the tumor.

Uterine size per se should not influence the management of patients who are operative candidates. Although stage I_b tumors are associated with a poorer overall survival then stage I_a, this results from the greater frequency of poorly differentiated and more deeply invasive tumors in larger uteri. When corrected for the histologic grade of tumor, uterine size alone does not appear to influence survival. This finding is not unexpected because uterine enlargement often can result from unrelated causes including uterine myomata, adenomyosis, and grand multiparity.

When intraperitoneal dissemination is found, operation should consist of total abdominal hysterectomy, bilateral salpingo-oophorectomy, and omentectomy. Ascites and bowel obstruction often accompany peritoneal seeding and can be prevented or postponed by omentectomy. Patients with dissemination by the peritoneal, hematogenous, or lymphatic routes also should be considered for adjuvant chemotherapy. Progestational agents should be administered (Kohorn 1976; Rozier and Underwood 1974) in addition to cytotoxic drugs including Adriamycin and cyclophosphamide (Muggia et al. 1977). Because long-term survivals have been reported in patients with tumor dissemination, an aggressive approach is warranted in treating them.

Conclusions

Optimal management of stage I endometrial cancer has not been defined; however, a rational approach to therapy can be based upon the patterns of dissemination and an understanding of risk factors associated with a poor prognosis. Risk factors that make patients likely to suffer recurrence include deep myometrial penetration and tumor dedifferentiation. Depth of invasion appears to assume a more important role, and therefore decisions about adjuvant therapy are best made when knowledge of myometrial invasion is assessed prior to administration of radiation. While superficial low-grade tumors are treated best with operation alone, all other patients should be managed with a combination of initial surgery followed by adjuvant radiation. The type of adjuvant radiation is determined by an assessment of the surgical and pathologic features influencing the biological patterns of spread.

References

Bickenbach, W, et al. Factor analysis of endometrial carcinoma in relation to treatment. *Obstet. Gynecol.* 29:632–636, 1967.

Boronow, R.C. Endometrial cancer: not a benign disease. *Obstet. Gynecol.* 47:630–634, 1976.

Brown, J.M, et al. Vaginal recurrence of endometrial carcinoma. *Am. J. Obstet. Gynecol.* 100:544–549, 1968.

Carmichael, J.A, and Bean, H.A. Carcinoma of the endometrium in Saskatchewan. *Am. J. Obstet. Gynecol.* 97:294–307, 1967.

Cheon, H. Prognosis of endometrial carcinoma. *Obstet. Gynecol.* 34:680–684, 1969.

Creasman, W.T, et al. The surgical pathological correlation in stage I endometrial cancer. Presented at the tenth annual meeting of the Society of Gynecologic Oncologists, Marco Island, January 1979.

De Muelenaere, G.F. The case against Wertheim's hysterectomy in endometrial carcinoma. *J. Obstet. Gynaecol. Br. Comm.* 80:728–734, 1973.

Dobbie, B.M.W; Taylor, C.W.; and Waterhouse, J.A.H. A study of carcinoma of the endometrium. *J. Obstet. Gynaecol. Br. Comm.* 72:659–673, 1965.

Fletcher, G.H. *Textbook of radiotherapy*, second ed. Philadelphia: Lea and Febiger, 1973.

Frick, H.C. II et al. Carcinoma of the endometrium. *Am. J. Obstet. Gynecol.* 115:663–676, 1973.

Graham, J. The value of preoperative or postoperative treatment by radium for carcinoma of the uterine body. *Surg. Gynecol. Obstet.* 132:855–860, 1971.

Homesley, H.D.; Boronow, R.C.; and Lewis, J.L., Jr. Treatment of adenocarcinoma of the endometrium at Memorial–James Ewing Hospitals, 1949–1965. *Obstet. Gynecol.* 47:100–105, 1976.

Homesley, H.D.; Boronow, R.C.; and Lewis, J.L., Jr. Stage II endometrial carcinoma—Memorial Hospital for Cancer, 1949–1965. *Obstet. Gynecol.* 49:604–608, 1977.

Hulbert, M. Adjunctive pelvic irradiation in carcinoma of the endometrium. *J. Obstet. Gynaecol. Br. Comm.* 76:624–630, 1969.

Javert, C.T. The spread of benign and malignant endometrium in the lymphatic system with a note on coexisting vascular involvement. *Am. J. Obstet. Gynecol.* 64:780–806, 1952.

Joelsson, I.; Sandri, A.; and Kottmeier, H.L. Carcinoma of the uterine corpus: a retrospective survey of individualized therapy. *Acta Radiol. [Suppl.]* 334:3–63, 1973.

Jones, H.W. III. Treatment of adenocarcinoma of the endometrium. *Obstet. Gynecol. Surv.* 30:147–169, 1975.

Kohorn, E.I. Gestagens and endometrial carcinoma. *Gynecol. Oncol.* 4:398–409, 1976.

Kottmeier, H.L. *Annual reports on the results of treatment in carcinoma of the uterus, vagina, and ovary,* vol. 16. Stockholm: Pago Print, 1976.

Landren, R.C. et al. Irradiation of endometrial cancer in patients with medical contraindications to surgery or with resectable lesions. *Am. J. Roentgenol.* 126:148–154, 1976.

Lees, D.H. An evaluation of treatment in carcinoma of the body of the uterus. *J. Obstet. Gynaecol. Br. Comm.* 76:615–623, 1969.

Lewis, B.V.; Stallworthy, J.A.; and Cowdell, R. Adenocarcinoma of the body of the uterus. *J. Obstet. Gynaecol. Br. Comm.* 77:343–348, 1970.

Malkasian, G.D. Carcinoma of the endometrium: effect of stage and grade on survival. *Cancer* 41:996–1001, 1978.

Morrow, C.P.; DiSaia, P.J.; and Townsend, D.E. The role of postoperative irradiation in the management of stage I adenocarcinoma of the endometrium. *Am. J. Roentgenol.* 127:325–329, 1976.

Muggia, F.M. et al. Doxorubicin-cyclophosphamide: effective chemotherapy for advanced endometrial adenocarcinoma. *Am. J. Obstet. Gynecol.* 128:314–319, 1977.

Ng, A.B.P., and Reagan, J.W. Incidence and prognosis of endometrial carcinoma by histological grade and extent. *Obstet. Gynecol.* 35:437–443, 1970.

Piver, S.M.; Vongtoma, V.; and Barlow, J.J. Para-aortic node irradiation for cervical carcinoma. Presented at the sixth annual meeting of the Society of Gynecologic Oncologists, Key Biscayne, Fla., January 1975.

Price, J.J.; Hahn, G.A.; and Rominger, C.J. Vaginal involvement in endometrial carcinoma, *Am. J. Obstet. Gynecol.* 91:1060–1065, 1965.

Rozier, J.C., Jr, and Underwood, P.B., Jr. Use of progestational agents in endometrial adenocarcinoma. *Obstet. Gynecol.* 44:60–64, 1974.

Rutledge, F. The role of radical hysterectomy in adenocarcinoma of the endometrium. *Gynecol. Oncol.* 2:331–347, 1974.

Sall, S.; Sonneblick, B.; and Stone, M.L. Factors affecting survival of patients with endometrial adenocarcinoma. *Am. J. Obstet. Gynecol.* 107:116–123, 1970.

Shah, C.A., and Green, T.H. Evaluation of current management of endometrial carcinoma. *Obstet. Gynecol.* 39:500–509, 1972.

Stander, R.W. Vaginal metastases following treatment of endometrial carcinoma. *Am. J. Obstet. Gynecol.* 71:776–779, 1956.

Truskett, I.D., and Constable, W.C. Management of carcinoma of the corpus uteri. *Am. J. Obstet. Gynecol.* 101:689–694, 1968.

Wade, M.E.; Kohorn, E.I.; and Morris, J.M. Adenocarcinoma of the endometrium. *Am. J. Obstet. Gynecol.* 99:869–876, 1967.

Wharton, J.T. et al. Preirradiation celiotomy and extended field irradiation for invasive carcinoma of the cervix. *Obstet. Gynecol.* 49:333, 1977.

Chapter 10

The Statistical Evaluation of Clinical Trials in Cancer: Use and Misuse

PERSPECTIVE:

Emmet J. Lamb

The randomized clinical trial is a prospective controlled experiment in which the therapies under study are allocated by a chance mechanism. It is the most effective way of determining the relative efficacy and toxicity of a new therapy. Recently, 10 experienced biostatisticians compiled for the British Medical Research Council a clear and succinct report written specifically to give physicians the statistical ideas and methods needed to design, carry out, and analyze clinical trials (Peto et al. 1976). By avoiding special statistical jargon, by including all necessary tables, and by using worked examples, they made it easy for nonstatisticians to obtain a working knowledge of three essential statistical techniques: (1) the life table method of estimating the survival (time-to-response) distribution of patients who have been observed over varying periods of time, (2) the log-rank procedure for obtaining P values from life tables to test for statistical significance of the differences between survival distributions, and (3) the retrospective stratification technique to account for prognostic variables during analysis so that one does not have to stratify for these variables among the patients admitted to the study. We will refer to this as the MRC report.

Basic Statistical Terms

Relative Risk

The investigator who has found out through an epidemiologic study which people were exposed and which were not exposed to an alleged causal factor may construct a 2×2 contingency table. Such a table (table 10.1) displays the

Table 10.1
The 2 × 2 Contingency Table and the
Formulae for Calculation of Risk Ratio, Odds
Ratio, and the Chi-Square Statistic

		Condition	
		+	−
Character	+	A	B
	−	C	D

$$\text{Odds ratio} = \frac{A/C}{B/D}$$

$$\text{Risk ratio} = \frac{A/(A+B)}{C/(C+D)}$$

$$\chi^2 = \Sigma \frac{(O-E)^2}{E}$$

$$\chi^2 = \frac{(A+B+C+D)\ (AD-BC)^2}{(A+B)\ (C+D)\ (A+C)\ (B+D)}$$

relationship between the independent variable, which can be any characteristic or risk factor, and the dependent variable, which can be any condition
or event, such as death. The investigator may express the end result as a risk
ratio, the ratio of the rate at which the event occurs in people exposed to the
factor divided by the rate at which it occurs in people not exposed. In table
10.2 the risk ratio of 1.47 was determined by obtaining the ratio of the 4.6%
occurrence rate in the exposed group (32 diseased people among 693 exposed)
to the 3.1% occurrence rate in the controls (21 diseased among 668). A ratio

Table 10.2
Cases of Breast Cancer Developing within 25
Years in Mothers Exposed and Not Exposed
to Diethylstilbestrol

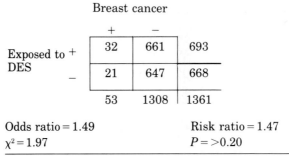

		Breast cancer		
		+	−	
Exposed to DES	+	32	661	693
	−	21	647	668
		53	1308	1361

Odds ratio = 1.49   Risk ratio = 1.47
$\chi^2 = 1.97$ $P = >0.20$

SOURCE: Bibbo et al. 1978.

above 1 means that the exposed group had a greater chance of having the disease. A ratio of 1 would have meant equal risks for each group.

Another ratio, the odds ratio, is especially useful for reports of case control studies (Freiman et al. 1978). In this type of study (table 10.3), the investigator has collected a group of people with the disease, the cases, and has selected a similar group, the controls, from available nondiseased people. The odds ratio, the ratio of the exposure rate in the cases divided by the exposure rate in the controls, may differ markedly from the risk ratio. When the disease is uncommon and both rates of occurrence are small, the odds ratio will closely approximate the risk ratio, table 10.2.

Significance Levels

Noting that the exposed group in table 10.2 appears to have become diseased more frequently than the control group, we must consider at least two possible reasons: (1) the factor, exposure to DES, had a real effect on outcome, the later development of breast cancer, or (2) the exposed group by chance contained disproportionately many patients who would have developed breast cancer anyway. The fundamental question a statistician asks is this: is a risk ratio of 1.47 significantly different from 1 for a study of this size? For data which can be displayed in a 2×2 contingency table, the statistical test of whether the relative risk differs from one is the chi-square (χ^2) test. The null hypothesis, that exposure had no effect on subsequent development of the disease and that the results observed occurred by chance variation alone, can be subjected to statistical testing. By use of the χ^2 test, one can calculate the probability of getting a difference at least as large as that observed by chance alone if the two groups were in fact equivalent. This state-

Table 10.3
Replacement Estrogen Use among Group
Health Women with Intact Uteri at Age
50–64 Years in 1972–75

		Endometrial cancer cases	Controls	
Current user	+	50	14	64
	−	17	60	77
		67	74	141

Odds ratio = 12.6	Risk ratio = 3.53
$\chi^2 = 44.0$	$P = <0.01$

SOURCE: Jick et al. 1979.

ment of probability, *P,* the significance level, is the end point for nearly all statistical tests.

At this point let us look at the results of a simple clinical trial (table 10.4). The distributions assumed for this fictitious study are those previously noted (table 10.3) in an actual epidemiologic study. In this new setting *P* less than 0.05 would mean this: Patients in treatment group A have fared better in terms of negative cultures than patients in group B. If there were no difference between the effects of the two treatments and the only cause of differences in outcome between the treatment groups were a chance allocation of more good-prognosis patients to one group than to the other, then the chance of one treatment group faring at least this much better than the other group would be less than 0.05, that is, less than one chance in 20.

The *Chi*-Square Test

The data used in calculating the χ^2 test statistic are the observed number (0) and the expected number (E) in each of the 4 cells A, B, C, D. If the null hypothesis were true, one would expect to have negative cultures among the 64 people who were treated with therapy A in about the same proportion as among the total, that is, 67 of 141 or 47.5%. Thus one would expect 30.4 people in cell A, 47.5% of 64. The difference between the observed number (0) and the expected number (E) in cell A is 50 minus 30.4, or 19.6. The value of $(O - E)$ could be determined for each cell and the χ^2 statistic obtained using one of the formulae shown in table 10.1. For manual calculations, one can use the formula shown on the right, which is mathematically equivalent to the one on the left. Comparison of the result with the values for χ^2 listed in the appropriate table tells us that the relative risk, 3.5, which we found does differ significantly from unity at the 5% level.

Alpha and Beta Errors

Two types of error are possible in decisions about the null hypothesis as tested by the χ^2 test or other statistical test of significance. A type I error,

Table 10.4
Vaginal Cultures after Two Weeks of
Therapy A or B in Women with Initially
Positive Cultures (Fictitious)

	Culture Negative	Culture Positive	
Therapy A	50	14	64
Therapy B	17	60	77
	67	74	141

$\chi^2 = 44.0;$ $\qquad\qquad P = < 0.01$ $R = 3.53$

rejecting the null hypothesis as false when it is really true, results in the investigator's attributing to the factor or drug an effect which it really does not have. Making this type of error is analogous to reporting a false positive Pap test. Custom, more than anything else, dictates that the probability, α, of committing an error of this type in reporting the results of a clinical trial be set at 0.05, the 5% significance level—at least for the initial testing. Events with P of 0.05, 1 chance in 20, are really not rare events. For example, throwing double sixes with a pair of dice (1 chance in 36) has P less than 0.05.

If the investigator cannot reject the null hypothesis, he concedes that the relative risk does not significantly differ from unity. This is not equivalent to concluding the absence of an effect. One must be concerned about missing an important therapeutic improvement. Accepting a false null hypothesis, that is, making a decision that no significant difference exists when there is a real difference in the effectiveness of the treatments, is a type II error, and the probability of erring in this way is indicated by β. The probability of disclosing a difference when one actually exists $(1-\beta)$ is called the power of the test. If a type I error (α) is analogous to a false positive Pap report, then a type II (β) error is analogous to a false negative Pap report.

It is a mistake to consider the identity of two treatments proven when no significant difference can be shown. Many trials end with a finding of no-difference-from-control because the sample size was not adequate. Thus therapies with clinically meaningful effects were discarded as ineffective after negative trials that included too few patients.

Confidence Intervals

When a report of a clinical trial lists a 90% or 95% confidence interval for the risk ratio, the difference is significant only if the interval does not include a risk ratio of 1. One can see that reporting a confidence interval conveys more information about the extent to which the two groups differ than reporting the P value alone. The latter directs all interest onto one boundary of the confidence interval. If the confidence interval includes the possibility of a strong effect, the study should not be classified as simply a negative study. A review of 71 randomized clinical trials reported as "negative" showed the confidence limit for most extending far into the territory of a definitely beneficial effect of treatment (fig. 10.1) (Freiman et al. 1978).

Planning a Clinical Trial

Randomization

Frugal investigators might consider it more efficient to place all their subjects on the study regimen and compare the outcome with that of historical controls, that is, subjects previously treated in a similar setting with a stand-

Figure 10.1

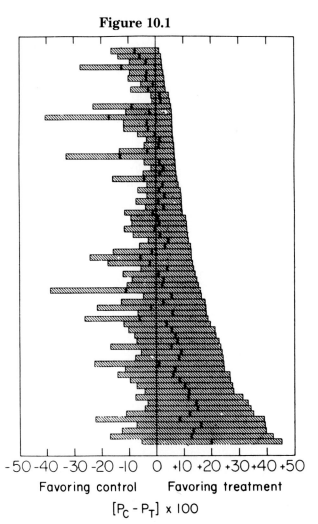

-50 -40 -30 -20 -10   0 +10 +20 +30 +40 +50

Favoring control   Favoring treatment

$[P_C - P_T] \times 100$

*Ninety percent confidence limits for the true
percentage difference for 71 trials. The vertical bar
in the center of each interval indicates the value of
the percentage difference between the event rate (P_1)
observed in the controls and the event rate (P_2)
observed in the treatment group. (Freiman 1978.
Reproduced with permission.)*

ard regimen. The advantage gained, however, having larger numbers of subjects in both the therapy and the control groups, would be more than offset by the strong possibility that systematic differences exist between the groups. These systematic differences could change the results to such an extent that an effect detected at the usual 5% significance level would be unconvincing.

236

Unless an experiment is constructed in such a way that a valid estimate of error is possible, it will be incapable of proving anything. To allow statistical evaluation of the results the process of randomization and, indeed, the rest of the elaborate machinery to avoid systematic sources of error are necessary. The MRC report lists simple and specific instructions for randomized allocation of patients to treatment groups (Peto et al. 1977).

The value of randomization was again demonstrated in a recent follow-up study of women who had participated many years before in a randomized clinical trial of interest to gynecologists (Bibbo et al. 1978). Mothers given diethylstilbestrol (DES) during pregnancy had an overall age-standardized relative risk of developing breast cancer during a 25-year follow-up period which substantially (risk ratio = 1.79) and significantly ($P < 0.01$) exceeded the baseline level for an historical control, the general population represented by the Connecticut Cancer Registry. When the DES-treated mothers were compared, however, with the control group from the original randomized clinical trial (table 10.2), the difference in cumulative rate of breast cancer between the treated group (4.6%) and the control group (3.1%) was not significant. The cause for the high incidence of breast cancer developing subsequently in this entire group of mothers is not known. Were it not for the set of controls, a conclusion that the incidence of breast cancer was increased after use of DES might have been drawn from this study.

Balance and Stratification

Information about factors that might affect prognosis, such as the stage of disease, sex, and age, should be obtained on all patients prior to their entry into the study. Retrospective stratification to detect and to correct for the effect of these covariates can be done during analysis of the data using the life table and log-rank methods of analysis. The authors of the MRC report argue persuasively that if these methods are used there is hardly ever need for stratification at entry. An overall estimate of the relative effects of treatments A and B adjusted for each of the initial prognostic factors is obtained by addition of the statistical indexes obtained by comparison of the outcome for patients within each of the strata. It is not necessary deliberately to balance the number of patients in each prognostic stratum between the two treatment groups. If a balance actually exists as a result of random allocation, the statistical tests are only slightly more sensitive. Moreover, the greater organizational complexity required to achieve the balance by stratification at entry may reduce the number of collaborators willing to participate.

Estimating Sample Size

The investigator who persists in a trial with virtually no chance of obtaining meaningful results wastes time and resources. During the planning phase before initiating the trial, the wise investigator can determine whether there is a reasonable chance of obtaining definitive results by addressing a few questions. Even if the results of the trial, carefully planned to have an adequate sample size, do not attain the 5% level of significance, they are likely to indicate the correct direction of the difference and to be close to significance. These are the questions to be answered during the early planning phase.

1. What cumulative event rate, P_1, do you expect at the time of analysis for the control group? To estimate the event rate (mortality rate, failure rate, and so on) for the control group, the investigator should take into consideration both unpublished and published opinions of other experts.

2. What cumulative event rate, P_2, do you expect for the treatment group given the greatest plausible effectiveness of the treatment? Investigators considering a clinical trial usually will be liberal in this estimate since they are likely to be convinced that the potential improvement from the new treatment is clinically important.

3. How many patients can you reasonably expect to randomize into the study? Investigators usually have a fairly good idea of the feasible sample size, at least in terms of the number of patients who could enter the study each year at their own centers. The desired sample size is one of the factors determining the duration of the intake phase.

4. What level of assurance, α, do you require that you will not report a difference due merely to the chance allocation of good-prognosis patients to one group rather than to the other? The probability, α, of rejecting a true null hypothesis is the desired level of significance. Customarily the probability is set at 0.05, or 1 chance in 20, of giving a false positive report, of making a decision that there is a difference in the effectiveness of two treatments when in reality there is no difference.

5. What level of assurance (β) do you need that you will not miss a real difference in effectiveness of the treatment? The probability, β, of accepting a false null hypothesis should be determined before the trial since one should be aware of the chance of missing a real therapeutic improvement. In practice values of 0.05, 0.10, or 0.20 are set for β. The probabilities α and β are closely related. If other conditions are the same, as β increases α decreases, and vice versa; however, β is not one minus α. The probability of making an error of either the first or second kind is decreased by increasing the sample size.

Making the First Estimate of Sample Size

From standard formulae in textbooks (Brown and Hollander 1977) one can determine the number of observations required to attain a certain level of assurance $(1 - \beta)$ of demonstrating a significant (α) difference in the outcome of two treatments with true event rates of P_1 and P_2. In practice, the value set for the probability α is almost always 0.05 and that for β 0.10 or 0.20 for the first run, to get a feeling for the sample sizes required to detect various differences, $(P_1 - P_2)$. A more helpful approach is to use an isograph of the sort shown in figure 10.2 to determine what difference, $(P_1 - P_2)$, the study can detect for a fixed α and β if n patients are entered per treatment group (Feigl 1978). Similarly, where the feasible sample size is roughly known, the detectable difference can be read directly from the graph.

As an example consider clinicians who wish to evaluate a new treatment for advanced ovarian cancer. They expect the mortality rate with the stand-

Figure 10.2

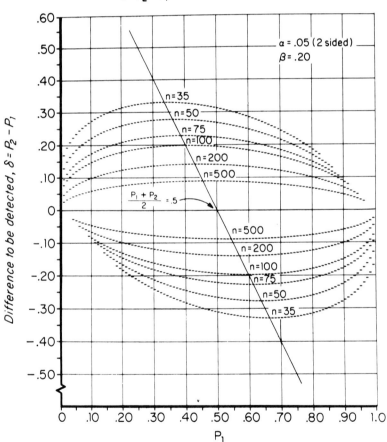

n = number of observations <u>per group</u>

$\delta = P_2 - P_1 = $ difference to be detected

Detectable differences between the event rate of the treatment group, P_2, and the event rate of the control group, P_1, required at various sample sizes, n, for an 80% probability of obtaining a significant result at the 5% level. (Feigl 1978. Reproduced with permission.)

ard treatment to be between 60% and 70% at the time of analysis and think it would be feasible to enter about 200 patients in a three-year period, enough for 100 in each treatment group. Of those entered, 75% would have died at the time of analysis. If these clinicians want to have an 80% level of assurance that they will not miss a real difference in effectiveness ($\beta = 0.20$) and they plan to test at the 5% level of significance ($\alpha = 0.05$), they could use the isograph shown in figure 10.2. From the graph we see that if P is between 0.60 and 0.70 and n is 100, the minimum difference (P_2 minus P_1) must be approximately 0.30. In other words, the mortality with the new treatment (P_2) must be in the range of 0.30 to 0.40 at the time of analysis. If it seems highly unreasonable that this rate could be achieved, then something must give. It will not be the mortality rate of the standard therapy, P_2, nor should it be the customary significance level, $P = 0.05$, necessary to avoid a false positive report.

Given the option of changing n or changing β, the prudent investigator will increase the sample size by prolonging the intake period or by enlisting the cooperation of collaborators. The investigator who selects the other path should do so consciously being aware of how much greater chance he is taking of missing a real difference in effectiveness. He should consult tables listing the sample size needed to achieve $\beta = 0.10$, 0.20, or 0.50 for $\alpha = 0.05$ or 0.01 at various proportions, P_1 and P_2. For instance, the clinicians in our example, finding that they would have a better than even chance ($\beta < 0.50$) of detecting a difference in proportions of 0.20 without any increase of sample size, might elect to proceed if they felt that that was a clinically meaningful difference. Any trial plan yielding less than a fifty-fifty chance of detecting a difference seems hardly worthwhile.

Life Table Methods

Survival Curves

Reporting only the number from each group who suffer the event is sufficient if the condition is an acute one, with most of the events occurring within a short time. On the other hand, if some of the events do not occur for some time, it is worthwhile plotting a survival curve to look at the times in which the events do occur.

First, let us consider how to calculate such a curve when we have reached the end of a period of observation (table 10.5). Had we followed continually and uniformly a group of 100 patients for five years, we could determine the overall mortality, 0.66, by counting the number who had died at the end of five years ($30 + 14 + 11 + 6 + 5$) and dividing by 100. By direct calculation of the cumulative percentage dead at the end of each yearly interval, we could obtain the points needed for the entire survival curve. To calculate the five-year survival curve in this way, we would have to continue

Table 10.5
Deaths during First Five Years in Group
with Standard Therapy (Fictitious)

Interval (Years)	Number at Risk at Start of Interval	Number of Deaths	
		Interval	Cumulative
0–0.9	100	30	30
1–1.9	70	14	44
2–2.9	56	11	55
3–3.9	40	6	61
4–4.9	25	5	66

the follow-up until all patients, including those admitted toward the end of the intake period, have been at risk for at least five years. We then would ignore some recent information about those survivors who had registered early and, therefore, had been followed for longer than the five-year period.

Probability of Death

From the data in table 10.5, we could determine for any interval after registration the sample proportions that are estimates of the conditional probability of death, that is, the probability of death during the interval for those who have survived the preceding interval. To die during the second year one must survive to the end of the first. In our table the probability of death during the first year is 0.30. Of the 70 alive at the beginning of the second year, 14 die during the ensuing year, and thus the conditional probability of death in the second year is 0.20. Similarly, for the group having not died by the end of any year the conditional probability of death during the subsequent year can be estimated as shown in table 10.6. The probability of surviving during the first year is 0.70 (1 − 0.30), and the probability of surviving during the second year if alive at the beginning of that year is 0.80 (1 − 0.20). The cumulative probability of surviving to the end of the second year is the product of these (0.80 × 0.70 = 0.56). Data for the entire curve could be obtained by the successive application of the probabilities of death during the interval to the number actually at risk of death during the interval.

Censored Observations

In practice we do not have a single group of patients all of whom have been continually followed for the same period of time. Patients enter the study one by one. Some die of the disease under study. Others, having survived varying periods, may die in an auto accident, may move away and become lost to fol-

Table 10.6
Life Table Estimates of Survival for the Two
Groups in Table 10.5

Group	Interval (Years)	Number at Risk at Start of Interval	Number of Terminations		Conditional Probability of Survival during Interval	Cumulative Probability of Survival to End of Interval
			Deaths	Censored		
Standard therapy	0–0.9	100	30	0	0.700	0.700
	1–1.9	70	14	0	0.800	0.560
	2–2.9	56	10	6	0.811	0.454
	3–3.9	40	5	10	0.857	0.389
	4–4.9	25	3	10	0.850	0.330
New therapy	0–0.9	100	9	10	0.905	0.905
	1–1.9	81	5	15	0.932	0.843
	2–2.9	60	4	6	0.930	0.784
	3–3.9	50	3	7	0.935	0.733
	4–4.9	40	2	12	0.941	0.690

low-up, or may still be alive at the time of analysis. All these situations in which the patient is no longer exposed to the risk of dying from the disease or in which we lack information about the patient's risk of dying yield incomplete observations called censored observations. Life table methods use all available follow-up information including censored observations and thus are more efficient and less subject to error due to incomplete follow-up than direct calculations whenever there are censored observations.

Methods of Analysis

Similar data are required for both methods in common use in estimating survival distribution (table 10.7). The actuarial life table estimate of Cutler and Ederer (1958) groups data by time intervals. The product-limit estimate of Kaplan and Meier (1958) examines individual survival times. The two methods are identical if the Kaplan-Meier method is thought of as a daily life table in which each interval contains only one observation. Although the calculations for both methods can be done by hand, computer programs are usually used. Copies of these programs can be obtained from several sources (Azen et al. 1976; Dixon and Brown 1978; Peto et al. 1976; Hull and Nie 1979).

In table 10.6 we use the fictitious data of table 10.5 to illustrate the life table method to calculate the probability of survival at the start of five annual intervals. The number exposed to risk at the start of each interval is obtained by subtracting from the number at risk (alive) at the beginning of the preceding interval the number dying or terminating for other reasons during the preceding interval. For example, at the start of the second interval, 1 to 1.9 years, only 70 subjects of the original 100 are still at risk. The proportion of deaths during the interval is obtained by dividing the number of deaths during the interval by the effective number exposed to the risk. In the third interval, there were 10 deaths. The effective number exposed to risk is obtained by subtracting from the number at risk at the start of the interval (56 in this instance) one-half of the censored observations occurring during the interval (6/2 = 3). The use of half the censored observations is based on the following reasoning: if one assumes that the dates of registration and the dates of the censoring events, such as loss to follow-up, are roughly equally distributed during the calendar year, then one can assume that those people composing the censored observations were exposed to risk for half the interval on the average. Thus the probability of dying during the third interval having survived the first two is 10 divided by 53, or 0.189. The probability of surviving the interval is obtained by subtraction from one. The probability of surviving to the end of any interval is obtained by successively multiplying the proportions surviving during each interval. For example, the probability of survival to the end of the third interval is .811 times 0.560, or 0.454. The figures in this last column are the points plotted on a survival curve. The survival curve for this data is shown in figure 10.3.

Table 10.7
Data Collection Format for Clinical Trials

Patient Identification Number	Type of Therapy*	Reason for Termination†	Date of Randomization	Date of Termination	Days of Exposure‡
1	2	1	01–01–78	02–10–78	41
2	2	2	02–12–78	12–31–80	749
3	1	1	02–14–78	11–15–80	1004
4	1	2	04–28–78	12–31–80	976
5	2	3	09–01–78	10–13–78	42
6	2	4	12–24–78	07–04–79	193

*Type of therapy: 1 standard therapy; 2 new therapy.
†Reasons for termination: 1 death from cancer; 2 alive on closing day of study; 3 lost to follow-up;
  4 deaths from causes other than cancer.
‡The length of the interval between the dates in the preceding two columns is obtained by calculation and is
  used in subsequent calculations for the Kaplan-Meier method of analysis.

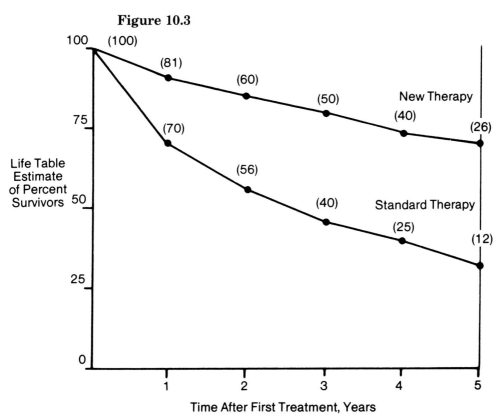

Figure 10.3

Life Table Estimate of Percent Survivors

Time After First Treatment, Years

Life table for patients randomly assigned to new therapy or standard therapy. Data from table 10.6. The numbers in parentheses indicate the number of patients at risk at the start of each interval.

Note that, in life table calculations, censored observations are not ignored but, on the other hand, influence the calculated rates only insofar as the information is available. Thus these methods allow maximum utilization of information. The event rates determined by either of these methods allow one to compare groups that vary in size, in relative magnitude of death rates during the intervals, and in completeness of follow-up. These methods allow comparison with the survival curve for a control group or for the general population.

A Summary *Chi*-Square Statistic

The statistical method used in comparison of survival curves is one based upon the χ^2 test. For any discrete interval in the life table graph, imagine that we construct a 2×2 contingency table comparing the two groups. From the observed number A, B, C, and D in each of the four cells and the marginal totals, we can determine E, the expected number if the null hypothesis were true, and then calculate the χ^2 statistics for that interval. Now, if we pass our observation window across the entire life table graph from the beginning, stopping at the end of each interval to accumulate the χ^2 statistics as we go, we derive a summary χ^2 statistic. The interval at which we stop may be the time when each event (death, loss of follow-up, and so on) occurs, as would be the case in the Kaplan-Meier estimate. The summary χ^2 is a measure of the significance of the difference between the two curves.

This summary *chi*-square technique is called the Mantel-Haenszel method of log-rank analysis (Mantel 1966). The name log-rank, like the name product-limit (used by Kaplan and Meier), refers to a statistical technicality which need not concern us. Using the Mantel-Haenszel technique it is possible to compare the probability of survival (of not suffering an event) among two, three, or more treatment groups. Because the *chi*-square statistics are added, it is possible to adjust during analysis for differences among subgroups in order to control for relevant prognostic factors such as age or stage of disease (Peto et al. 1977).

Applications of These Methods

These methods for planning and analysis are applicable to a variety of clinical studies. The event need not be death but can be any other time-related variable such as the appearance of metastases, the occurrence of infection, or even conception (Azen et al. 1976; Lamb and Leurgans 1979). The conditions compared need not be a new drug and a standard drug but may be a drug and no therapy or surgery and radiation.

Life table methods can be used in follow-up studies that do not include randomized assignment (Lamb and Leurgans 1979). In clinical trials, however, valid use of these methods requires randomization to eliminate bias in the initial assignment of patients to treatment groups. Moreover, randomization is the best way to balance unknown covariates as well as known ones. Because of these considerations, a strong argument can be made that all clinical trials should include random assignment and that journal editors should avoid publishing reports of clinical trials that were not randomized. Ethical considerations in the design and conduct of randomized clinical trials are discussed both in the MRC report and in the editorials accompanying a recent proposal for a new experimental design in which patients are randomly assigned to standard or new treatment groups before their consent is obtained (Zelen 1979).

246

References

Azen, S.P. et al. Some suggested improvements to current statistical methods of analyzing contraceptive efficiency. *J. Chronic Dis.* 29:649–666, 1976.

Bibbo, M. et al. A twenty-five year follow-up study of women exposed to diethylstilbestrol during pregnancy. *N. Engl. J. Med.* 298:763–767, 1978.

Brown, B.W., and Hollander, M. *Statistics, a biomedical introduction.* New York: John Wiley & Sons, 1977.

Cutler, S.J., and Ederer, F. Maximum utilization of the life table method in analyzing survival. *J. Chronic Dis.* 8:699–713, 1958.

Dixon, W.J., and Brown, M.B. *BMDP-77. Biomedical computer programs, P-series.* Berkeley: University of California Press, 1977.

Feigl, P. A graphical aid for determining sample size when comparing two independent proportions. *Biometrics* 34:111–122, 1978.

Freiman, J.A. et al. The importance of beta, the type II error and sample size in the design and interpretation of the randomized control trial. Survey of 71 "negative" trials. *N. Engl. J. Med.* 299:690–694, 1978.

Hull, C.H., and Nie, N.H. *Statistical package for the social sciences. SPSS update: new procedures and facilities for releases 7 and 8.* San Francisco: McGraw-Hill, 1979.

Jick, H. et al. Replacement estrogens and endometrial cancer. *N. Engl. J. Med.* 300:218–222, 1979.

Kaplan, E.L., and Meier, P. Nonparametric estimation from incomplete observations. *J. Am. Stat. Assoc.* 53:457–481, 1958.

Lamb, E.J., and Leurgans, S. Does adoption affect subsequent fertility? *Am. J. Obstet. Gynecol.* 134:138–144, 1979.

Mantel, N. Evaluation of survival data and two new rank order statistics arising in its consideration. *Cancer Chemother. Rep.* 50:163–170, 1966.

Peto, R. et al. Design and analysis of randomized clinical trials requiring prolonged observation of each patient. I. Introduction and design.
II. Analysis and examples. *Br. J. Cancer* 34:585–612, 1976; 35:1–39, 1977.

Zelen, M. A new design for randomized clinical trials. *N. Engl. J. Med.* 300:1242–1245, 1979.

PART V

CARCINOMA OF THE OVARY

Five chapters are devoted to ovarian carcinoma. This reflects increasing frustration on the part of those involved in the management of patients with this disease as little impact on survival has been achieved in the past three decades. This is true in spite of a dramatic increase in the understanding of the pathophysiology of ovarian carcinoma; an array of cytotoxic drugs which are active against this disease; sensitivity of ovarian cancer to ionizing radiation; and the recognition that an interdisciplinary approach to the management of these patients is required. Dr. Carter, in his painstaking review of the single agent and combination chemotherapy regimens that have shown activity in epithelial ovarian carcinoma, critically analyzes the data from single institution and cooperative group trials. It becomes apparent that although many drugs and combinations of drugs can cure selected patients, the criteria for their selection are difficult to analyze and even more difficult to reproduce. Although combination chemotherapy appears superior to single alkylating agents, the argument for combination therapy must be viewed in the context of palliation or cure as the goal of treatment. The role of cytoreductive operation is alluded to by both Drs. Carter and Thigpen in relation to its positive effect on subsequently administered chemotherapy. This topic is discussed in detail by Drs. Clark and Homesley, who describe the technique of exploratory laparotomy in patients with ovarian carcinoma (Dr. Clark) and critically analyze that data that suggest that reduction of tumor burden is truly meaningful (Dr. Homesley).

Dr. Kagan cautions that aggressive radiotherapy in patients with ovarian carcinoma without precise attention to staging is fraught with serious complications. In selected groups of patients, however, data are available that suggest a role for external beam therapy and the administration of intraperitoneal radioactive isotopes (Dr. Martinez).

With the advances in combination chemotherapy discussed in Chapter 11 have come an increasing number of patients in whom a complete clinical response to treatment has been achieved. Many women now are being subjected to a "second look" operation to document the pathologic completeness of this response, identify those who are cured, and withhold additional chemotherapy. Dr. Castaldo presents a critical overview of this procedure and places it in its proper historical perspective. Based on a careful review of existing literature, both he and Dr. Schwartz emphasize the role of appropriate second look operations in patients who are free of clinically measurable tumor.

A chapter on dysgerminoma (Chapter 15) is included because of the consideration of the preservation of reproductive function in young women afflicted with this disease. Dr. Krepart analyzes the experience at the M. D. Anderson Hospital and defines those criteria by which patients may be selected for conservative therapy.

Chapter 11

The Chemotherapy of Epithelial Ovarian Cancer

PERSPECTIVE:

Stephen K. Carter

Chemotherapy has several possible roles to play in epithelial ovarian cancer. These include (1) palliation of advanced or recurrent disease; (2) adjuvant use after surgery and/or radiation for early stage disease; (3) curative intent treatment as part of a multidisciplinary approach to primary advanced disease. This chapter will attempt to review the following areas: the single-agent drug data in advanced or recurrent disease; the question of whether combinations are superior to single-agent treatment in this setting; the question of drug plus radiation in the advanced setting; and the data for adjuvant use of chemotherapy in early stage and whether drugs are a viable alternative to radiation after optimal surgical therapy.

Four classes of drugs have established single-agent activity in advanced epithelial ovarian cancer. These are the alkylating agents, hexamethylmelamine, Cis-diamminedichloroplatinum (II), and Adriamycin. There is evidence for activity for 5-fluorouracil as well. In all probability methotrexate and actinomycin D, which have been included in some combination regimens, are not significantly active to the same degree based on available data.

Single-Agent Chemotherapy

Alkylating Agents

For a long period of time single-agent therapy has dominated chemotherapy literature discussing stages III and IV disease, found in many cases in patients who either failed initial radiotherapy or who were felt to be too ill or otherwise unsuitable for radiotherapy. The alkylating agents were the most commonly used drugs, especially L-phenylalanine mustard (L-PAM), cyclophosphamide, thiotepa, and chlorambucil. The historical results with the alkylating agents, summarized in table 11.1, are derived from a review by Young (1975). Recognizing heterogeneity inherent in the data, the meaningful activity of alkylating agents is still apparent. In addition, there does not appear to be any definite advantage for one alkylating agent over the other or for one type of schedule over the other. Prospective randomized studies comparing alkylating agents have not been common.

The Southwest Oncology Group (Rossof et al. 1976) did compare melphalan 6 mg/m², days 1 to 6 every 6 weeks to chlorambucil 6 mg/m² daily for 6 weeks followed by 4 mg/m² daily thereafter. The melphalan gave a low response rate of only 12.5% (3 of 24), as compared to 21.7% for chlorambucil (5 of 23). On the other hand, the median survival was 68 weeks in the melphalan group and only 38 weeks in the chlorambucil group.

The National Cancer Institute (Young et al. 1970) has reported perhaps the best response rates with single alkylating agent therapy. In one study they randomized 24 previously untreated, fully staged (III or IV) patients to receive either melphalan 0.2 mg/kg orally daily for 5 days repeated every 4 or 5 weeks or cyclophosphamide at a dose of 40 mg/kg every 12H IV twice every 3 to 4 weeks. Most of the patients had considerable tumor left behind after surgery. Nine (64%) of the 14 patients receiving melphalan responded, and 2 had a complete remission confirmed by peritoneoscopy. The median duration for all remissions was six months. Six of 10 (60%) patients treated with cyclophosphamide responded, with again 2 patients achieving a complete remission. The median duration of response was five months. The median duration of survival for all patients treated with melphalan was 14 months, as compared to 15 months for high-dose cyclophosphamide. Since the high-dose cyclophosphamide was significantly more toxic it was discarded.

Several variables have been shown to be important in terms of alkylating agent response. Prior radiotherapy tends to lower the drug response rate. Beck and Boyes (1968) reported that 75% of patients without prior radiation responded to cyclophosphamide, as compared to only 42% who had been previously irradiated. The histologic type does not appear to be important, with roughly equivalent response rates being seen for serous, mucinous or undifferentiated lesions. In Smith's (1970) large experience with L-PAM, the undifferentiated lesions did have a lower complete response rate (13%) when compared to the other types (22%). In addition, the median duration of complete response was shorter for those with undifferentiated histology (16.5 months) than for those achieving a similar response with serous (20 months) or mucinous (46.5 months) tumors.

Hreshchyshyn (1973) has reviewed retrospectively his experience with 257 patients with extrapelvic spread of ovarian cancer treated either with drug alone (150 patients) or in combination with radiation (107 patients). A good response was defined as regression of the tumor mass, 25% measurable or 50% palpable in one diameter, lasting more than 3 months, and associated with symptomatic improvement. Anything less was called some response. In this analysis only the alkylating agents showed any meaningful response

Table 11.1
Alkylating Agents in Ovarian Carcinoma
(Single-Agent Data)

Year	Drug / Reference	Schedule	No. of Patients	Overall Response Rate in %	Median Survival (Mos)			% Alive 5 Years
					All Patients	Responders	Nonresponders	
1970	L-PAM Smith and Rutledge	0.2 mg/kg/d ×5 po or IV every 3–5 weeks	494	47 (20% complete)	14	22	8	9
1968	Cyclophosphamide Beck and Boyes	50–150 mg/day po	126	49	—	20	13	—
1968	Cyclophosphamide Decker et al.	400 mg/day ×4 IV then 50–150 mg/day po	104	37	—	—	—	—
1965	Thiotepa Wallach et al.	10 mg/day ×15 IV	144	49	13	17	10	6
1965	Chlorambucil Masterson and Nelson	0.2 mg/kg/d po	280	50	—	—	—	—
1975	Chlorambucil Young	—	26	—	21	—	—	—
1970	Mechlorethamine Parker and Wilbanks	0.2 mg/kg/d ×2 IV then chlorambucil 8–14 mg/d po	81	35	10	—	—	5

rate, but they were the only drugs used as primary drug treatment. The alkylating response rates were as follows:

	Number of Patients	Good Response	Some Response	% Response
Thiotepa	92	12	21	36
Cyclophosphamide	12	2	3	42
Chlorambucil	9	1	2	33
Melphalan	4	0	2	50
Nitrogen mustard	7	1	2	42

It was found that the amount of tumor removed just prior to chemotherapy affected both response and survival. Patients with more than 75% of the tumor removed generally responded better and survived longer. A serous and poorly differentiated carcinoma was more likely to respond to drugs than a mucinous and well-differentiated tumor. The overall survival for these factors, however, was exactly opposite. Factors such as stage and previous radiation had no impact on response.

In advanced disease, there have been several studies in the last 10 to 15 years which have looked at the combination of single alkylating agent treatment with radiation. Analyzing these studies is fraught with difficulty since they vary as to stages, histologic types, histologic grades, and previous therapy.

Kottmeier (1978) has reported a study in which patients with stage III disease were prospectively randomized to total abdominal radiotherapy with or without thiotepa. The median survival for the combined modality group was 13 months, as compared to 7 months for those treated with radiation alone. At the Mayo Clinic (Decker et al. 1967) a similar study was performed, with cyclophosphamide being the drug. In this study the combined group's superiority was 14 months, as compared to 8 months for radiotherapy only. In both studies the patients failing on radiation alone received chemotherapy. Johnson and associates (1972) have compared the use of cyclophosphamide alone to the use of the same drug in conjunction with total abdominal radiotherapy. In this study, there was no statistically significant difference in median survival, which was 10.5 months for drug alone and 14 months for the combined modalities. Smith and associates (1972) from M. D. Anderson have compared the addition of radiation therapy after a melphalan induced remission to melphalan maintenance. No advantage for the radiotherapy maintenance approach could be demonstrated. The data for all of these studies would indicate that chemotherapy and radiation are roughly comparable for stage III disease and that there may be some advantage to combining the two, but, as tested so far, this advantage is not dramatic.

The Eastern Cooperative Oncology Group (Miller et al. 1965) compared 3500 rad abdominal radiotherapy midplane to chlorambucil alone (0.2 mg/kg/ daily x 8 weeks) and to the combination. All patients had previously untreated stage III disease. The clinical response rates were similar, with drug alone being 50% (9 of 18), radiation alone being 52% (9 of 17), and the combination 69% (11 of 16). Median survivals were 94.9 weeks, 33.5 weeks, and 42.2 weeks, respectively. The numbers in this study are too small to make it helpful.

Hexamethylmelamine

Hexamethylmelamine is a substituted melamine derived from cyanuric chloride. Its mechanism of action is unclear. Structurally it resembles triethylenemelamine (TEM), but unlike TEM it does not react as a classical alkylating agent. Clinically, it is not cross-resistant with alkylating agents. In early studies, the cumulative response rate for hexamethylmelamine was 39% (21 of 54) (Legha, Slavik, and Carter 1976).

The National Cancer Institute (NCI) has studied hexamethylmelamine in 21 patients with previous alkylating agent therapy (Johnson et al. 1978). Sixteen had stage III disease and five stage IV. The drug was given on two schedules. The first 18 patients received 8 mg/kg daily until dose-limiting toxicity developed. The last three patients were treated with intermittent 14-day courses at a dose of 8 mg/kg/day. Six patients (28%) showed objective tumor response with no complete responders. All responders had stage III serous cystadenocarcinoma. Only four patients had a true partial response (> 50% shrinkage). The median overall survival of all patients from start of hexamethylmelamine therapy was seven months. Ninety percent of all patients required some degree of dose modification because of toxicity, including nausea and vomiting (57%) and neurologic (28%) and bone marrow (29%) toxicity.

The M. D. Anderson group (Smith and Rutledge 1975) has looked at hexamethylmelamine alone against previously untreated (with drugs) patients in two sequential studies. In the first, the drug at a dose of 8 mg/kg/d by mouth was compared to melphalan or 5-fluorouracil. Hexamethylmelamine brought an overall response rate of 45% (10 of 22), with 70% of the responses being complete (CR). Melphalan was somewhat lower at 30% (15 of 50–11 CR) and 5-fluorouracil was the lowest at 16% (4 of 24), although all the responses were complete. In a second study (McGuire and Young 1978) hexamethylmelamine and melphalan at identical doses were compared again, with a third arm being Adriamycin alone (60 mg/m^2 every 3 weeks) and fourth arm being hexamethylmelamine 4 mg/kg/d × 14 combined with cyclophosphamide 250 mg/m^2/d × 5 every 4 weeks. The results of this study were as follows:

1. Hexamethylmelamine   7 of 33 (22%) with 1 CR
2. Melphalan   10 of 33 (30%) with 4 CR
3. Adriamycin   10 of 34 (29%) with 4 CR
4. Combination   17 of 32 (53%) with 10 CR

When the two protocols are combined, the cumulative response rate for hexamethylmelamine is 17 of 55 with 8 complete responses, as compared to 25 of

83 with 15 for melphalan. The two drugs would seem to be roughly comparable. The reason why the CR rates fell in the second study is that second look surgery was used to document a complete response in the latter study.

The current dosage of hexamethylmelamine recommended by the NCI in its guidelines for clinical use is 8 mg/kg/day (300 mg/m^2) x 90 or indefinitely if tolerated. The total dose is usually divided into four equal parts and given after meals and at bedtime. Antiemetics may be of help in reducing gastric upset. The major toxicities with the drug are gastrointestinal, hematologic, and neurologic. Anorexia, nausea, and vomiting, occasionally accompanied by abdominal cramps and diarrhea, have been reported in 50% to 70% of those treated. Patients do appear to develop some tolerance to these effects after they have received the drug for about three weeks. A moderate degree of myelosuppression occurs in 20% to 40%. About 5% to 10% of patients will have white cell counts reduced to around 2000/mm^3. Thrombocytopenia is usually less pronounced. Neurologic toxicity is less frequent and involves either parasthesias and numbness or a central effect expressed as sleep disturbance, hallucinations, and depression.

Cis-diamminedichloroplatinum (II)

Cis-diamminedichloroplatinum has shown activity as both a single agent and as a part of combination regimens. Wiltshaw and Kroner (1976) at the Royal Marsden Hospital have studied platinum as a single agent on two dosage schedules. An initial study used a low dose of 30 to 50 mg/m^2 every 3 to 4 weeks. In 52 patients the complete response rate was 15.4%, with an overall response rate of 31%. A second study administered a high dose to 29 patients of 100 mg/m^2 every four weeks with hydration and mannitol diuresis. Thirty-one percent achieved a complete response, with 52% responding overall. Bruckner and associates (1978a, 1978b) from Mt. Sinai Hospital in New York, treated 19 patients with 50 mg/m^2 as an intravenous bolus injection every 3 weeks. In this study, six patients objectively responded. Piver and associates (1978) saw only one complete remission in 20 extensively pre-treated patients who received 50 to 100 mg/m^2.

Bruckner and associates compared platinum alone to platinum plus Adriamycin or thiotepa plus methotrexate. All patients were previously untreated. The single-agent response rate was 41%, with 18% being complete. There were 6 complete remissions (33%) and an overall response rate of 67% to platinum plus Adriamycin. The alkylating agent with methotrexate resulted in a 12% complete remission and overall a 35% response rate. The platinum combination had the best survival, with 50% still alive 18 months after beginning therapy. In previously treated patients the response rate to platinum and Adriamycin was lower. The response rate was only 38% in 20 such patients reported by Briscoe and associates (1978).

The official recommended dose level for cis-platinum as a single agent is 50 mg/m^2 once every three weeks. Higher doses can be given, with pretreatment hydration being used to prevent renal toxicity. Dose-related and cumulative renal insufficiency are the major dose-limiting factors. After a first single dose of 50 mg/m², this will occur in nearly one-fourth of the cases but will be reversible. It will be first noted during the second week after drug administration and will be manifested by an elevated blood urea nitrogen and creatinine, hyperuricemia, and/or a decreased creatinine clearance. The renal toxicity becomes more prolonged and severe with repeated courses of drug.

Adriamycin

Adriamycin is an anthracycline antitumor antibiotic and has a wide spectrum of activity against both solid tumors and hematologic malignancies (Carter 1975). It has been shown to inhibit DNA-dependent RNA synthesis as a result of its intercalation between the base pairs of DNA, but whether this totally explains its antitumor effect is now a subject of controversy. In earlier studies, when used against predominantly previously treated cases, the drug gave a 38% response rate in 48 cases. In the M. D. Anderson study, discussed earlier in the hexamethylmelamine section, it gave activity in previously untreated cases equivalent to that observed with melphalan and hexamethylmelamine.

Combination Chemotherapy

With at least four drug classes showing meaningful activity, it would seem that ovarian cancer should respond to successful combination regimens. The success of a combination would be manifest initially as a higher complete response rate and ultimately as increased disease-free and overall survival. The literature now contains six studies of combinations compared to melphalan or cyclophosphamide (table 11.2). In only one of these is a superiority for the combination established. It is interesting to note that in five studies using melphalan as the control, the response rates have ranged from 11% to 54%. The response rate of 54% with melphalan in the National Cancer Institute series is higher than the response rates reported for all the other combinations reported except their own. This is indicative of heterogeneity of the chemotherapy data in this disease.

The ACTFUCY regimen had shown a response rate of 38%, with 9% being complete, in patients failing on melphalan (Smith, Rutledge, and Wharton 1972). In previously untreated patients, however, it could not be demonstrated to be superior to the alkylating agent in efficacy, and in terms of toxicity it was inferior. In the Eastern Cooperative Group also the combination used could not be shown to be superior overall, with toxicity again being more severe with multiple drugs (Bruckner et al. 1978). Both of these studies compared melphalan to combinations in which the dose of an alter-

Table 11.2
Combination Chemotherapy vs Single-Agent
Trials in Ovarian Cancer

Reference	Group	Regimens	Number Evaluation	Number Response	% Response
Smith, Rutledge, and Wharton 1972	M. D. Anderson	ACTFUCY actinomycin D 5-fluorouracil cyclophosphamide vs	47	21	45
		melphalan	50	21	42
McGuire and Young 1978	Eastern Cooperative Oncology Group	CMF cyclophosphamide methotrexate 5-fluorouracil vs	53	20	38
		melphalan	50	14	28
Young et al. 1978	National Cancer Institute	hexaCAF hexamethylmelamine cyclophosphamide methotrexate 5-fluorouracil vs	45	30	75 (33% CR*)
		melphalan	37	20	54 (16% CR*)
Edmonson et al. 1979	Mayo Clinic	cyclophosphamide Adriamycin vs	36	13	45
		cyclophosphamide	35	11	32
Ehrlich et al. 1979	Eastern Cooperative Oncology Group	thiotepa methotrexate vs	72	11	15
		CAF cyclophosphamide Adriamycin 5-fluorouracil vs	71	21	30
		TSPA-MTX alternating with CAF vs	62	13	21
		melphalan	70	8	11
	NCI, Canada	HDMTX-CF 5-fluorouracil melphalan vs	53	25	47
		melphalan→ 5-fluorouracil→ HDMTX	50	30	60

*CR = complete response.

nate alkylating agent had to be lowered to accommodate other myelo-suppressive drugs with much lower single-agent response rates.

The hexaCAF regimen of the National Cancer Institute (Young et al. 1978) appears to be the first combination demonstrating some superiority to melphalan in a controlled fashion. The hexaCAF regimen resulted in 30 of 45 (75%) patients responding, with 13 (33%) achieving complete response. In comparison, the melphalan gave a 54% response rate, with responses being observed in 20 of 37 and 6 (16%) achieving complete status. The median duration of complete remission for the six in the melphalan group was 25 months while in the hexaCAF group the median has not been reached, inasmuch as only 4 of 13 have relapsed. The median will exceed 30 months, however. The overall median survival of the hexaCAF group was 29 months, as compared to 17 months for the patients receiving the single alkylating agent. Thirty percent of patients treated with hexaCAF remain alive more than three years after initial therapy. With either treatment arm, patients documented to have complete remission by restaging procedures had a median survival in excess of three years. The median survival was 16 months for those with partial remission and only 7 months for those with no objective response.

The toxicity of the hexaCAF was more formidable than it was with melphalan. Twenty-eight percent of patients treated with the combination experienced severe myeolosuppression (WBC < 1200 or platelets < 50,000), as compared to 13% with melphalan. Other toxicities more common with the combination included nausea and vomiting (68%), alopecia (50%), and mucositis (15%).

An important observation in this study is that patients with minimal residual disease (< 2 cm) had a response rate of 85%, while it was 53% with larger amounts of residual disease ($P < 0.05$). This would be a response equivalent to what could be achieved with radiation. For eight patients with < 2 cm residual disease treated with hexaCAF, the complete remission rate was 100%.

The Mayo Clinic (Edmonson et al. 1979) executed a controlled comparison of cyclophosphamide alone at a dose 1 gm/m^2 or in combination with Adriamycin (40 mg/m^2) at a dose of 500 mg/m^2 every 3 to 4 weeks. At the time of progressive disease the two regimens were crossed over. Eighty-two patients with stage III$_b$ and IV advanced disease were entered, and 71 were evaluable. With cyclophosphamide alone 11 of 35 responded, as compared to 13 of 36 with the combination. As cross-over the single agent gave 2 of 20 responses while the combination gave only 1 of 21 responses. Time to progression curves were nearly identical for the two primary treatment regimens. Similarly, survival curves for the two treatments were also nearly identical, with the median being 12 months for both.

The same randomization was also made for patients with minimal residual disease staged as either FIGO II or III. This group had surgical excision of all tumors greater than 2 cm in diameter at the time of surgery and had no residual disease greater than 2 cm. In this group the median survival was approximately 21 months. Both the time to progression and survival curves favor the combination but do not reach the traditional P-value of less than 0.05.

The discovery of the significant activity with cis-platinum has lead to a range of new combinations with exciting induction rates (table 11.3). All of these combinations combine platinum with Adriamycin alone or with the addition of hexamethylmelamine, cyclophosphamide, and 5-fluorouracil. For the first time high response rates are being reported in patients failing on alkylating agent therapy. The controlled studies do not exist to establish clearly the superiority of these regimens over single-agent therapy. The oncologic community appears so convinced at this time by these high response rates that such studies may well not be undertaken.

Ehrlich et al. (1979) has studied a three-drug combination of platinum, Adriamycin, and cyclophosphamide (PAC) in 39 women previously untreated with chemotherapy. In 35 evaluable cases the complete response rate was 37% and the partial response rate was 31.5%. The interval to response was 4 to 12 weeks. In women with postoperative tumors less than 3 cm, 46% achieved a complete response and 5 of these had their complete response documented by a second look laparotomy. This treatment was toxic, with 3 treatment-related deaths. Two were due to sepsis and one to a pulmonary embolus.

Vogl and associates (1979) have reported on a four-drug regimen called CHAD. This regimen consists of cyclophosphamide 600 mg/m^2, Adriamycin 25 mg/m^2, and platinum 50 mg/m^2, all given on day 1. In addition, hexamethylmelamine is given on days 8 to 22 at a dose of 150 mg/m^2. The cycle is repeated on day 29. Thirty patients, without prior chemotherapy or whole abdominal irradiation, were treated with CHAD. Of 21 evaluable for response, 20 responded, 10 of whom were clinically complete. At this point in time it is too early to speak about duration and survival. The regimen was well tolerated.

Chemotherapy and/or Radiation after Surgery for Stage I–III Disease

An area for continued investigation is combined drug and x-ray for early stage disease. Smith, in 1970, in a study discussed earlier for stage III disease, also reported on the same approach for stages I and II disease. The comparison was surgery and additional radiotherapy versus additional single-agent melphalan. The patients all had complete surgical resection or debulking such that no patient had residual disease greater than 2 cm. Patients were stratified according to age and histologic type but not histologic grade or stage. The radiation consisted of abdominal strip at a dose of 2600 to 2800 rad midplane and a pelvic boost of 2000 rad midpelvis. In stage I pa-

Table 11.3 Some Recent Combinations Involving Cis-platinum

Reference	No. of Patients Evaluated	Prior Chemotherapy	No. Complete Response	No. Partial Response	% Response	Regimen
Einhorn Ehrlich et al. 1979	35	no	37%	31.5%	68.5%	PAC platinum Adriamycin cyclophosphamide
Southwest Oncology Group	29	yes (alkylating agent only)	2	12	48	platinum Adriamycin HXM 5-FU
Alberts et al. 1979	74	yes (alkylating agent + Adriamycin)	0	23	31	platinum HXM 5-FU
Central Pennsylvania Oncology Group Kane et al. 1979	35	yes	7 (20%)	10	49	CHAP cyclophosphamide HXM Adriamycin platinum
Eastern Cooperative Oncology Group	22	yes	4	10	63	HAD HXM Adriamycin platinum
Vogl et al. 1979	21	no	10 (47.6%)	9	90	CHAD cyclophosphamide HXM Adriamycin platinum
Mt. Sinai Hospital (NYC) Bruckner et al. 1978	30	no	11	13	80	Adriamycin + platinum
CALGB Briscoe et al. 1978	24	yes	4	5	38	Adriamycin + platinum

tients, the long-term disease-free survival was 90% in 28 patients treated with melphalan, as compared to 85% in 14 patients irradiated. In stage II, drug gave 58% ($n = 29$) while irradiation gave 55% ($n = 37$). There were no statistically significant differences in these data. Berkson-Gage projections of five-year survivals show a trend in favor of radiotherapy in stage I and drug in stage II.

The Gynecologic Oncology Group (Hreschchyshyn 1976) has reported results of a study in stage I disease in which surgery patients were randomized either to observation, pelvic irradiation (5000 rad midpelvis), or melphalan 0.2 mg/kg/daily × 5 every 4 weeks × 18 cycles. The recurrence rate so far is 17% (5 of 29) with observation, 36% (8 of 22) with x-ray, and 10% (3 of 30) with drug. The smaller number of patients in the radiotherapy arm is due to the high numbers of protocol deviations requiring exclusion from the study.

The Princess Margaret trial (Dembo et al. 1979) (table 11.4) indicates the superiority of total abdominal irradiation over pelvic radiation alone or

Table 11.4
Princess Margaret Hospital Ovarian
Cancer Study

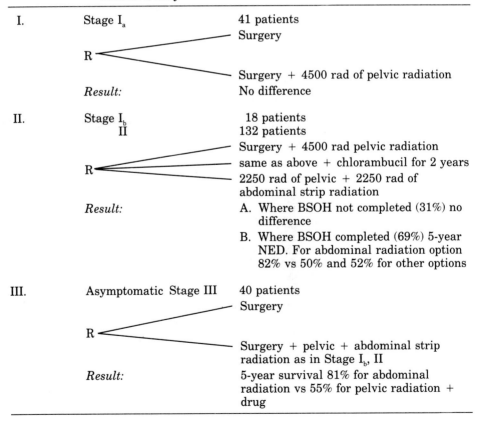

I.	Stage I$_a$	41 patients
		Surgery
	R	
		Surgery + 4500 rad of pelvic radiation
	Result:	No difference
II.	Stage I$_b$ II	18 patients 132 patients
		Surgery + 4500 rad pelvic radiation
	R	same as above + chlorambucil for 2 years
		2250 rad of pelvic + 2250 rad of abdominal strip radiation
	Result:	A. Where BSOH not completed (31%) no difference
		B. Where BSOH completed (69%) 5-year NED. For abdominal radiation option 82% vs 50% and 52% for other options
III.	Asymptomatic Stage III	40 patients
		Surgery
	R	
		Surgery + pelvic + abdominal strip radiation as in Stage I$_b$, II
	Result:	5-year survival 81% for abdominal radiation vs 55% for pelvic radiation + drug

combined with chlorambucil for patients with stage I_b, II, and asymptomatic III disease. This superiority only exists when the hysterectomy and bilaterial salpingo-oophorectomy (BSOH) could be completed. The relapse patterns show that the total abdominal radiation prevents abdominal recurrence outside of the pelvis, which the adjuvant chlorambucil, as given, could not accomplish. This study indicates that the ability to complete BSOH is a much more potent prognostic variable than stage within the range of stage I_b to III disease. It is clear that pelvic radiation alone is no longer adequate treatment for these stages and that newer approaches with extended irradiation and/or drugs are needed.

Currently, the National Cancer Institute (table 11.5) and the European Organization for Research on the Treatment of Cancer (EORTC) (table 11.6) are sponsoring controlled trials for early stage ovarian cancer testing the value of adjuvant melphalan after surgery and/or radiation.

Chemoimmunotherapy

The Southwest Oncology Group (Alberts et al. 1979a, 1979b) is studying the role of chemoimmunotherapy in the treatment of advanced ovarian carcinoma. The chemotherapy chosen is the combination called ACe, which consists of Adriamycin 40 mg/m² on day 1, followed by cyclophosphamide 200 mg/m²/d on days 3 to 6. The courses of ACe are repeated every 3 to 4 weeks. In a pilot study at the University of Arizona this combination was reported to achieve a 61% response rate. The immunotherapy chosen was BCG from the Pasteur Institute 6×10^8 viable organisms given by scarification on days 8 and 15 of each ACe course. The study involves a randomization of stage III or IV cases, without prior exposure to cytotoxic drugs, to chemo-

Table 11.5
National Cancer Institute Sponsored Trials
for Ovarian Cancer

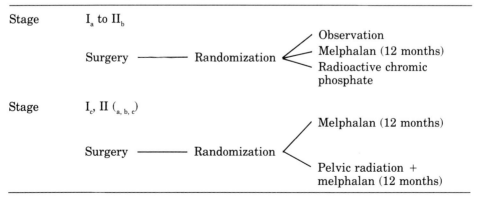

Table 11.6
EORTC Sponsored Protocols for Ovarian
Cancer

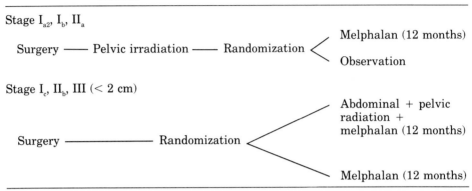

Stage I_{a2}, I_b, II_a

Surgery —— Pelvic irradiation —— Randomization — Melphalan (12 months) / Observation

Stage I_c, II_b, III (< 2 cm)

Surgery ———————— Randomization — Abdominal + pelvic radiation + melphalan (12 months) / Melphalan (12 months)

therapy alone, or to chemoimmunotherapy. The ACe regimen alone in 61 evaluable cases has resulted in only 1 complete response and 21 partial responses for a 36% overall response rate. The complete response is low because of the requirement of second look confirmation before this status is recorded. The chemoimmunotherapy in 57 cases has achieved 7 complete responses and 23 partial responses, for an overall response rate of 52.7%. If improvements are added the total benefit rate is 52.4% for ACe and 59.7% for ACe plus BCG. The median duration of response is 9.5 months for drug plus BCG versus 7.0 months for drug alone. The median survival fror the start of chemotherapy is 23.5 months for the ACe plus BCG, as compared to 13.5 months for ACe by itself. After 36 months, 33 (54%) of the patients treated with drug alone and only 22 (39%) of those given drug plus BCG have died. At this preliminary point in time chemoimmunotherapy does not appear to increase response or duration meaningfully but does appear to influence survival. Further follow-up and analysis will be required to determine the meaning of this result.

Conclusion

The chemotherapy literature for epithelian ovarian cancer has become massive, and interpretation is fraught with great difficulty. Wide extremes in complete and overall response rates with both single agents and combination regimens can be observed. These differences are due to variabilities in patient selection factors, aggressiveness of therapy, response criteria, and data analysis techniques which are nearly impossible to delineate fully from the existing literature. Despite these problems of analysis some conclusions can be drawn from the existing data base.

The first is that combination chemotherapy with the existing active drugs will almost surely be superior to the use of sequential single agents. With the exception of the hexaCAF study from the National Cancer Institute all prospectively randomized studies of combinations versus single alkylating agent therapy have failed to demonstrate an advantage for the aggressive approach. Few of these, however, have used the newer combinations with platinum and Adriamycin as their core. The data for these platinum-anthracycline combinations are so impressive that it is hard to conceive that they will not be superior in initial inducing ability to studied single-agent treatment. What needs to be emphasized, however, is that if palliation is the goal of therapy then the critical analysis concerns overall survival and its quality. Using these criteria the arguments for combinations may be less persuasive. The critical element to study will be the achievement of pathologic complete response, since this has always been the benchmark of a true progress with cancer chemotherapy as ultimately reflected in meaningful survival gain. Future therapy for advanced stage ovarian cancer may well be a combination of drug, surgery, and x-ray with curative intent. Within this framework the achievement of a high initial induction with combination chemotherapy will be highly important.

The existing data show that useful response to any chemotherapy is dramatically reduced if patients have failed previous irradiation or drug treatment. This is a major prognostic variable which must be taken into account in making comparative analysis of the worth of various regimens. Studies including both untreated and previously treated patients are virtually uninterpretable. There is now convincing evidence that chemotherapy is more successful when minimal residual disease is present. The data from the National Cancer Institute with hexaCAF and from the Mayo Clinic with Adriamycin plus cytoxan are particularly persuasive in this regard. This opens up the potential of combining chemotherapy with reductive surgery in advanced disease. If surgery can leave a minimal residual disease situation, then the potential for drugs to achieve a complete remission is dramatically enhanced.

There appears to be a substantial difference between the survival impact of a pathologically documented complete response and a clinical complete response. Studies using the former will report lower complete response rates than studies using the clinical criteria only. In the future, pathologic complete response will become increasingly important, and should be kept in mind today in making comparative analysis. Recently a new format for response criteria reporting in ovarian cancer has been proposed by Wharton of M. D. Anderson and published by Young of the National Cancer Institute (1979) (table 11.7). Such an approach, if widely accepted, would be extremely helpful in achieving comparability in the literature.

267

Table 11.7
Ovarian Carcinoma Response Criteria

Response Status	Definition
I. Complete	
1. Clinical	Complete regression of all evaluable tumor for 1 month
2. Surgical	No clinically recognizable tumor at restaging
A. Laparoscopy	
L (−)	Biopsies and washings negative for tumor
L (+)	Biopsies and/or washings microscopically positive for tumor
B. Laparotomy	
S (−)	Biopsies and washings negative for tumor
S (+)	Biopsies and/or washings microscopically positive for tumor
II. Partial	
1. Clinical	50% reduction in sum of the cross-sectioned diameters of the largest tumor lasting for 2 months
2. Surgical	50% reduction in sum of the cross-sectioned diameters at second look at tumor reduction surgery

It should be remembered that response rate alone is not adequate to evaluate fully the value of a drug regimen. It is only an initial evaluation. More important in the long run will be median duration of remission and survival data with a regimen. One should avoid the premature assumption that a particular regimen with a high clinical response rate will ultimately be better than one with a lower response rate confirmed by surgical restaging, one for which survival information is already available.

The question of chemotherapy versus total abdominal irradiation after surgery for stage I to III disease is a difficult one. Two prospectively randomized series fail to give a clear answer to the question. The M. D. Anderson series comparing melphalan to total abdominal irradiation shows no difference in five-year overall survival rate for patients with stage I to III disease. The toxicities, while different, appear to be comparable. The Princess Margaret Hospital study indicates that, in a carefully selected subset of patients with stage I_b, II, and asymptomatic III disease, a uniquely designed radiation approach was more successful than either pelvic irradiation alone or pelvic irradiation with chlorambucil. This approach of 2250 rad total abdominal irradiation, without shielding the liver and the superior parts extending above the dome of the diaphragm, has significantly reduced the frequency of abdominal relapse. It must be emphasized that this can be said only for patients with minimal residual disease.

The Gynecologic Oncology Group study for stage I_a and I_b has shown that surgery plus melphalan has a lower relapse rate (2 of 30) than does pelvic irradiation (8 of 22) or no further treatment (5 of 24). It is clear that pelvic irradiation is inadequate, but the question of total abdominal irradiation versus drug is still open. The future, however, will most likely see some combination of both modalities to achieve a result superior to any that either could accomplish alone.

References

Alberts, D.S. et al. Combination chemotherapy for alkylator-resistant ovarian carcinoma: a preliminary report of a Southwest Oncology Group trial. *Cancer Treat. Rep.* 63:301–305, 1979a.

Alberts, D.S. et al. Randomized study of chemoimmunotherapy for advanced ovarian carcinoma: a preliminary report of a Southwest Oncology Group study. *Cancer Treat. Rep.* 63:325–331, 1979b.

Beck, R.E. and Boyes, D.A. Treatment of 126 cases of advanced ovarian cancer with cyclophosphamide. *Cancer Med. Assoc. J.* 98:539–541, 1968.

Briscoe, K. et al. Cisdiamminedichloroplatinum (II) and Adriamycin treatment of advanced ovarian cancer. *Proc. AACR-ASCO* 19:378, 1978.

Bruckner, H.W. et al. Treatment of advanced ovarian cancer with cis-dichlorodiammineplatinum (II); poor-risk patients with intensive prior therapy. *Cancer Treat. Rep.* 62:555–558, 1978a.

Bruckner, H.W. et al. Cis-platinum for combination chemotherapy of ovarian cancer: improved response rates and survival. *Proc. AACR-ASCO* 19:373, 1978b.

Carter, S.K. Adriamycin—a review. *J Natl. Cancer. Inst.* 55:1265–1274, 1975.

Decker, D.G. et al. Adjuvant therapy for advanced ovarian malignancy. *Am. J. Obstet. Gynecol* 97:171–180, 1967.

Decker, D.G. et al. Cyclophosphamide in the treatment of ovarian cancer. *Clin. Obstet. Gynecol.* 11:382–400, 1968.

Dembo, A.J. et al. The Princess Margaret Hospital study of ovarian cancer: stages I, II and asymptomatic III presentations. *Cancer Treat. Rep.* 63:249–254, 1979.

Edmonson, J.H. et al. Different chemotherapeutic sensitivities and host factors affecting prognosis in advanced ovarian carcinoma versus minimal residual disease. *Cancer Treat. Rep.* 63:241–247, 1979.

Ehrlich, C.E. et al. Chemotherapy for stage II–IV epithelial ovarian cancer with cis-dichlorodiammineplatinum (II), Adriamycin, and cyclophosphamide: a preliminary report. *Cancer Treat. Rep.* 63:261–288, 1979.

Hreshchyshyn, M.M. Single drug therapy in ovarian cancer. *Gynecol. Oncol.* 1:220–232, 1973.

Hreshchyshyn, M.M. Results of the gynecologiconcology group trials on ovarian cancer: preliminary report. *Natl. Cancer Inst. Monogr.* 42:155–165, 1976.

Johnson, B.L. et al. Hexamethylmelamine in alkylating agent resistant ovarian carcinoma. *Cancer* 42:2157–2161, 1978.

Johnson, E.C. et al. Advanced ovarian cancer: therapy with radiation and cyclophosphamide in a random series. *Am. J. Roentgenol.* 114:136–141, 1972.

Kane, R. et al. Phase II trial of cyclophosphamide, hexamethylmelamine, Adriamycin and cis-dichlorodiammineplatinum (II) combination chemotherapy in advanced ovarian cancer. *Cancer Treat. Rep.* 63:307–309, 1979.

Kottmeier, H.L. Treatment of ovarian cancer with thio-tepa. *Clin. Obstet. Gynecol.* 11:428–438, 1978.

Legha, S.S.; Slavik, M; and Carter, S.K. Hexamethylmelamine. An evaluation of its role in the therapy of cancer. *Cancer* 38:27–35, 1976.

Masterson, J.G., and Nelson, J.H. The role of chemotherapy in the treatment of gynecologic malignancy. *Am. J. Obstet. Gynecol.* 93:1102–1111, 1965.

McGuire, W.P., and Young R.C. Ovarian cancer. In *Randomized trials in cancer: a critical review by sites,* ed. M.J. Staquet. New York: Raven Press, 1978.

Miller, S.P. et al. Comparative evaluation of combined radiation, chlorambucil treatment of ovarian cancer. *Cancer* 36:1625–1630, 1965.

Parker, R.T; Parker C.H; and Wilbanks, G.D. Cancer of the ovary: survival studies based upon operative therapy, chemotherapy and radiotherapy. *Am. J. Obstet. Gynecol.* 108:878–888, 1970.

Piver, M.S. et al. Cis-dichlorodiammineplatinum (II) as third-line chemotherapy in advanced ovarian adenocarcinoma. *Cancer Treat. Rep.* 62:559–560, 1978.

Rossof, A.H. et al. Randomized evaluation of chlorambucil and melphalan in advanced ovarian cancer. *Proc. AACR-ASCO* 17:300, 1976.

Smith, J.P., and Rutledge, F. Chemotherapy in the treatment of cancer of the ovary. *Am. J. Obstet. Gynecol.* 107:691–703, 1970.

Smith, J.P., and Rutledge, F. Random study of hexamethylmelamine, 5-fluorouracil and melphalan in treatment of advanced carcinoma of the ovary. *Natl. Cancer. Inst. Monogr.* 42:169–172, 1975.

Smith, J.P; Rutledge, F; and Wharton, J.T. Chemotherapy of ovarian cancer. New approach to treatment. *Cancer* 30:1565–1571, 1972.

Vogl, S.E. et al. The CHAD and HAD regimens in advanced ovarian cancer: combination chemotherapy including cyclophosphamide, hexamethylmelamine, Adriamycin and cis-dichlorodiammineplatinum (II). *Cancer Treat. Rep.* 63:311–317, 1979.

Wallach, R.C. et al. Thio-tepa chemotherapy for ovarian carcinoma influence of remission and toxicity on survival. *Obstet. Gynecol.* 25:475–478, 1965.

Wiltshaw, E., and Kroner, T. Phase II study of cis-dichlorodiammineplatinum (II) (NSC–119875) in advanced adenocarcinoma of the ovary. *Cancer Treat. Rep.* 60:55–60, 1976.

Young, R.C. Chemotherapy of ovarian cancer: past and present. *Semin. Oncol.* 2:267–276, 1975.

Young, R.C. Ovarian carcinoma: an optimistic epilogue. *Cancer Treat. Rep.* 63:333–337, 1979.

Young, R.C. et al. Chemotherapy of advanced ovarian carcinoma: a prospective randomized comparison of phenylalanine mustard and high dose cyclophosphamide. *Gynecol. Oncol.* 2:489–497, 1974.

Young, R.C. et al. Advanced ovarian adenocarcinoma—a prospective clinical trial of melphalan (L-PAM) versus combination chemotherapy. *N. Engl. J. Med.* 299:1261–1266, 1978.

PERSPECTIVE:

The Chemotherapy of Epithelial Ovarian Cancer

Tate Thigpen

Cancer of the ovary is the leading cause of death among gynecologic malignancies and the fourth most common cause of cancer death in women. These neoplasms accounted for 17,000 new cases of cancer and 10,800 deaths in 1977 (Seidman, Silverberg, and Holleb 1976). In comparison with other gynecologic malignancies, a greater percentage of ovarian cancers, in fact 60% to 70%, present with advanced disease because the tumor remains asymptomatic until it becomes quite large (Day and Smith 1975). This tendency accounts for the higher frequency of death among these patients as compared to patients with other gynecologic cancers and explains the greater interest in the use of chemotherapy to treat ovarian cancer.

Studies of the use of chemotherapy in the treatment of ovarian cancer have concerned for the most part epithelial neoplasms of the ovary since these tumors account for 80% to 90% of ovarian cancer (Barber and Kwon 1976). In regard to these ovarian adenocarcinomas, information from clinical research deals with five important aspects: (1) the importance of proper evaluation of the patient; (2) the activity of single agents in treating advanced disease; (3) combination therapy in the management of advanced disease; (4) treatment of advanced disease after optimal cytoreduction; and (5) possible roles of adjuvant therapy in early ovarian adenocarcinoma. This discussion will center on these five aspects of the management of adenocarcinomas of the ovary.

Evaluation of the Patient with Ovarian Adenocarcinoma

Proper assessment of patient characteristics influencing prognosis is essential to proper therapeutic decision making and necessary if studies of therapeutic alternatives are to be meaningful. From recent studies, the degree of histologic differentiation (Malkasian, Decker, and Webb 1975; Decker, Malkasian, and Taylor 1975; Ozols et al. 1979) and the extent of disease (Griffiths 1975; Brady et al. 1979; Young et al. 1978) would appear to be the two most important patient characteristics in the determination of prognosis and response to therapy. Other patient characteristics such as age and pattern of histology have not been shown definitely to relate to patient prognosis.

With regard to histologic grade or degree of differentiation, two different grading systems are employed by various centers: Broders' system (1926) designates grade by the percentage of undifferentiated cells present as grade 1 (0% to 25%) through grade 4 (75% to 100%), while a pattern grading system defines well-differentiated, moderately well-differentiated, and poorly differentiated neoplasms. In each case, survival, stage by stage, can be shown to correlate with the histologic grade; the more undifferentiated the tumor, the worse the survival. Furthermore, as will be discussed later, grade might provide a clue as to the type of chemotherapy needed in advanced cases (Young et al. 1978).

In the case of extent of disease, the FIGO staging classification (Day and Smith 1975) expresses those factors in regard to extent of disease that most influence prognosis (table 11.8) and the expected five-year survival for each subset (table 11.9) (Tobias and Griffiths 1976). In recent literature, two modifications of this system have been suggested. The first proposes that stage I_a and I_b lesions should be subdivided into those lesions with an intact capsule and no tumor on the external surface (intracystic lesions, subset i) and those lesions with capsular rupture and/or tumor present on the external surface (extracystic lesions, subset ii). Support for this modification is found in a study of stage I grade 1 ovarian carcinomas in which patients with intracystic lesions had a 90% five-year survival as opposed to 68% for extracystic lesions and 56% for patients with ruptured cysts (Webb, Decker, and Mussey 1973). The second modification proposes that patients with stage III disease be divided into an optimal group, in whom adequate cytoreductive surgery can be carried out, and a suboptimal group, in whom a significant bulk of disease remains after surgery. The definition of adequate bulk reduction has varied from study to study (Brady et al. 1979; Young et al. 1978; Griffiths, Parker, and Fuller 1979; Edmonson et al. 1979); minimal residual or optimal disease has been defined as patients with no remaining nodules greater than 1.5 cm, 2 cm, or 3 cm in diameter. Regardless of definition, survival and response to chemotherapy of optimal patients in each study was superior to that of suboptimal patients with bulky disease present after surgery.

The specific characteristics of stage and grade thus must be identified and considered in any comparative study of therapeutic alternatives before study results can be considered meaningful. Furthermore, these characteristics have specific implications with regard to the therapeutic decisions which will be discussed.

Table 11.8
International Federation of Gynecology and
Obstetrics (FIGO) Staging Classification for
Epithelial Ovarian Cancer with Modifications

Stage	Description
I	Growth limited to ovaries
a	Growth limited to one ovary; no ascites
i	No tumor or external surface; capsule intact
ii	Tumor on external surface or capsule ruptured or both
b	Growth limited to both ovaries; no ascites
i	No tumor on external surface; capsule intact
ii	Tumor on external surface or capsule ruptured or both
c	Tumor stage I_a or I_b plus ascites or malignant cells in peritoneal washings
II	Growth involving one or both ovaries with pelvic extensions
a	Extension or metastases or both to uterus or tubes or both
b	Extension to other pelvic tissues
c	Tumor stages II_a or II_b plus ascites or malignant cells in peritoneal washings
III	Growth involving one or both ovaries with intraperitoneal metastases outside pelvis or positive retroperitoneal nodes or both
Optimal	All remaining nodules ≤ 3.0 centimeters in diameter
Suboptimal	All remaining nodules > 3.0 centimeters in diameter
IV	Distant metastases
	Pleural effusion must contain malignant cells.
	Parenchymal liver metastases indicate stage IV

Management of Advanced Ovarian Adenocarcinoma

Single Agent Chemotherapy

A majority of the literature on chemotherapy of ovarian carcinoma concerns the use of single agents to treat advanced disease. The most commonly used agents are alkylating agents. Collected data from multiple studies (DeVita et al. 1976; Young 1975) reveal five such agents used in a sufficient number of patients to evaluate activity (table 11.10). All five drugs appear to be active, with a 50% or greater reduction in disease volume in 35% to 64% of patients. Certain other agents have also been evaluated in an adequate number of patients to determine activity (table 11.11) (DeVita et al. 1976; Young

Table 11.9
Expected Five-Year Survival by FIGO Stage

Stage	5-Year Survival (%)
I	61
a	62
b	59
c	53
II	39
a	62
b	39
III	7
IV	0

1975; Baker, Izbicki, and Vaitkevicius 1976; Baker, Samson, and Izbicki 1976; Falkson and Falkson 1976). These data suggest that, in addition to alkylating agents, 5-fluorouracil, methotrexate, hexamethylmelamine, Adriamycin, porfiromycin, and mitomycin-C are also active in the treatment of advanced ovarian adenocarcinoma.

More recently, an orderly approach to the evaluation of new drugs as single agents in the treatment of advanced ovarian adenocarcinoma no longer responsive to first-line chemotherapy has been undertaken by the Gynecologic Oncology Group in an effort to identify still other active drugs (table 11.12) (Omura et al. 1977; Thigpen, Dolan, and Morrison 1978; Thigpen, Lagasse, and Bundy 1979; Slayton, Petty, and Blessing 1979; Lewis 1979). To date, five agents have been evaluated, with one, cis-platinum, showing significant activity at a dose of 50 mg per meter square intravenously every three weeks (Thigpen 1979). The results with cis-platinum corroborate ear-

Table 11.10
Results from Multiple Trials of Use of
Alkylating Agents Alone in the Treatment of
Advanced Ovarian Adenocarcinoma

Agent	Number of Patients	Response (%)
Melphalan	494	47
Chlorambucil	280	50
Thiotepa	144	64
Cyclophosphamide	126	49
Mechlorethamine	81	35

Table 11.11
Results from Multiple Trials of the Use of
Nonalkylating Agents in the Treatment of
Advanced Ovarian Adenocarcinoma

Drug	Number of Patients	Response (%)
5-FU	81	32
Methotrexate	16	25
Hexamethylmelamine	53	41
Adriamycin	33	36
Porfiromycin	12	42
Mitomycin-C	11	27
Progestins	50	10
6-MP	19	5
Vincristine	17	0
Vinblastine	16	13
Cytembena	19	0

lier reports of response rates of 26% (Wiltshaw and Kroner 1976) and 32% (Bruckner et al. 1978) with the same or higher doses of the drug. Similarly, the negative result with VP-16 agrees with an earlier report of no responses in 14 patients with the agent (Edmonson et al. 1978). Continuation of these single-agent trials of new drugs will hopefully add to the present therapeutic armamentarium with current trials of maytansine, Baker's Antifol, ICRF-159, AMSA, and Yoshi 864 (Lewis 1979).

Alkylating agents, among these various active drugs, have generally been accepted as the drugs of choice in the systemic treatment of ovarian adenocarcinoma. Melphalan, as the most commonly used agent, has been re-

Table 11.12
Results of Recent Single-Agent Trials of the
Gynecologic Oncology Group in Patients Who
Have Received Prior Chemotherapy

Drug	Number of Patients	Complete Response	Partial Response	Response (%)
Nitrosoureas	57	0	0	0
Piperazinedione	35	0	1	2.9
Cis-platinum	34	2	6	23.5
VP-16	24	0	2	8.3
Galactitol	38	0	4	10.5

276

garded as easy to administer and relatively free of those adverse effects such as nausea and vomiting which are of most concern to patients. The frequency of response has often been reported at excessively inflated levels; and, coupled with negative comparative trials of some combinations of drugs (Smith, Rutledge, and Wharton 1972; Blom, Park, and Blessing 1978), this fact has led to a reluctance on the part of many physicians to consider a potential for improved results with combination chemotherapy and a willingness to become satisfied with what in reality may be less than optimal therapy. A critical examination of response data on melphalan may hopefully shed some light on this difficult problem.

A review of the literature on melphalan in the treatment of advanced ovarian adenocarcinoma shows response rates that vary from 12%, reported by the Southwest Oncology Group (Rossof et al. 1976), to 54%, reported by the National Cancer Institute (Young et al. 1978). To some extent, this can be explained by a variable number of stage III optimal cases in the study population, a variable number of patients with prior radiotherapy and/or chemotherapy, and possibly variable absorption of melphalan (Alberts, personal communication). Unfortunately, the higher response rates reported produce a false impression of the efficacy of melphalan. To determine as realistic a view of the efficacy of melphalan as is feasible, a consideration of the Gynecologic Oncology Group experience with melphalan in patients with stage III suboptimal and stage IV disease in three separate studies is illuminating (table 11.13) (Brady et al. 1979; Blom, Park, and Blessing 1978; Omura 1979). Response rates over these three studies, each using a standard five-day regimen of melphalan 0.2 mg per kg per day, are remarkably consistent (32%, 28%, and 36%), as is the frequency of complete response (12%, 16%, and 17%). The facts that the patient population in each of these studies is well described and includes no optimal stage III patients and no patients with prior chemotherapy, that the number of patients in each study is relatively large, and that the criteria for response are strict and uniform from study to study suggest that the observed response rates of 30% to 35% accurately reflect the true level of efficacy of melphalan in advanced ovarian adenocarcinoma. Median response duration ranged from five to seven months for the

Table 11.13
Response Rates to Therapy with Melphalan
in Three Different Studies by the Gynecologic
Oncology Group

Study	Number of Patients	Complete Response	Partial Response	Response (%)
Protocol 2	40	5	8	32.5
Protocol 3	93	15	12	28.1
Protocol 22	60	10	12	36.7

three study populations, while median survival ranged from 9.8 to 12.7 months. These data, while suggesting significant activity for melphalan in advanced ovarian adenocarcinoma, reflect considerable room for improvement. Attempts to achieve an improved response rate for alkylating agents by employing high-dose regimens of cyclophosphamide have not succeeded in improving frequency of response when compared with melphalan (Young et al. 1974), reports of extremely high responses in nonrandomized trials of high-dose cyclophosphamide notwithstanding (Buckner et al. 1974; Geisler, Minor, and Eastland 1976).

Combination Chemotherapy

The less than optimal efficacy of single-agent therapy taken together with the relatively large number of nonalkylating agents (seven) with activity against advanced ovarian adenocarcinoma logically leads to an evaluation of combination chemotherapy. In view of the variable response rates reported for single agents such as melphalan, no conclusion about the relative merits of combination versus single-agent therapy can be drawn from nonrandomized trials. For this reason, only such trials will be considered to evaluate the relative merits of combination chemotherapy.

Early studies (Smith, Rutledge, and Wharton 1972; Blom, Park, and Blessing 1978; Barlow and Piver 1977) of combination chemotherapy focused on regimens which included an alkylating agent, 5-fluorouracil, and actinomycin-D, the latter an agent with no clearly demonstrated activity in ovarian adenocarcinoma (table 11.14). Two of these studies demonstrated no ther-

Table 11.14
Early Trials of Combination Chemotherapy in Ovarian Adenocarcinoma Reveal No Statistical Advantages for Combination

Study	Number of Patients	Response (%)
GOG Protocol 3		
Melphalan	93	28
Melphalan + 5-FU	71	30
Melphalan + 5-FU + actinomycin-D	67	36
Cyclophosphamide + 5-FU + actinomycin-D	38	26
Roswell Park		
Melphalan	49	35
Cyclophosphamide + 5-FU + actinomycin-D	49	37
M.D. Anderson		
Melphalan	50	42
Cyclophosphamide + 5-FU + actinomycin-D	47	45

apeutic advantages for the combination regimens as compared to a standard regimen of melphalan, while a third study showed a significantly lower progression rate (32% versus 55%, $P = 0.025$) for patients receiving a combination of actinomycin-D, 5-fluorouracil, and cyclophosphamide as compared to those receiving melphalan. Even in the last study, however, no difference in response rates was noted, nor was median duration of response significantly different. In each instance, the combination regimens were more toxic. These trials thus suggested no advantage for combination chemotherapy.

The subsequent identification of three additional active agents, Adriamycin, hexamethylmelamine, and cis-platinum, led to the development of newer combination regimens which have been tested in recent randomized trials. Investigators at the National Cancer Institute selected four drugs with significant activity, differing mechanisms of action, and slightly different patterns of organ toxicity and evaluated this combination, hexaCAF (table 11.15), in a randomized comparison to melphalan alone (Young et al. 1978). Approximately 25% of the patients in the trial had stage III optimal disease while the rest had either stage III suboptimal or stage IV disease. Slightly more patients with low-grade neoplasms and optimal stage III disease received melphalan. The results of the trial (table 11.16) showed the combination regimen to be significantly superior to melphalan in overall response rate ($P < 0.05$) and survival ($P < 0.05$) and to produce twice as many documented complete responses, although this latter difference was not sta-

Table 11.15
Hexa CAF Regimen

Drug	Dose	Route	Days
Hexamethylmelamine	150 mg/m^2	po	1–14
Cyclophosphamide	150 mg/m^2	po	1–14
Methotrexate	40 mg/m^2	IV	1 and 8
5-Fluorouracil	600 mg/m^2	IV	1 and 8
	No therapy on days 15–28		

Table 11.16
Results of NCI trial of Hexa CAF vs Melphalan

Parameter	Melphalan		HexaCAF
Patients	37		40
CR	6	$P = 0.08$	13
PR	14		17
CR + PR	54%	$P < 0.05$	76%
Response duration	17 months	$P < 0.05$	29 months

tistically significant ($P = 0.08$). As in the case of other such trials, the combination regimen was more toxic, with 28% of patients developing severe or life-threatening myelosuppression, as compared to only 13% with melphalan, and 68% of patients on hexaCAF experiencing nausea and vomiting versus 28% on melphalan. Two additional important observations in this trial concern the significance of histologic grade and of bulk of disease in relation to response to therapy. Using Broders' system, too few grade 1 cases were identified to draw any conclusions. Grade 4 cases did not fare well regardless of therapy, but grade 2 and 3 lesions survived significantly longer with the combination than with the single agent (Ozols et al. 1979). With regard to bulk of disease, patients with optimal stage III disease (all nodules less than 2 cm in diameter) had a significantly better response rate to chemotherapy than those with suboptimal stage III and stage IV disease (16 of 19, or 84%, versus 31 of 58, or 53%, $P < 0.05$).

A second recent trial of combination chemotherapy, undertaken by the Gynecologic Oncology Group, compared melphalan to two combinations, Adriamycin plus cyclophosphamide and melphalan plus hexamethylmelamine (table 11.17). All patients entered on this trial had suboptimal stage III or stage IV disease. An updated analysis of this recently closed trial (table 11.18) (Omura et al. 1979) reveals that a significantly greater percentage of patients on the combinations achieved a clinically complete response than did so on the single agent (37% and 32% versus 17%, $P = 0.047$). Differences in overall response rate and median survival, though favoring the combination regimens, are not as yet significant; follow-up, however, continues. As with other trials of combination chemotherapy, adverse effects were more common with the multidrug regimens, particularly in reference to severe or life-threatening leukopenia and to nausea and vomiting.

These two studies make a reasonable case for the superiority of combination chemotherapy over a single alkylating agent in one or more respects. The three combination regimens evaluated in these trials produced similar results in terms of complete responses. The higher overall response and

Table 11.17
Regimens Studied by the Gynecologic
Oncology Group in a Recent Randomized
Trial

Regimen I	Melphalan 7 mg/m² po days 1–5, repeat every 28 days
Regimen II	Adriamycin 50 mg/m² IV, repeat every 21 days Cyclophosphamide 500 mg/m² IV, repeat every 21 days
Regimen III	Melphalan 7 mg/m² po days 1–5, repeat every 28 days
	Hexalamethylmelamine 150 mg/m² po days 1–14, repeat every 28 days

Table 11.18
Results of a Recent Analysis of an Ongoing
Gynecologic Oncology Group Randomized
Trial Showing That Both Combinations Are
Significantly Superior to Melphalan in the
Induction of Complete Responses (P = 0.047)

	Melphalan	Adriamycin + Cyclophosphamide	Melphalan + Hexamethylmelamine
Patients	60	52	60
Complete response (%)	17	37	32
Complete + partial response (%)	37	54	54
Median survival	12.7 months	15.2 months	15.1 months

longer median survival seen with hexaCAF in comparison with the other two combinations is difficult to assess since the hexaCAF study population included patients with minimal residual disease. Three recent studies, however, direct attention in particular to the Adriamycin-cyclophosphamide combination and possibilities of further enhancement of therapeutic benefit. In a trial of cis-platinum added to Adriamycin-cyclophosphamide (table 11.19) (Ehrlich et al. 1979), high overall and complete response rates were observed. Follow-up is not sufficiently long to permit an analysis of response duration and survival. The addition of both cis-platinum and hexamethylmelamine to Adriamycin-cyclophosphamide would appear to yield even higher complete and overall response rates, as observed in two other trials (Vogl, Greenwald, and Kaplan 1979; Bruckner et al. 1979). One of these in particular, a pilot study of the Eastern Cooperative Oncology Group, resulted in an overall response rate exceeding 90% and a clinically complete response rate approaching 50% (table 11.20). Again, follow-up is as yet too short to permit an evaluation of response duration and survival. These trials do not establish that the three- and four-drug regimens are superior to Adriamycin-cyclophosphamide, but do suggest that these regimens should be evaluated in comparison with the two-drug combination.

Chemoimmunotherapy

Concomitant with the increasing interest in combination chemotherapy, attention has been directed to possible combination of chemotherapy with immunomodulating agents such as BCG, *Corynebacterium parvum,* and levamisole. Interest was stimulated by observations in animal tumor models suggesting synergism between alkylating and immunopotentiating agents (Fisher, Wolmark, and Saffer 1975) and by identification of human ovarian

Table 11.19
Results of a Limited Trial of Cis-platinum, Adriamycin, and
Cyclophosphamide in Advanced Ovarian Adenocarcinoma

Regimen	Drugs	Patients	Complete Response %	Complete Response + Partial Response (%)
PAC-1	Cis-platinum 50 mg/m^2 day 1 every 3 weeks Adriamycin 50 mg/m^2 day 1 every 3 weeks Cyclophosphamide 750 mg/m^2 day 1 every 3 weeks	18	39	61
PAC-5	Cis-platinum 20 mg/m^2 days 1–5 every 4 weeks Adriamycin 50 mg/m^2 day 1 every 4 weeks Cyclophosphamide 750 mg/m^2 day 4 every 3 weeks	17	35	76
	Total	35	37	68

Table 11.20
Results of an Eastern Cooperative Oncology
Group Pilot Study in Ovarian
Adenocarcinoma

Drug	Dose	Route	Schedule
Cyclophosphamide	600mg/m^2	IV	Day 1, repeat every 3 weeks
Adriamycin	25mg/m^2	IV	Day 1, repeat every 3 weeks
Cis-platinum	50mg/m^2	IV	Day 1, repeat every 3 weeks
Hexamethylmelamine	150mg/m^2	po	Days 8–22, repeat every 3 weeks

Results

Total patients	21
Complete response (%)	48
Partial response (%)	43

282

tumor antigens (DiSaia, Sinkovics, and Rutledge 1972; Gall, Walling, and Pearl 1973). As a result of these data, two member institutions of the Gynecologic Oncology Group studied 45 patients with stage III ovarian adenocarcinoma treated with a combination of melphalan and *Corynebacterium parvum,* an immunopotentiating agent. (Creasman et al. 1979). When compared with a nonrandomized but concomitantly studied control group treated with melphalan alone (table 11.21), the combination regimen yielded a superior response rate (53% versus 29%), a better progression-free interval (12 months versus 6 months), and a longer median survival (24 months versus 11.7 months). This result, of course, must be accepted cautiously since the comparison was not randomized, even though the two groups were reasonably well balanced in regard to such factors as histologic grade and amount of residual disease postoperatively.

The apparent superiority of the melphalan–*C. parvum* combination in the nonrandomized pilot study prompted the Gynecologic Oncology Group (GOG) to undertake a randomized comparison of the two regimens in optimal stage III patients based on an expectation that patients with minimal residual disease would in theory be more likely to benefit from immunotherapy. This trial is still accruing patients, with no discernible difference between the two treatment arms as yet (Lewis 1979). It is simply too early to draw any conclusions from this randomized study.

A recently completed randomized trial of advanced ovarian adenocarcinoma conducted by the Southwest Oncology Group does, however, support the results of the nonrandomized GOG pilot in demonstrating a positive and significant influence of an immunopotentiating agent, BCG, on patient survival. This study compared a combination of Adriamycin plus cyclophosphamide to the same regimen plus BCG by escarification (table 11.22). A recently updated analysis (Alberts et al. 1979) reveals statistically significant

Table 11.21
Results of a Gynecologic Oncology Group
Pilot Study of Chemoimmunotherapy in
Patients with Advanced Ovarian
Adenocarcinoma

Regimen	Number of Patients	Complete Response + Partial Response (%)	Progression-Free Interval	Survival
Melphalan	63	29	6 months	11.7 months
Melphalan + *C. parvum*	45	53	12 months	24 months

NOTES: Historical control: Melphalan 0.2 mg/kg/day for 5 days by mouth every 4 weeks.

Study regimen: Melphalan as above plus *Corynebacterium parvum* 4 mg/m^2 IV on day 7 after start of melphalan; repeat every 4 weeks.

Table 11.22
Results of Southwest Oncology Group
Randomized Trial of Chemotherapy with or
without Immunotherapy in Advanced
Ovarian Adenocarcinoma ($P < 0.004$)

Regimen	Number of Patients	Complete Response + Partial Response (%)	Response Duration	Survival
AC	61	36	7 months	13.1 months
AC + BCG	57	53	9.5 months	23.5 months

NOTES: Regimen I: Adriamycin 40 mg/m^2 IV day 1; Cyclophosphamide 200 mg/m^2 po days 3–6; repeat every 3 to 4 weeks.
Regimen II: Same as Regimen I plus BCG (scarification) days 8 and 15.

improvement in survival (23.5 months versus 13.1 months, $P < 0.004$) for those patients receiving BCG as a part of this regimen. Although response rate (53% versus 36%) and response duration (9.5 months versus 7 months) were greater for the immunotherapy arm of the study, the differences were not statistically significant. An evaluation of prognostic factors showed good balance between the two regimens with regard to histologic grade and bulk of residual disease. All patients had stage III or IV disease.

Conclusions

Data reviewed herald an increasingly optimistic outlook for the patient with advanced ovarian carcinoma. In addition to an expectation for an increased frequency of response to therapy and an improved median survival, the increasing percentage of clinically complete responders provides hope for a growing number of long-term survivors and possibly even cures in this group of patients for whom the outlook previously was uniformly dismal. Specific conclusions which can be drawn from current information on the management of advanced disease are several: (1) Studies of single-agent therapy suggest that at least seven nonalkylating agents and five alkylating agents possess significant activity against ovarian adenocarcinoma. (2) Response rates of 30% to 35%, response duration of 5 to 7 months, and survival of 9 to 12 months can be expected from the use of traditional therapy with single alkylating agents such as melphalan. (3) Combination chemotherapy in well-done trails using newer active agents such as hexamethylmelamine and Adriamycin yields a greater frequency of clinically complete responses, an improved overall response rate, and possibly prolonged survival. (4) Immunopotentiating agents, when combined with chemotherapy, may favorably influence survival, although this as yet has been documented in only one randomized trial.

While it is clear that chemotherapy, and in particular combination chemotherapy, is of significant benefit to the patient with advanced ovarian adenocarcinoma, further research is needed to improve the still guarded prognosis of these patients. Future directions suggested by data to date include: (1) A continued effort to identify new active drugs in those patients failing on primary therapy is needed to enlarge therapeutic options. Such an effort continues in at least two major cooperative research groups. (2) Efforts are needed to improve further combination drug regimens by the addition of agents with different mechanisms of action and adverse effects to current combinations. The Adriamycin-cyclophosphamide combination provides an ideal opportunity for such efforts, as suggested by nonrandomized trials adding cis-platinum or cis-platinum plus hexamethylmelamine to Adriamycin-cyclophosphamide. (3) The possible role of immunotherapy, as suggested by the Southwest Oncology Group trial, must be confirmed or denied in further randomized studies. Well-controlled, randomized, large trials with careful patient evaluation are required if reliable conclusions in regard to each of these three points are to be reached.

Management of Early Ovarian Adenocarcinoma

The role of chemotherapy in the management of early ovarian adenocarcinoma falls into two categories, the adjuvant therapy of patients with no evidence of gross disease after operation and treatment of patients with minimal residual gross disease after surgical bulk reduction. The case for chemotherapy in each category is not at all clear because of a lack of well-done trials, but certain directions for future research can be discerned by a review of available data.

Adjuvant Chemotherapy

Patients with stage I ovarian adenocarcinoma can virtually always be rendered free of gross disease with resection. Patients can then be grouped into those at low risk for recurrences and those at high risk (Webb, Decker, and Mussey 1973). Low-risk patients are those with stage I, grade 1 ovarian adenocarcinoma with an intact capsule and no tumor on the external surface. Such individuals have a five-year survival of 90% and hence little need for further therapy after resection. High-risk stage I patients are those with higher-grade lesions or with either capsular rupture or tumor growing on the external surface of the capsule. Such patients have a five-year survival of less than 70% and possibly as low as 50%. This substantial increase in risk for recurrence raises the question of a potential role for adjuvant therapy, either chemotherapy or radiotherapy or a combination of the two.

No well-controlled and well-executed trials with adequate patient numbers have been successfully completed in an effort to define the role of adjuvant therapy in stage I ovarian adenocarcinomas. Two attempts to answer the question regarding the role of adjuvant therapy have yielded inconclusive results. The first study randomized patients with stage I disease to receive either melphalan or whole abdominal radiation by a moving strip technique plus a pelvic boost (Smith, Rutledge, and Delclos 1975). A nontreatment control arm was not included, nor were patient groups compared as to histologic grade and stage I subgroup. The number of patients on each arm was small (14 treated with radiotherapy, 28 with chemotherapy), and the observed difference (85% of irradiated patients alive at two years versus 90% of those treated with chemotherapy) was not significant. No conclusions can be drawn as to whether either therapy was better than no adjuvant treatment.

The second trial of adjuvant therapy for stage I ovarian adenocarcinoma was undertaken by the Gynecologic Oncology Group and randomized patients to receive no further treatment, pelvic radiation, or melphalan (table 11.23) (Hreshchyshyn and Norris 1977). The study dealt with stage I_a and I_b cases only, and the three arms were reasonably well balanced with regard to histologic grade and stage I subgroup. Although the trial accrued too few patients to answer definitively the question of which approach was best, those patients which were entered and evaluable were of sufficient numbers to suggest that melphalan was statistically significantly superior to pelvic radiation as an adjuvant treatment ($P = 0.047$).

Another approach to adjuvant treatment which has been reported is the use of intraperitoneal radioisotopes such as chromic phosphate (^{32}P) or radiogold following resection. No trials comparing this approach to no further therapy or to other therapeutic alternatives have been reported as yet. Reports of five-year survival exceeding 90% in stage I patients receiving radioisotopes recommend this approach for direct comparison with other alternatives (Buchsbaum, Keetel, and Latourette 1975).

Two studies currently being conducted jointly by the Gynecologic Oncology Group and the Ovarian Cancer Study Group are seeking to answer both the therapeutic questions noted above and questions regarding adequate staging of such patients. After a thorough exploratory laparotomy and multiple blind biopsies, patients with stage I, grade 1, subset i, a and b lesions are randomized to receive either melphalan or no further therapy in an attempt to determine whether melphalan will improve on the expected 85% to 90% five-year survival of these patients. For patients with high-risk stage I cases, randomization between melphalan and intraperitoneal chromic phosphate ($Cr^{32}PO_4$) bypasses the question of whether either approach is better than no further therapy and seeks to determine which therapy is superior. Because of the rigorous but necessary requirements for patient assessment prior to entry (Young et al. 1979), accrual on these trials is slow and time to

Table 11.23
Results of Gynecologic Oncology Group Trial
in Stage I Ovarian Adenocarcinoma

Regimen I	No therapy
Regimen II	Pelvic radiation 5000 rad in 5 to 6 weeks at daily dose 160 to 200 rad 5 days/week
Regimen III	Melphalan 0.2 mg/kg po days 1–5 Repeat every 4 weeks for 18 months

Results

Regimen	Number of Patients	Recurrences (No./%)
No therapy	29	5/17%
Radiation	23	7/30%
Melphalan	34	2/6%

NOTE: Radiation is significantly inferior to melphalan in this study ($P = 0.047$), but no conclusion can be drawn that melphalan is superior to no treatment.

completion of the studies very long. Until these questions are dealt with, however, progress in the management of stage I ovarian adenocarcinoma will be minimal.

Minimal Residual Disease

Patients with stage II and optimal stage III ovarian adenocarcinoma represent a group of individuals in whom the expected five-year survival is at best less than 40%. Following maximum surgical effort, most will have evidence of residual disease; and, in fact, most with an adequate exploratory laparotomy will prove to have stage III disease even though they may have been clinically assigned to stage II. Several approaches have been employed in the postoperative management of these patients; but, as in the case of stage I disease, no definitive study has been carried out.

Three significant attempts at randomized trials to evaluate the relative roles of radiation therapy and chemotherapy have been reported (Brady et al. 1979; Welander, Kjorstad, and Kolstad 1978; Miller et al. 1975). The Gynecologic Oncology Group, in a four-arm study, compared whole abdominal radiation versus pelvic radiation either preceded or followed by melphalan versus melphalan alone in a population of patients with stage III ovarian adenocarcinoma and noted no significant difference in progression-free interval (6.8 to 12.5 months) or survival (16.7 to 20 months) among the four arms (Brady et al. 1979). A Norwegian study (Welander, Kjorstad, and Kolstad 1978) randomized patients to treatment with either whole abdominal radiation at a dose of 5000 rad or a reduced, 3000 rad course of whole abdominal radiation followed by thiotepa. Again, no significant difference in survival was noted between the two treatment groups. Finally, the Eastern Cooperative Oncology Group conducted a small trial comparing, in a randomized study, whole abdominal radiation to 3500 rad versus chlorambucil for eight weeks versus a combination of the two. Small numbers (17, 18, and 16 patients on each arm) and suboptimal chemotherapy cloud conclusions drawn from this trial, but no differences were noted among the three regimens except for an improved survival in ambulatory patients who received radiation alone (eight patients with median survival of 94 weeks versus 33 and 42 weeks among patients with similar performance ratings on the other two regimens). In patients with poorer performance ratings, no advantage for radiation alone could be discerned.

These three trials display no significant advantage for one approach over the other except for a possible but inconclusive survival advantage in ambulatory patients who receive whole abdominal radiation alone. The technique of whole abdominal radiation employed in each trial was a single-field approach. More recently, a study using a moving strip technique for whole abdominal radiation plus a pelvic boost demonstrated superiority for this approach over pelvic radiation plus chlorambucil in a group of stage I_b, II, and asymptomatic III patients (Dembo et al. 1979). Actuarial five-year survival rates were 81% for whole abdominal plus pelvic radiation and 55% for chlorambucil plus pelvic radiation. The two study populations were balanced for stage and grade, and the survival differences were significant ($P = 0.02$). Interpretation of these results is clouded by the lack of definition of bulk disease in the asymptomatic stage III patients, the failure to include an arm for chemotherapy alone, and the choice of suboptimal chemotherapy. This latter flaw is particularly emphasized by the results of two recent studies (Griffiths, Parker, and Fuller 1979; Edmonson et al. 1979) which suggest that a combination of Adriamycin plus cyclophosphamide yields a significantly better survival than a single alkylating agent in the treatment of minimal residual (stage II and optimal III) disease.

Although no dogmatic statements can be made about the current best approach to minimal residual ovarian adenocarcinoma, studies cited do suggest two positive findings. Both whole abdominal radiation and combination chemotherapy may offer a survival advantage over pelvic radiation and/or single alkylating agents. Further investigation of these alternatives will be required before solid recommendations can be made.

Conclusion

The role of chemotherapy in early ovarian adenocarcinoma is not clear at the present time. Data suggest that single-agent chemotherapy can enhance the survival of stage I, high-risk patients when used as an adjuvant following resection of all gross disease. Combination chemotherapy appears to offer a better outlook for the patient with minimal residual stage II and III disease when compared with single-agent chemotherapy. The relative role of radiation therapy, radioisotopes, and chemotherapy either alone or in combination is completely unsettled. Further studies in patients with early ovarian adenocarcinoma should emphasize (1) the role of chemotherapy relative to no further treatment or radioisotopes intraperitoneally in stage I, high-risk disease; (2) the relative roles of whole abdominal radiation alone and chemotherapy alone in minimal residual stage II and III disease; and (3) the possible role of immunotherapy in these patients if the positive findings in advanced disease are corroborated.

Summary and Recommendations

Despite a growing body of literature on the role of chemotherapy in the management of ovarian adenocarcinoma, no conclusive statements can be made regarding the proper therapeutic approach for each stage of the disease. Treatment recommendations, however, can and should be made to serve as guides to proper therapy based on current knowledge. These recommendations, though defensible with data, reflect a personal interpretation of a complex subject.

For patients with suboptimal stage III and stage IV disease, combination chemotherapy is indicated. Adriamycin plus cyclophosphamide is the preferred regimen since it includes agents which are commercially available and manifests superiority over single alkylating agents in at least one large study. The addition of BCG should await confirmation of the Southwest Oncology Group observations. For patients with cardiac problems, in particular congestive heart failure, treatment with melphalan plus hexamethylmelamine is indicated if the latter agent is available. Should hexamethylmelamine not be available, single alkylating agent treatment is appropriate.

Recommendations for patients with early ovarian adenocarcinoma are more difficult to make and much more open to criticism. Patients with stage I, low-risk ovarian adenocarcinoma (stage $I_a i$ and $I_b i$, grade 1 lesions) should receive no further therapy after resection of all gross disease. All other patients with stage I disease should probably receive adjuvant therapy with a single alkylating agent. Patients with minimal residual stage II and stage III disease should receive combination chemotherapy with Adriamycin plus cyclophosphamide following maximum resection, although a case can be made for the use of whole abdominal radiation plus a pelvic boost in lieu of the chemotherapy.

Major alterations in these recommendations may become necessary as results of current trials become available in the next two to three years. Furthermore, issues of paramount importance such as the role of second look laparotomy to document response, the proper length of treatment in responders, and the need for maintenance therapy have been too inadequately examined to permit any recommendations at present. These facts dictate that the physician responsible for the care of the patient with ovarian adenocarcinoma retain an open mind and critically read reports on current and ongoing clinical trials. With this kind of approach, the physician will be able to offer the patient with ovarian carcinoma an increasingly optimistic outlook for long-term survival.

References

Alberts, D. et al. Randomized study of chemoimmunotherapy for advanced ovarian carcinoma: a preliminary report of a Southwest Oncology Group study. *Cancer Treat. Rep.* 63:325–331, 1979.

Baker, L.; Izbicki, R.; and Vaitkevicius, V. Phase II study of porfiromycin versus mitomycin-C utilizing acute intermittent schedules. *Med. Pediatr. Oncol.* 2:207–213, 1976.

Baker, L.; Samson, M.; and Izbicki, R. Phase I and II evaluation of cytembena in disseminated epithelial ovarian cancers and sarcomas. *Cancer Treat. Rep.* 60:1389–1391, 1976.

.Barber, H., and Kwon, T. Current status of the treatment of gynecologic cancer by site: ovary. *Cancer* 38:610–619, 1976.

Barlow, J., and Piver, S. Single agent versus combination chemotherapy in the treatment of ovarian cancer. *Obstet. Gynecol.* 49:609–611, 1977.

Blom, J.; Park, R.; and Blessing, J. Treatment of women with disseminated and recurrent ovarian carcinoma with single and multichemotherapeutic agents. *Proc. AACR-ASCO* 19:338, 1978.

Brady, L. et al. Radiotherapy, chemotherapy and combined therapy in stage III epithelial ovarian cancer. *Cancer Clin. Trials* 2:111–120, 1979.

Broders, A. Carcinoma: grading and practical application. *Arch. Pathol.* 2:376–380, 1926.

Bruckner, H. et al. Treatment of advanced ovarian cancer with cis-dichloro-diammineplatinum (II): poor-risk patients with intensive prior therapy. *Cancer Treat. Rep.* 62:555–558, 1978.

Bruckner, H. et al. Prospective controlled randomized trial comparing combination chemotherapy of advanced ovarian carcinoma with Adriamycin and cis-platinum ± cyclophosphamide and hexamethylmelamine. *Proc. AACR-ASCO* 20:414, 1979.

Buchsbaum, H.; Keetel, W.; and Latourette, H. The use of radioisotopes as adjunct therapy of localized ovarian cancer. *Semin. Oncol.* 2:247–251, 1975.

Buckner, D. et al. Intermittent high-dose cyclophosphamide (NSC-26271) treatment of stage III ovarian carcinoma. *Cancer Chemother. Rep.* 58:697–703, 1974.

Creasman, W. et al. Chemoimmunotherapy in the management of primary stage III ovarian cancer: a Gynecologic Oncology Group study. *Cancer Treat. Rep.* 63:319–323, 1979.

Day, T., Jr., and Smith, J. Diagnosis and staging of ovarian carcinoma. *Semin. Oncol.* 2:217–222, 1975.

Decker, D.; Malkasian, G., Jr.; and Taylor, W. F. Prognostic importance of histologic grading in ovarian carcinoma. *Natl. Cancer Inst. Monogr.* 42:9–11, 1975.

Dembo, A. et al. The Princess Margaret Hospital study of ovarian cancer: stages I, II, and asymptomatic III presentations. *Cancer Treat. Rep.* 63:249–254, 1979.

291

Devita, V., Jr. et al. Perspectives and research in gynecologic oncology. *Cancer* 38:509–525, 1976.

DiSaia, P.; Sinkovics, J.; and Rutledge, F. Cell-mediated immunity to human malignant cells. *Am. J. Obstet. Gynecol.* 114:979–989, 1972.

Edmonson, J. et al. Phase II evaluation of VP-16-213 (NSC-141540) in patients with advanced ovarian carcinoma resistant to alkylating agents. *Gynecol. Oncol.* 6:7–9, 1978.

Edmonson, J. et al. Different chemotherapeutic sensitivities and host factors affecting prognosis in advanced ovarian carcinoma versus minimal residual disease. *Cancer Treat. Rep.* 63:241–248, 1979.

Ehrlich, C. et al. Chemotherapy for stage III–IV epithelial ovarian cancer with cis-dichlorodiammine-platinum (II), Adriamycin, and cyclophosphamide: a preliminary report. *Cancer Treat. Rep.* 63:281–288, 1979.

Falkson, H., and Falkson, G. Phase II trial of cytembena in patients with advanced ovarian and breast cancer. *Cancer Treat. Rep.* 60:1655–1658, 1976.

Fisher, B.; Wolmark, N.; and Saffer, E. Inhibiting effect of prolonged *Corynebacterium parvum* and cyclophosphamide administration on the growth of established tumors. *Cancer* 35:134–143, 1975.

Gall, S.; Walling, J.; and Pearl, J. Demonstration of tumor-associated antigens in human gynecologic malignancies. *Am. J. Obstet. Gynecol.* 115:387–393, 1973.

Geisler, H.; Minor, J.; and Eastland, M. The treatment of advanced ovarian carcinoma with high dose, intravenous cyclophosphamide. *Gynecol. Oncol.* 4:43–52, 1976.

Griffiths, T. Surgical resection of tumor bulk in the primary treatment of ovarian carcinoma. *Natl. Cancer Inst. Monogr.* 42:101–104, 1975.

Griffiths, T.; Parker, L.; and Fuller, A., Jr. Role of cytoreductive surgical treatment in the management of advanced ovarian cancer. *Cancer Treat. Rep.* 63:235–240, 1979.

Hreshchyshyn, M., and Norris, H. Postoperative treatment of women with resectable ovarian cancer with radiotherapy, melphalan, or no further treatment. *Proc. AACR-ASCO* 18:195, 1977.

Malkasian, G., Jr.; Decker, D.; and Webb, M. Histology of epithelial tumors of the ovary: clinical usefulness and prognostic significance of the histologic classification and grading. *Semin. Oncol.* 2:191–201, 1975.

Miller, S. et al. Comparative evaluation of combined radiation-chlorambucil treatment of ovarian carcinomatosis. *Cancer* 36:1625–1630, 1975.

Omura, G. et al. Chemotherapy for mustard-resistant ovarian adenocarcinoma: a randomized trial of CCNU and methyl-CCNU. *Cancer Treat. Rep.* 61:1533–1535, 1977.

Omura, G. et al. A randomized trial of melphalan versus melphalan plus hexamethylmelamine versus Adriamycin plus cyclophosphamide in advanced ovarian adenocarcinoma. *Proc. AACR-ASCO* 20:358, 1979.

Ozols, R. et al. Histologic grade in advanced ovarian cancer. *Cancer Treat. Rep.* 63:235–264, 1979.

Rossof, A. et al. Randomized evaluation of chlorambucil and melphalan in advanced ovarian cancer. *Proc. AACR-ASCO* 17:300, 1976.

Seidman, H.; Silverberg, E.; and Holleb, A. Cancer statistics, 1976. *Cancer* 26:2, 1976.

Slayton, R.; Petty, W.; and Blessing, J. Phase II trial of VP-16 in treatment of advanced ovarian adenocarcinoma. *Proc. AACR-ASCO* 20:190, 1979.

Smith, J.; Rutledge, F.; and Delclos, L. Results of chemotherapy as an adjunct to surgery in patients with localized ovarian cancer. *Semin. Oncol.* 2:277–281, 1975.

Smith, J.; Rutledge, F.; and Wharton, T. Chemotherapy of ovarian cancer. *Cancer* 30:1565–1571, 1972.

Thigpen, T.; Dolan, T.; and Morrison, F. Phase II trial of piperazinedione in treatment of advanced ovarian adenocarcinoma. *Proc. AACR-ASCO* 19:332, 1978.

Thigpen, T.; Lagasse, L.; and Bundy, B. Phase II trial of cis-platinum in treatment of advanced ovarian adenocarcinoma. *Proc. AACR-ASCO* 20:84, 1979.

Tobias, J., and Griffiths, T. Management of ovarian carcinoma: current concepts and future prospects. *N. Engl. J. Med.* 294:818–823, 877–882, 1976.

Vogl, S.; Greenwald, E.; and Kaplan, B. The CHAD regimen (cyclophosphamide, hexamethylmelamine, Adriamycin, and diammine-dichloroplatinum) in advanced ovarian cancer. *Proc. AACR-ASCO* 20:384, 1979.

Webb, M.; Decker, D.; and Mussey, E. Factors influencing survival in stage I ovarian cancer. *Am. J. Obstet. Gynecol.* 116:222, 1973.

Welander, C.; Kjorstad, K.; and Kolstad, P. Postoperative irradiation and chemotherapy in patients with advanced ovarian cancer. *Acta Obstet. Gynecol. Scand.* 57:161–164, 1978.

Wiltshaw, E., and Kroner, T. Phase II study of cis-dichlorodiammine platinum (II) (NSC-119875) in advanced adenocarcinoma of the ovary. *Cancer Treat. Rep.* 60:55–60, 1976.

Young, R. Chemotherapy of ovarian cancer: past and present. *Semin. Oncol.* 2:267–276, 1975.

Young, R. et al. Chemotherapy of advanced ovarian carcinoma: a prospective randomized comparison of phenylalanine mustard and high dose cyclophosphamide. *Gynecol. Oncol.* 2:489–497, 1974.

Young, R. et al. Advanced ovarian adenocarcinoma: a prospective clinical trial of melphalan (L-PAM) versus combination chemotherapy. *N. Engl. J. Med.* 299:1261–1266, 1978.

Young, R. et al. Staging laparotomy in early ovarian cancer. *Proc. AACR-ASCO* 20:399, 1979.

Chapter 12

*The Role of
Radiation Therapy
in the Treatment of
Epithelial Ovarian Cancer*

PERSPECTIVE:

A. Robert Kagan

The modern oncologist whose goal is to find a single treatment for epithelial malignancy of the ovary is engaged in oncology's oldest exercise, that is, the search for a superior moral justification for egoism. It is an exercise that always involves a certain number of internal contradictions and unfortunately even a few absurdities.

Munnell (1968) showed that radiation increased the five-year survival in the operative treatment of ovarian carcinoma stage II and III, while Maier (1978) stated that radiation was only of value in stage II. Brady (1978) wrote: "It is an accepted fact that ovarian cancer is radioresponsive, but the role of radiation therapy in the primary management of ovarian cancer is at this point, unclear. In those studies of therapy in which external radiation sources are utilized, the fields irradiated have varied in size and shape, as well as in time-dose relationships. Often the volumes irradiated did not include the potential areas of tumor extent."

Does Maier (1978) agree or disagree with Brady when he says: "Unfortunately, the time-dose relationship for ovarian tumor sterilization is poorly understood. . . . Data on the exact amounts of dosage required for sterilization are quite lacking. Thus, the doses employed for such tumors have been somewhat dictated by the limits of tolerance of the normal tissues encompassed by the required treatment volume. To further complicate matters, the necessary treatment volume is not always clear-cut because of our inability to correctly identify the location of the tumor target volume"?

No matter what side of an argument one is on in the treatment of ovarian cancer, one always finds some people on one's side who one wishes were on the other side. Although Maier and Brady, early on, tend to take courage with the minority opinion (mine) that radiation has little to offer in epithelial malignancy of the ovary, in the end they join the majority in favor of radiation for most stages.

Are all facts created equal?

Is it correct to say that the only physician who can change his or her mind is one who has one?

The chief value in treating epithelial tumors of the ovary (with the exception of pelvic irradiation for stage II) is that it is the only way to learn that it does not really matter. Brady has identified and assessed this subject: "In large measure the multiple studies reviewed fail to indicate the benefit of radiotherapy in ovarian cancer."

In my opinion, to understand radiocurability, one must have a mass that one can feel or see on an imaging study. Comparing patients who have received adjuvant therapy for suspected or unpalpable disease with those who have not received similar adjuvant therapy leads most frequently to statistical gamesmanship. Fuks (1975) reviewed the results in the literature. He found that 70% (270 of 389) stage I, 21% (22 of 103) stage II, and 5% (14 of 280) stage III survived when treated by surgery alone. The results for surgery and external irradiation were 57% (375 of 657) stage I, 30% (185 of 607) stage II, and 10% (88 of 909) stage III.

Hintz (1975) has recently reported 76% survival for 30 stage I patients, 56% for 62 stage II patients, and 16% for 55 stage III patients. Delclos and Smith (1973) reported 57% with no evidence of disease (NED) for stage III when the operative procedure had removed all visible tumors, 27% when 2 cm tumor remained, 17% for 2 to 4 cm, and 10% for 4 to 6 cm.

Staging with biopsy or peritoneoscopy or lymphography have demonstrated that 20% of patients with clinical stage I and II are, in fact, stage III. Surgery has become more aggressive, with more total hysterectomies and bilateral salpingo-oophorectomies, omentectomies, and bowel surgery now being performed. A "maximum surgical effort" in the pelvis and upper abdomen can more than double survival at five years. The difficulties proposed by grade and staging prevent adequate comparison of data. Low malignant potential stage I cancers have double the survival at five years when compared to frank stage I carcinomas or stage I carcinomas with ascites. The survival in stage I in relation to histologic types at five years can range from 30% to 98%, with a median of 70% (Delclos and Smith 1973; Aure, Hoeg, and Kolstad 1971).

Since staging and surgical extirpation are becoming more sophisticated, it appears to me that it is intellectually impossible to attribute a better survival to the increased role of radiation where survival can simply be increased markedly by selectivity. Looking at the role of external radiation in epithelial tumors of the ovary is akin to looking at a painting. Physicians see mostly what they already know. In brief, the treatment of epithelial carcinoma is not the treatment of a single disease. Sharing a common organ of origin does not make these cancers homogeneous. Ironically the reason we succeed so well on the one hand and fail so miserably on the other may be due to selection and categorization rather than our cleverness or competence in designing or executing treatment regimens. The scientific atmosphere generated by discussing the treatment of ovarian carcinoma is talkative, critical, restless, and sometimes even tiresome because of the insoluble problems involved.

Can these problems be solved by randomized studies? Unlikely. To know ovarian cancer is perhaps to know something about medicine itself. Successes and failures go together.

Dr. Franz Buschke is fond of telling neophytes: "So you want to become famous. Good! Review the literature 30 years ago and reinvent it." Dr. Buschke perhaps was thinking of the bewildering scientific behavior of the enthusiasts for the use of isotopes in ovarian carcinoma. Del Regato and Spjut (1977) have summarized the use of ^{198}Au in ovarian cancer in the following manner:

> Injection of radioactive gold into the peritoneal cavity is advocated as a substitute for postoperative roentgentherapy. . . . Radiations from Au^{198} have a very limited penetrability of a few millimeters. Thus, they cannot attain in fruitful amounts the neoplastic cells that are imbedded in the tissue and nodes. . . . The value of intraperitoneal radioactive gold treatments as a routine postoperative procedure would be difficult to prove unless it is by a remarkable improvement of results that cannot be expected. . . . We question that the cost and risk of this approach is justified by the result.

Del Regato's scepticism of the efficacy of ^{198}Au can also be assigned to colloidal ^{32}P, although the hazards to personnel and possibly the patient are less with ^{32}P.

My experience with isotope therapy is limited. We have seen patients with recurrence after ^{198}Au with severe obstruction due to recurrent tumor, where the operative skill of the surgeon was severely tested against the chronic peritonitis and serositis caused by poor and unpredictable distribution of the radioactive particles. Perhaps these sticky serosal surfaces can be avoided by the use of intraoperative catheters. Some have advocated isotope therapy and external radiation. This therapy is overzealous, and the risks of fistula outweigh the benefits.

Previously our policy was to give total abdominal radiation for stage I$_c$, II$_o$, and III. Pelvic radiation was delivered in stage II, and chemotherapy was added in stage III. Presently our policy is to give external irradiation only for stage II disease followed by alkeran administration. We limit our port size to the true and false pelvis. Chemotherapy is given for high-risk stage I, with a second look at the end of 12 to 16 courses of alkeran, followed by localized radiation if persistent disease is uncovered. Stage III is treated by chemotherapy and second look when indicated.

The most important prognostic factor for survival is not the adjuvant treatment but whether the tumor can be completely removed at the initial operative procedure. Despite directed irradiation at second look for minimal disease in stage I and selected stage III, the majority of these patients have succumbed to abdominal carcinomatosis.

The second important factor for survival is whether patients can fully sustain the adjuvant treatment. Daily low-dose chlorambucil for one year combined with total abdominal radiation or 12 courses of pulse alkeran (with or without pelvic radiation) cannot be completed by all patients. Patients whose tumors can be totally removed and who can tolerate a complete course of adjuvant therapy survive a longer length of time. Miliary tumors and abundant ascites are more important than size of residual tumor. One large residual tumor is better than a dozen small tumors.

Treatment of the upper abdomen by irradiation is not recommended. An adequate dose cannot be given because of the intolerance of kidneys, liver, and gastrointestinal tract. It is difficult to visualize how any radioactive material could be guided to defy the natural fluid currents which favor the pelvis instead of the subdiaphragmatic region.

In summary, the only completely beneficial treatment for cancer of the ovary is surgery for stage I. Adjuvant therapy has yet to demonstrate survival advantage independent of selectivity. Series which seem to prove the benefit of adjuvant therapy do so, by and large, by the process of selection, which includes rigorous staging. Mrs. Robert A. Taft summed up, in my mind, what I hesitantly suggest may be applied to statistics in ovarian carcinoma: "I always find that statistics are hard to swallow and impossible to digest; the only one I can even remember is that if all the people who go to sleep in church were laid end to end they would be a lot more comfortable." The attitude that more and more treatment is one of the natural pleasures of oncologists brings with it, like everything else, the complications and side effects. The weighing of each ingredient in a treatment regimen does present insuperable difficulties that are unlikely to be resolved by randomization. There is no question that ovarian cancer is evil, but our overzealous meddling with isotopes and external irradiation will not make it good except for our colleagues in hyperalimentation.

References

Aure, J.C.; Hoeg, K.; and Kolstad, P. Clinical and histologic studies of ovarian carcinoma. *Obstet. Gynecol.* 37:1, 1971.

Brady, L.W. Cancer of the ovary. In *Modern radiation oncology*, eds. H.A. Gilbert, and A.R. Kagan. Hagerstown, Maryland: Harper & Row, 1978.

Delclos, L., and Smith, J.P. Tumors of the ovary. In *Textbook of radiotherapy*, ed. G.H. Fletcher. Philadelphia: Lea & Febiger, 1973.

Del Regato, J.A., and Spjut, H.J. *Cancer.* St. Louis: C.V. Mosby, 1977.

Fuks, Z. External radiotherapy of ovarian cancer. Standard approaches and new frontiers. *Semin. Oncol.* 2:253–266, 1975.

Hintz, B.L. et al. Results of postoperative megavoltage radiotherapy of malignant surface epithelial tumors of the ovary. *Radiology* 114:675–700, 1975

Maier, J.G. Radiotherapy treatment of ovarian cancer. In *Gynecologic oncology*, ed. L. McGowan. New York: Appleton-Century-Crofts, 1978.

Munnell, E.W. The changing prognosis and treatment in cancer of the ovary. *Am. J. Obstet. Gynecol.* 100:790–805, 1968.

PERSPECTIVE:

The Role of Radiation Therapy in the Treatment of Epithelial Ovarian Cancer

Alvaro Martinez

Ovarian carcinoma is the leading cause of death from gynecologic cancers, representing the third most common malignancy of Müllerian origin. It is also the fourth leading cause of death from cancer in North American women, following colon, breast, and lung cancer. Survival rates are low and have improved little over the last two decades. Perhaps this could be changed if present knowledge were uniformly applied by the surgeon at the time of laparotomy and if the principles of management were understood by all physicians responsible for the care of these patients.

The most common ovarian cancers are the epithelial types. They tend to invade and break through the capsule, particularly the serous variety, which is associated with papillary excrescences on the surface. Thus a high proportion of epithelial ovarian cancers are found to have spread intraperitoneally, involving the pelvic and abdominal viscera and/or the peritoneal surface. In the Stanford series published by Fuks and Bagshaw (1975), 16 of 32, or 50% of the patients with stage I disease and 44 of 75 (60%) of the stage II patients had gross and/or microscopic tumor excrescences on the tumor capsule. Lymphatic and vascular spread does occur but is less dominant. Bilaterality is often seen, particularly in the serous type, but also, less frequently, in endometrioid and mucinous carcinomas.

Information obtained at the initial laparotomy is of critical importance to successful therapy planning. After careful exploration, the surgeon must determine the exact extent of the disease process, obtain an adequate sample for documentation of histologic type, and estimate the volume, if any, of unresectable cancer. The pathologist analyzes the resected tissues, providing us with vital information regarding sites of involvement, cell type, and cell differentiation, the latter being an extremely important prognostic indicator (Ozols et al. 1980).

This chapter presents an overview of the role of radiotherapy in the treatment of epithelial ovarian cancer. It reviews the Stanford, the M. D. Anderson, and the Princess Margaret hospitals' experiences in this subject. It also describes the current philosophy practiced at the Division of Radiation Therapy of the Stanford University Medical Center, including a new radiotherapy technique presently used for the treatment of ovarian carcinoma.

Staging

The FIGO staging classification adopted in October 1974 is the system currently employed. It is based on both clinical and operative findings. No classification of ovarian cancer is ideal because of the multiplicity of cell types and variability in natural history; however, its use is essential to assess and compare results. Staging should be supplemented by an exact record of cell type, histologic grade of malignancy, and the adequacy of surgical exploration and resectability, including careful description of any gross residual disease. Although none of these parameters is included in the FIGO staging classification, their availability is important for appropriate therapy planning.

Pattern of Spread

Ovarian cancer is a disease of the entire abdominal cavity. Once it has penetrated the ovarian capsule, carcinoma tends to involve multiple sites in the pelvis and abdomen. All four classical methods of cancer spread apply to ovarian cancer. These include vascular and lymphatic spread, local extension, and peritoneal seeding. Local extension to contiguous structures such as tube, uterus, bladder, rectosigmoid, pelvic peritoneum, and omentum is a common finding.

The role of lymphatic spread is less well appreciated. The ovary has a dense lymphatic network which converges upon the hilus to form the subovarian lymphatic plexus (Cordier 1959). The plexus is drained by large collecting trunks that ascend bilaterally with the ovarian blood vessels and terminate on the left in the paraaortic group of lymph nodes between the bifurcation of the aorta and the renal pedicles and on the right in the precaval nodes. Accessory efferent vessels (Rouviere 1932), seen in less than 50% of females, course within the broad ligament toward the lateral and posterior pelvic wall and terminate in the high external iliac nodes or, less commonly, in the hypogastric chain. Still another efferent group runs along the round ligament, draining into the external iliac and inguinal group (Eichner and Bove 1954), explaining the rare but clinically significant incidence of inguinal node metastasis. Most of the ovarian lymph node drainage is opacified following bipedal lymphangiography. Our data (Fuks 1975) showed a high incidence of positive lymphograms (21%) in stages I and II disease. Unfortunately, histologic correlation has not always been available.

Another major route of spread in ovarian carcinoma is through the peritoneal cavity, particularly if there are papillary excrescences on the ovarian capsule. Even in early stages free tumor cells can frequently be collected from the peritoneal cavity by peritoneal washings. These cells have a tendency to implant. Peritoneal fluid, which has a high rate of turnover, is drained through lymphatic channels located in the diaphragms (Feldman and Knapp 1974). Its movement is directed by changes in intraperitoneal hydrostatic pressures (Meyers 1970). During respiration, the hydrostatic pressure in the subphrenic compartments of the peritoneal cavity falls with inspiration (creating a negative pressure under the diaphragms) and rises with expiration. Consequently, the undersurface of the diaphragm serves as a pump to drain peritoneal fluid and cells from the lower compartments. The fluid and cells, having reached the diaphragmatic leafs, are collected into a rich network of lymphatics located underneath the mesothelial cell lining of the undersurface of the diaphragm (French, Florey, and Morris 1960). This mechanism accounts for more than 80% of the drainage from the peritoneal cavity. The remainder of the drainage is into the upper paraaortic nodes. Often multiple small nodules found on the surface of the dome of the liver, on the subdiaphragmatic peritoneum, or in the lateral colic gutter represent the only clinical evidence of metastasis to the abdominal cavity.

Peritoneal cytology may reveal clusters of malignant cells after a clinically negative exploration. Specimens are obtained by lavaging the areas lateral to the ascending and descending colon, undersurface of the diaphragms, and pelvis with isotonic saline solution.

Therapy Selection

Epithelial ovarian malignancies respond to both radiation and chemotherapy. Careful treatment selection is essential if the full potential of either modality is to be realized. By determining the exact location and extent of intraabdominal disease, the surgeon supplies necessary information for this selection. External beam radiotherapy will be less effective if tumor implants are present either on the liver or on the peritoneum covering the kidneys because irreversible damage to these organs will occur at doses below the level required to control tumor implants.

One of the basic concepts of curative radiotherapy implies the use of tumoricidal doses in an attempt to induce a permanent control of treated areas. The assessment of tumoricidal dose levels requires a knowledge of the time-dose relationship for tumor sterilization and the acceptable limits of normal tissue tolerance. Since the details of time-dose relationship for ovarian tumors are unknown, the dose level employed in patients with carcinoma of the ovary has been governed by the limits of tolerance of the normal tissues encompassed by treatment fields. Based on our own experience, patients with multiple nodules exceeding 2 cm in greatest diameter are poor candidates for radiotherapy.

Ascitic fluid facilitates a free flow of malignant cells through the peritoneal cavity. Lead blocks used to shield the liver and kidneys from high-dose irradiation provide a potential sanctuary for these free-floating cells. Ascitic patients with large daily variation in abdominal girth may be technically difficult to treat. Patients with symptomatic ascitis are, in our experience, also poor candidates for curative radiotherapy, even though in some instances palliation could be obtained.

At Stanford, patients are selected for curative radiotherapy if they meet the following criteria: (1) stages I, II, and selected III disease with optimal surgical exploration and tumor masses no larger than 2 cm in greatest diameter; (2) no evidence of metastatic deposits on the peritoneum of the liver and kidneys; (3) no symptomatic ascites; (4) no evidence of distant metastasis; (5) no history of prior abdominal irradiation; and (6) no history of prior malignancy during the last five years.

Radiation Therapy

General Aspects

It has been estimated that approximately 75% of the patients with ovarian carcinoma will have neoplasm outside of the ovary at the time of initial exploration. These patients need some type of additional treatment postoperatively. Irradiation is often chosen, but its role has been the subject of considerable controversy. Radiotherapists do not agree about the need for upper abdominal treatment in addition to pelvic irradiation in patients with stages I and II cancers, nor is there a standard form for treatment fields, dose rate, total dose, or use of megavoltage equipment when irradiation to the entire peritoneal cavity is to be administered. It is currently accepted in most institutions where a large experience has accumulated that patients selected for irradiation should receive treatment to the entire abdomen and pelvis. This treatment plan is based on the concept that ovarian cancer is a disease of the entire abdomen. Cells that escape from the primary ovarian tumor circulate thoughout the entire abdominal cavity and, obviously, cannot be reached if treatment is directed to the pelvis only. This concept is supported by the fact that 25% to 30% of patients with stage 1 cancer will recur intraperitoneally if treated with surgery alone. Dembo and colleagues (1979) analyzed the patterns of failure in patients with stage I and II disease treated with a pelvic field at the Princess Margaret Hospital in Toronto. They describe a 29% incidence of abdominal failure despite a pelvis clear of tumor. Rosenoff and colleagues (1975) reviewed a group of patients with ovarian cancer in whom peritoneoscopy was done within one month of exploratory laparotomy. Six of the seven patients who were thought to have ovarian carcinoma localized to the pelvis (stages I, II) were found upon peritoneoscopy to have disease in the subdiaphragmatic area. Metastatic diaphragmatic involvement was found in 77% of the 30 patients studied. It should be clear from all this evidence that if postoperative radiotherapy is to be used with curative intent in stage I and II disease, the entire abdomen and pelvis must be treated. Anything less is doomed to fail.

Types of Radiation

External beam irradiation and installation of radioisotopes are both utilized in the postoperative treatment of ovarian cancer. External beam is best delivered with megavoltage equipment such as linear accelerators and Betatron units with energies of at least 6 Mv to obtain a homogeneous and acceptable depth dose distribution. These beams are well collimated and sharply defined, minimizing the problems associated with the penumbra from cobalt units or kilovoltage equipment. This allows precise blocking of kidneys and liver without underdosage of surrounding tissues due to penumbra. The high dose rates of the megavoltage units decrease the daily treatment time and minimize the influence of patient movement on treatment. External beam is best used as postoperative therapy for ovarian cancer two to four weeks after surgery.

Because the entire peritoneal cavity is known to be at risk in ovarian cancer, the Stanford philosphy has been to treat the entire abdomen with boost to the paraaortic and diaphragmatic lymphatics and the pelvis. Our current technique has been used for two years and represents an attempt to maximize the dose to high-risk areas, limit the exposure to sensitive organs, and provide a tolerable course of therapy for the patient (fig. 12.1).

Treatment is divided into three phases. All treatment is via AP opposed technique treating two fields per day. Initially the true pelvis is irradiated (from L4–5 to the obturator foramina) to 900 rad in one week at 180 rad/fraction. The field is then opened to include the entire abdominal and pelvic peritoneum and extend from 1 cm above the domes of the diaphragms to the obturator foramina. Treatment is continued at 150 rad per day to a dose of 3000 rad. One hundred percent posterior kidney blocks are introduced at 1000 rad and 50% transmission blocks shield the liver anteriorly and posteriorly for the last 1500 rad. At this point the pelvis has received 3900 rad, upper abdomen 3000 rad, kidneys 2000 rad, and liver 2250 rad. A planned one-week rest period is given for recovery of bone marrow and gastrointestinal toxicity. The third and last phase involves treatment to the paraaortic "T" and pelvis. The vertical part of the "T" covers the paraaortic nodes. The horizontal part covers the medial half of each diaphragm, 1 cm above the domes. The pelvic field is identical to the initial one, covering only the true pelvis. This region is treated to an additional 1200 rad in 150 rad fractions,

Figure 12.1

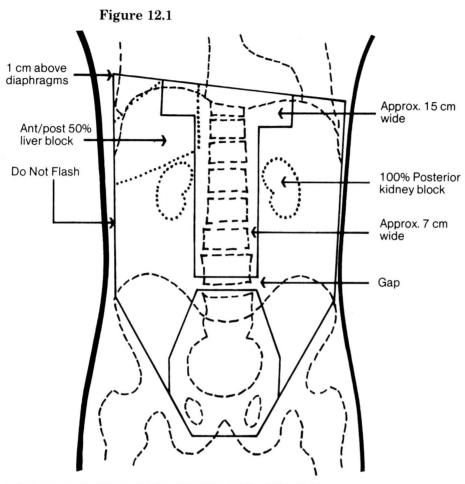

Port	Daily Dose	Pelvis	Abdomen	T-P.A.	
Pelvis	180 × 5	900			
Pelvis and T	150 × 8	1200		1200	
Abdomen-pelvis	150 × 20	3000	3000	3000	K-B- 1000 r L-B- 1500 r
Totals		5100	3000	4200	

Whole abdominopelvic and T boost technique for ovarian cancer.

yielding a total of 4200 rad to the paraaortic "T" and 5100 rad to the pelvis. If residual disease is known to have been left in the pelvis postoperatively, a boost of up to 900 rad may be given to a cone-down field in fractions 180 rad.

We have treated several patients with this aggressive technique, and comparison with the previously published technique by Glatstein, Fuks, and Bagshaw (1977) showed that the presently used one is much better tolerated with less gastrointestinal and liver toxicity. The follow-up is too short to assess the impact on survival with this new technique.

Intraperitoneal installation of radioisotopes has been widely used in ovarian cancer. They only penetrate a few millimeters into the tissues and can only treat cancers as free cells within the peritoneal cavity or as very small peritoneal surface implants. Two isotopes are frequently used, radioactive gold (^{198}Au) and radioactive chromic phosphate (^{32}P). Colloidal ^{198}Au emits 90% beta rays and is a 10% gamma emitter. The half-life is 2.7 days. The colloid is taken up by serosal macrophages and 90% of its ionizing radiation is absorbed within the first few millimeters of the peritoneal surface. Muller (1968) has estimated that 150 mCi of ^{198}Au delivers approximately 6000 to 7000 rad, with an additional 750 gamma component. The poor penetration of gold and frequent complications such as intestinal obstruction and dense peritoneal fibrosis have limited its usefulness. Colloidal ^{32}P is a pure beta emitter with a maximum energy of 1.7 Mv and effective range from 4 to 6 mm of tissue. Its half-life is 14.2 days. The colloid is removed from the fluid soon after the injection and is fixed on or near the surface of the lining of the peritoneal cavity, partly within phagocytes and partly absorbed on these surfaces. It is not systemically absorbed sparing radiation dose to intraabdominal organs and bone marrow. No major adverse effects have been seen and it is better tolerated than ^{198}Au.

Radiotherapy Results

Pezner and associates (1978) reported 95 cases with stages I and II epithelial carcinoma of the ovary who received intraperitoneal radiocolloids. Forty-nine of these patients also received external beam irradiation to the pelvis. The actuarial survival at five years was 95% for 20 patients with stage I_{ai}, 82% for 23 patients with stage I_{aii}, 70% for 30 patients with stages I_b, I_c, and 67% for 18 patients with stage II_a and II_b without gross residual tumor. Piver (1972) describes a 94% (17 of 18) survival in stage I_a patients after surgery plus installation of a radioactive colloid. In a smaller group of patients with stage I_a treated by surgery alone, the survival was not as good. Hilaris and Clark (1971) reported a five-year survival in 57 stage I_{a-b-c} patients with and without ^{32}P to be 92% (24 of 26 patients) and 64% (20 of 31 patients), respectively. All of these authors reported an absence of major adverse effects, either in the postoperative period or at a later date attributable to the installation of ^{32}P.

306

At Stanford University Medical Center, 153 patients with stages I, II, and III epithelial ovarian cancer were treated prior to April 1977. Of these patients, 102 received lower abdominal radiotherapy, while the remaining patients were almost equally divided between either a pelvic-paraaortic or pelvic and upper abdominal field. The overall relapse-free survival at 10 years for stages I, II, and III patients was 83%, 60%, and 22%, respectively. The amount of residual disease left after surgery was analyzed as a single variable. The 153 patients were divided into three groups: gross residual disease (grd) when masses larger than 2 cm were left either in the pelvis and/or abdomen, 54 patients; minimal residual disease (mrd) when masses up to 2 cm in largest dimension were left, 50 patients; and no residual disease (nrd) when an optimal surgical procedure was performed, and no evidence of macroscopic residual disease was noted, 49 patients. The 10-year relapse-free survival for the nrd group was 75%, mrd 54%, and grd 18%. The difference between nrd and mrd was not statistically significant ($P = 0.07$). The differences, however, between these two groups and the grd group were highly significant ($P < 0.0005$). These data support our contention mentioned previously in Therapy Selection that external beam irradiation is effective in controlling residual disease up to 2 cm in largest dimension. When analyzing the first site of relapse, 75% of the upper abdominal failures occurred in patients where the upper abdomen was not irradiated. This single factor explains the improved results seen in the Princess Margaret series where whole abdominal-pelvic irradiation was used.

Smith, Rutledge, and Delclos (1975), from the M.D. Anderson Hospital, reported their experience with 149 patients with epithelial ovarian cancer treated between 1969 to 1974. Patients were randomized postoperatively between abdominopelvic irradiation (70 patients) and systemic chemotherapy (79 patients). Although the groups are comparable in terms of histology, better prognostic indicators such as a grade of the tumor, type of surgical procedure, and extent of residual disease are not reported. Unfortunately, no attempt was made to stratify the treatment groups by stage and this resulted in a larger percentage of patients with stage I cancer being treated with chemotherapy, and a larger number of stage II$_b$ patients treated with irradiation. Patients treated with irradiation received treatment to the whole abdomen by the moving strip technique as described by Delclos. Chemotherapy consisted of melphalan, at a dosage of 0.2 mg/kg/day for five days. These five-day cycles were repeated every four weeks for a minimum of twelve cycles. It is clear that the two groups of patients cannot be compared and that crucial information regarding several prognostic indicators is not reported. Nevertheless, the authors show no difference in five-year survival of the patients by treatment modality (71% for the irradiated group and 72% for the chemotherapy group). An important finding was reported: the five-year survival rate by the Berkson-Gage method in stage I cancer patients treated with irradiation alone was 100%, in contrast to only 86% for the chemotherapy group. Few of the chemotherapy treated patients have developed leukemia.

Of great concern are the recent reports of acute leukemia following alkylating-agent therapy for ovarian cancer. Reimer and associates (1977) published a 36-fold increase over expected level for patients receiving chemotherapy, which rose to a 171-fold increase level for those surviving two years.

Bush and associates (1977), of the Princess Margaret Hospital in Toronto, published the preliminary results of a randomized clinical trial for stages I, II, and asymptomatic III epithelial ovarian carcinoma treated by either whole abdominal and pelvic radiation with the strip technique, or pelvic irradiation and chlorambucil. For stages I and II disease only a third arm was included using pelvic irradiation alone. Two hundred seventy-nine patients were included in the study from April 1971 to April 1975. At the time of publication in April 1977, two important findings were apparent: (1) when the overall survival rate in this prospective clinical trial was compared to the retrospective series, it was found to be significantly higher for the current trial, and (2) the completeness of the initial operation was correlated with an improved survival.

Recently, Dembo and associates (1979a; 1979b) have updated the Princess Margaret Hospital's results. Bilateral salpingo-oophorectomy and hysterectomy was performed in 132 patients with stages I_b to, II, and asymptomatic III cancers. Thirty-six percent of these patients had known gross residual disease less than 2 cm in diameter. The follow-up period of these patients ranged from 3 to 7.7 years, with a median follow-up time of 5.2 years. Prior to randomization, the patients were stratified by age, stage, and tumor type and grade. For stages I_b and II cancers, pelvic irradiation to 4500 rad in 20 fractions was designated as the standard postoperative treatment. The objective was to determine if survival could be improved significantly by addition of either 6 mg daily of chlorambucil for two years, or irradiation to the upper abdomen. Patients with stages I_b and II disease were randomized between all three therapies. Stage III patients were randomized between pelvic radiation plus chlorambucil and pelvic plus abdominal irradiation. In the latter, pelvic radiation of 2250 rad was followed by a downward moving strip delivering 2250 rad to the whole abdomen and pelvis. The upper margin was radiologically verified to be at least 1 cm above the dome of the diaphragms, and no liver shielding was used. These two factors distinguish the technique from the moving strip described by Delclos and Smith (1973). Pelvico-abdominal irradiation was found to improve survival significantly as compared with the other two therapies. The five-year actuarial survival was 38% for the pelvic irradiation group, 44% for the pelvic irradiation and chlorambucil group, and 77% for the pelvic and abdominal irradiation group. This difference is statistically significant at a P value less than 0.01 and reflects better control of occult upper abdominal disease. The upper abdominal failure rate in patients with a controlled pelvis was 26% for the pelvic irradiation group, 29% for the pelvic irradiation and chlorambucil group, and 2% for the pelvic plus upper abdominal irradiation group. This is statistically highly significant at a P value of less than 0.001.

There was also a strong correlation between tumor grade and treatment failures. In patients with well-differentiated tumors, the risk of relapse is less than in poorly differentiated tumors ($P = 0.05$). Adjuvant pelvic and upper abdominal irradiation significantly reduces the risk of relapse in patients with poorly differentiated histologies. Three out of 23 patients with poorly differentiated tumors in the irradiated group failed, compared with 12 of 18 patients treated with chlorambucil ($P = 0.001$). Young and associates (1978) also reported poor results to single agent and combination chemotherapy in patients with poorly differentiated tumors.

This study clearly demonstrated that abdominopelvic irradiation improves survival in patients with stages I, II, and asymptomatic III disease when careful radiotherapy techniques encompassing the entire peritoneum are utilized. Other drugs are now known to be more effective than single agents in treatment of ovarian cancer. The study demonstrates excellent five-year actuarial survival but does not answer the question regarding the superiority of adjuvant radiotherapy over more effective and currently utilized chemotherapeutic agents.

In an attempt to (1) reproduce the Princess Margaret Hospital results with radiotherapy and (2) to study the efficacy of adjuvant combination chemotherapy, a randomized prospective clinical trial will soon be initiated at Stanford. It will compare whole abdominal and pelvic irradiation (with the technique described in this chapter) to pelvic irradiation followed by Adriamycin and cyclophosphamide, two drugs known to be highly effective in the treatment of ovarian cancer.

References

Bush, R.S. et al. Treatment of epithelial carcinoma of the ovary: operation, irradiation and chemotherapy. *Am. J. Obstet. Gynecol.* 127:692–704, 1977.

Cordier, G. Quelques precisions sur la vascularisations et sur l'anatomie des lymphatique de l'ovaire. *Bull. Fed. Soc. Gynecol. Obstet. Fr.* 11:109–129, 1959.

Delclos, L., and Smith J.P. Tumors of the ovary. In *Textbook of radiotherapy*, ed. G.H. Fletcher. Philadelphia: Lea and Febiger, 1973.

Dembo, A.J. et al. The effectiveness of adjuvant abdominopelvic irradiation in ovarian cancer. In *Adjuvant therapy for cancer II,* eds. S.E. Salmon and S.E. Jones. New York: Grune and Stratton, 1979a.

Dembo, A.J. et al. Ovarian carcinoma: improved survival following abdominopelvic irradiation in patients with a completed pelvic operation. *Am. J. Obstet. Gynecol.* 134:793–800, 1979b.

Eichner, E., and Bove, E.R. In vivo studies on the lymphatic drainage of the human ovary. *Obstet. Gynecol.* 3:287–297, 1954.

Feldman, G.B., and Knapp, R.C. Lymphatic drainage of the peritoneal cavity and its significance in ovarian cancer. *Am. J. Obstet. Gynecol.* 119:991–994, 1974.

French, J.E.; Florey, H.W.; and Morris, B. The absorption of particles by the lymphatics of the diaphragm. *Q. J. Exp. Biol.* 45:88–103, 1960.

Fuks, Z. External radiotherapy of ovarian cancer: standard approaches and new frontiers. *Semin. Oncol.* 2:253–266, 1975.

Fuks, Z., and Bagshaw, M.A. The rationale for curative radiotherapy for ovarian carcinoma, *Int. J. Radiat. Oncol. Biol. Phys.* 1:21–32, 1975.

Glatstein, E.; Fuks, Z.; and Bagshaw, M.A. Diaphragmatic treatment in ovarian carcinoma: a new radiotherapeutic technique. *Int. J. Radiat. Oncol. Biol. Phys.* 2:357–362, 1977.

Hilaris, B., and Clark, D. The value of postoperative intraperitoneal injection of radiocolloids in early cancer of the ovary. *Am. J. Roentgenol.* 112:749–754, 1971.

Meyers, M.A. The spread and localization of acute intraperitoneal effusions. *Radiology* 95:547–554, 1970.

Muller, J.H. Intraperitoneal colloidal radiogold [198]Au therapy in ovarian cancer. In *Ovarian cancer,* UICC monograph series, vol. 2. Berlin: Springer-Verlag, 1968.

Ozols, R.F. et al. Advanced, ovarian cancer. Correlation of histological grade with response to therapy and survival. *Cancer* 45:572–581, 1980.

Pezner, R. et al. Limited epithelial carcinoma of the ovary treated with curative intent by the intraperitoneal instillation of radio colloids. *Cancer* 42:2563–2571, 1978.

Piver, S. Radioactive colloids in the treatment of stage I_a ovarian cancer. *Obstet. Gynecol.* 40:42–44, 1972.

Reimer, R. et al. Acute leukemia after alkylating-agent therapy of ovarian cancer. *N. Engl. J. Med.* 297:177–181, 1977.

Rosenoff, S. et al. Peritoneoscopy: a valuable staging tool in ovarian carcinoma. *Ann. Intern. Med.* 83:37–41, 1975.

Rouviere, H. *Anatomic des lymphatiques de l'homme.* Paris: Mason, 1932.

Smith, J.P.; Rutledge, F.; and Delclos, L. Results of chemotherapy as an adjuvant to surgery in patients with localized ovarian cancer. *Semin. Oncol.* 2:227–281, 1975.

Webb, M.J. et al. Factors influencing survival in stage I ovarian cancer. *Am. J. Obstet. Gynecol.* 116:222, 1973.

Young, R. et al. Advanced ovarian adenocarinoma a prospective clinical trial of melphalen versus combination chemotherapy. *N. Eng. J. Med.* 299:1261–1266, 1978.

310

Chapter 13

The Appropriate Extent of Bulk Resection in Advanced Ovarian Cancer

PERSPECTIVE:

Donald G. C. Clark

The clinical problems associated with advanced ovarian cancer are among the most challenging presented to the gynecologic oncologist. The mortality rate in ovarian cancer is the highest of any gynecologic cancer in the United States, and two-thirds of the patients with ovarian cancer are diagnosed at an advanced stage and develop complications associated with massive disease such as the malnutrition which is well illustrated by the drawing of the typical patient shown at the beginning of Barber's monograph on ovarian cancer (1978).

In the experimental animal the therapeutic results obtained by chemotherapy are in inverse proportion to the tumor load the animal has at the time of treatment, and there is increasing evidence that this inverse relationship holds true in the human patient. Bulk resection of the tumor, therefore, may be justified on the basis of an anticipated improvement in the response to subsequent chemotherapy or radiotherapy (Griffiths 1975; Hudson and Chir 1973; Symmonds 1975; Tobias and Griffiths 1976; Puck et al. 1957) and may also be of benefit in the immediate relief of symptoms produced by the tumor or its associated ascitic or pleural effusion. Bulk resection may also be accomplished with secondary benefit in patients who are explored for the relief of other problems such as intestinal or urinary tract obstruction.

Bulk reduction in tumor may not only result in a better response to secondary therapy as noted above but may in itself improve the immunologic status of the patient by reversing the possibly immunosuppressant effect of the tumor and allowing the host immune response to function better since acquired immunologic tolerance may result from antigens produced by such large bulk of disease.

In summary, bulk resection (perhaps more elegantly phrased as cytoreductive surgery) is indicated for the following reasons: (1) patient's psychologic benefit from the removal of the obviously bulky disease with associated ascites; (2) relief of discomfort associated with tumor; (3) improved response to subsequent chemotherapeutic or radiotherapeutic measures; and (4) possible reversal of immunologic depression.

Patient Evaluation

At the time of admission to the hospital many of these patients are in extremely poor general condition as the result of weeks or months of inadequate alimentation and, in addition, to the direct metabolic effects of the tumor. This poor general status is reflected in the associated anemia, hypoproteinemia, and other abnormalities associated with specific organ dysfunction. Dehydration is a common problem and, until recently, operation on such patients was hazardous and carried a hospital mortality rate from 5% to 25%, depending on the selection of patients and the magnitude of the operation performed. Since the development of total parenteral nutrition, however, it has been possible, in a reasonable period of time, to bring these patients into a much better physiologic state prior to anesthesia and operation. At the time of admission these patients should have a thorough medical evaluation, including a chest film, electrocardiogram, intravenous pyelogram, and barium enema, while upper gastrointestinal series and bone scan or other specialized studies should be employed as indicated.

Intestinal obstruction, or ileus, which is frequently associated with advanced disease, should be treated initially by long-tube intestinal intubation while the patient's general condition is improved by blood transfusion, if indicated, and total parenteral nutrition. The past history of the patient, with particular reference to prior treatment of the ovarian cancer, should be investigated thoroughly, and before aggressive surgical management is pursued, the previous surgical findings and likelihood of further response to chemotherapy or radiotherapy should be evaluated. These factors are important since the response rate to chemotherapy at the time of initial treatment has been reported as 45% to 65%, while the response rate of patients who have failed chemotherapy is much less (Hreshchyshyn 1973; Beck and Boyes 1968; Young, Hubbard, and DeVita 1974). Each patient consequently must be treated as an individual, and preoperative, intraoperative, and postoperative management must be designed carefully to suit the problems at hand. When the decision to operate has been reached, the patient should be placed on appropriate bowel preparation with the administration of laxatives and limitation of residue in the diet, and the use of intestinal antibiotics such as neomycin and erythromycin base.

In the management of these problems, it is of great importance that the surgeon, chemotherapist, and radiotherapist act as a team so that the skills of all these disciplines may be brought to bear on the problem at the appropriate time. The presence of the radiotherapist in the operating room, for example, can be of great value in the selection of the best mode of therapy. Preoperative preparation of the patient must also include consultation with the anesthetist and evaluation of the patient's respiratory and cardiac function. Thoracentesis for removal of large pleural effusion the night before surgery should be done for cytologic study and improvement in respiratory reserve. Insertion of a central venous line for monitoring is mandatory, since marked hemodynamic alterations associated with the removal of massive amounts of ascitic fluid and blood loss may occur and may present a life-threatening problem. The cooperation of an experienced and competent anesthesia staff and availability of a recovery room and intensive care unit have proven invaluable.

Surgical Techniques

The first principle in the treatment of ovarian cancer, regardless of extent of tumor, is that of adequate exposure. A mid-line or paramedian incision should be used in every case, and indeed, such an incision may extend from the xiphoid to the pubis to obtain adequate exposure of the entire abdominal cavity. The patient's abdomen should be prepared and draped accordingly. It is the author's preference to use a paramedian incision, initially extending from a point about 4 cm above to 10 cm below the umbilicus. This limited incision can be carried down to the peritoneum, which is then opened with a small incision and any ascitic fluid can be removed by an aspirator, initially fairly slowly. Following this, the peritoneum can be opened to the length of the incision to allow complete aspiration to be carried out. This limited incision is used to determine whether or not significant bulk resection is indeed feasible, and, if the findings contraindicate further operation, appropriate biopsies can be taken and the abdomen closed. Such a decision might be based, for example, on the finding of diffuse tumor spread over the entire peritoneal surface (both parietal and visceral), where almost no normal organ can be detected and where no mass of tumor lends itself to resection. Such cases are often associated with massive ascites and with intestinal dysfunction described by Brunschwig as carcinomatous ileus. In such cases, no surgical attack has been of any value. Even such a palliative procedure as a decompressive jejunostomy in an attempt to remove the nasal gastric tube has been of no avail. Following this exploration, if the presenting features indicate the feasibility of a significant bulk resection, the abdominal incision may be extended easily to allow adequate exposure in the pelvis and upper abdomen.

As a general rule in the bulk removal of ovarian cancer, it is wise to avoid resection of intestine or enterotomy unless indicated by concomitant intestinal obstruction, since the incidence of subsequent fistula is significant.

The common mode of spread of ovarian cancer is by intraperitoneal seeding, and much of this secondary growth is frequently found in the omentum. The second route is by the retroperitoneal lymph nodes along the infundibulopelvic and periaortic node chains. As a consequence of this unusual type of spread, it is found in many cases that the bulk of the tumor involves the ovaries, the intervening uterus, and the greater and lesser omenta, and it is often possible, therefore, to remove a large amount of tumor by resecting these organs. Furthermore, it is not uncommon to open the peritoneum and be able to see nothing but gross cancer, which, however, may be only malignant infiltration in the omentum, and by adequate exposure and evaluation it may be found that underlying intestine is relatively unaffected. If the bulk of tumor in the omentum is not too marked, a simple excision of the greater omentum, removing it from the transverse colon, together with a bilateral oophorectomy, may provide a very adequate bulk excision. If the infiltration of the omentum is extensive, however, it is often preferable to continue the dissection upward, removing the omentum from the colon, and entering the lesser sac to extend the removal to the greater curvature of the stomach. In many cases, despite massive infiltration of the greater or lesser omentum, the adjacent transverse colon and stomach are surprisingly little involved, although a small amount of tumor may be left on one or both organs. Care must be taken during such surgery to avoid injury to the middle colic artery and spleen or splenic pedicle, and a close evaluation of these must be carried out at the conclusion of such resection. If injury to the spleen is noted, a splenectomy should be done. In the pelvis, removal of the affected ovaries alone may be of value, but probably such cases benefit by a significant removal of bulk of tumor as recommended by Munnell, Jacox, and Taylor (1957). A frequent finding is the involvement of the uterus together with the adnexal tumor masses, and its removal may well be indicated; in such a situation it is advisable to do a supracervical hysterectomy, since a total hysterectomy would frequently entail entering the vagina through gross tumor with the probability of subsequent tumor growth into the vagina. In our experience, this problem has been more hypothetical than real, but in view of the patient's probable limited life span, removal of the cervical stump is hardly necessary, and since these tumors are often associated with an abnormal course of the ureter, it may be wise to limit the resection.

Following the above procedures, inspection of the abdomen may reveal further tumor masses which can be removed with relative facility. Again, attention should be directed to the careful preservation of the integrity of the intestine for the reasons outlined above. A thorough evaluation of the remaining tumor extent should be carried out, with inspection of the subdiaphragmatic spaces on both sides, paracolic gutters, and the retroperitoneal area. Hemostasis should be as complete as possible, with appropriate ligation or suture ligation and electrocauterization where indicated. The abdomen should be closed tightly, without drainage. The writer's preference is for a Tom Jones type of suture with No. 28 or No. 30 stainless steel wire. When recurrence of ascites is expected, a similar type of closure reinforced by retention sutures may be indicated. Postoperatively the nasogastric or Cantor tube, Foley catheter, and central venous line are maintained until the patient's status is stable and intestinal function has returned. It is worth noting that an omentectomy is often associated with a prolonged ileus, and delayed return of intestinal function for five to seven days is not uncommon. Total parenteral nutrition should be maintained until the patient's oral intake is adequate. Antibiotics are employed intraoperatively, and since these patients are classically at high risk for subsequent phlebitis, they are kept on miniheparin, 5000 units, every eight hours from the time of operation until they are fully ambulatory.

Special Problems

Patients explored for bulk resection of tumor frequently have other problems associated with their disease which require surgical correction. The commonest and the most significant of these are obstruction of the intestinal and/or urinary tracts and ascites. Intestinal obstruction is perhaps one of the most difficult to handle and requires a careful evaluation of the patient and mature surgical judgment. The majority of these patients have recurrent or persistent cancer, and their nutritional status is frequently very poor as a result of both tumor and toxicity associated with treatment. The first decision to be made is whether or not immediate operation is required. This may be indicated by questionable viability of the intestine or impending rupture. Such problems must be estimated by careful examination of the abdomen, appropriate x-ray studies, and such other indicators as fever or leukocytosis. In the absence of these indications, and they are relatively uncommon, a more conservative approach may be appropriate.

Intestinal Obstruction and Fistula

When operation for bulk reduction is not indicated by physical examination or history of recent exploration, it may still be necessary for obstruction. At such a time it is usually advisable to pass a long nasointestinal tube to relieve the patient's immediate symptoms, and follow this with appropriate correction of the patient's nutritional status, dehydration, and electrolyte imbalance. In a few cases, such measures may result in relief of the obstruction, with subsequent removal of the tube; the patient's chemotherapy and radiotherapy may then be reinstituted. On the other hand, if operation is still necessary, the patient is in a much better physical condition to withstand it.

Before the development of total parenteral nutrition, the surgical attack on obstructed intestine in the presence of abdominal carcinomatosis was frequently followed by the development of intestinal fistula. In our hands, at that time, the fistula rate was over 30%. With parenteral nutrition, however, healing appears to be improved and, in recent years, the fistula rate has been markedly reduced. At the time of laparotomy, the hope is that the obstruction may be caused by adhesions, secondary to previous operation, or by a small amount of obstructing tumor, either of which can be relieved readily with a rather minimal procedure. Indeed, such cases do occasionally occur, but most often one finds abdominal carcinomatosis with more than one area of partial obstruction, perhaps complicated by infiltration of the mesentery, which may require multiple areas of resection or bypass, or extensive excision of the small intestine. It is our feeling that, in patients with such findings, the least extensive procedure to relieve the obstruction should be carried out, and frequently this would be done by ileotransverse colostomy, end to side, with the proximal end of the defunctionalized ileum brought out as a mucous fistula. When feasible, a side-to-side ileoileostomy or ileotransverse colostomy may be considered. Whenever possible, massive resection of bowel should be avoided, unless the evaluation of the involved intestine indicates the probability of a subsequent blind loop obstruction. When anastomoses are carried out, the intestine should be carefully inspected to try to obtain an anastomosis in an area uninvolved by tumor. In our experience, a classic two-layer anastomosis has been the practice, although in recent years a staple type of resection and anastomosis has been done with excellent results. A frequent problem with obstruction is the spontaneous or iatrogenic formation of an intestinal fistula and, in such cases, the need for surgery must be based on the patient's life expectancy, the leak's site in the intestine, and the patient's general medical status. Such evaluation would follow the steps outlined above for intestinal obstruction, and the surgical correction of the fistula is done essentially in the same way, with the exception, of course, that the fistulized loop must be isolated entirely from the reconstructed gastrointestinal tract. In general, the deliberate formation of a mucous fistula from this isolated bowel is not necessary, since the already established fistula serves this purpose quite adequately.

The above surgical procedures are frequently followed by prolonged periods of ileus, and consequently long tube intubation and parenteral nutrition must be continued in the postoperative phase. Peri-operative antibiotics and mini-heparin prophylaxis are used routinely, although the heparin may be discontinued during operation if much friable tumor with copious bleeding is noted.

Urinary Tract Obstruction

Urinary tract obstruction is more common than was previously thought, and often can only be detected with the routine use of an intravenous pyelogram as part of the patient's preoperative evaluation. In the very advanced case with extensive cancer, in whom the primary modes of therapy have failed, and in the absence of specific symptoms, no treatment may be indicated, but where an adequate trial of surgery and chemotherapy has not been given, or where supervening infection with pyelonephritis is present, operative intervention may be required. In obstructive pyelonephritis, adequate drainage must be obtained either by appropriate pyelostomy or nephrostomy, and, in cases of long standing, a nephrectomy may be necessary. For obstruction with accompanying uremia, careful consideration must be given to the quality of the remaining life of the patient before surgical relief is attempted. A hopeless situation should be discussed with the family and, if indicated, with the patient. When active treatment is indicated, an initial trial should be made to pass a retrograde catheter through the ureters and, although this is rarely successful, it does work sufficiently often to warrant the attempt. If this fails, dialysis may be indicated as a temporary measure prior to corrective operation. At operation, the ideal situation occurs when the ureter or ureters can be reimplanted directly into the bladder, but this is often not feasible because of involvement by tumor or damage by prior radiation. Similarly the formation of an ileal conduit may be contraindicated, in which case cutaneous ureterostomy, pyelostomy, or nephrostomy may be the only procedure available.

Ascites

Ascites is a very common finding with cancer of the ovary and may be distressing indeed. This often does not respond to the usual medical management of ascites secondary to cardiac or hepatic disease. Abdominal paracentesis may be carried out for the immediate relief of distress or to obtain fluid for cytologic evaluation but in general is contraindicated because such fluid rapidly reforms with concomitant loss of protein and electrolyte. The relief of ascites may be the most important secondary benefit of bulk resection, and a rather modest reduction in the amount of tumor may be enough to restore the normal fluid balance in the abdominal cavity. The instillation of chemotherapeutic agents or a radioisotope into the abdominal cavity is often of little avail, per se, but in conjunction with bulk resection of the tumor, these added agents may be of value. It is worth noting that, in patients with ascites and accompanying pleural effusion, when the ascites can be controlled in the abdomen, the pleural effusion may disappear or may not recur after removal by thoracentesis.

References

Barber, H.R.K. *Ovarian carcinoma.* New York: Masson, 1978.

Beck, R.E., and Boyes, D.A. Treatment of 126 cases of advanced ovarian carcinoma with cyclophosphamide. *Can. Med. Assoc. J.* 98:539–541, 1968.

Griffiths, C.T. Surgical resection of tumor bulk in the primary treatment of ovarian cancer. *Nat. Cancer Inst. Monogr.* 42:101–104, 1975.

Hreshchyshyn, M.M. Single drug therapy in ovarian cancer—factors influencing response. *Gynecol. Oncol.* 1:220–232, 1973.

Hudson, C.N., and Chir, M. Surgical treatment of ovarian cancer, *Gynecol. Oncol.* 1:370–378, 1973.

Munnell, E.W.; Jacox, H.W.; and Taylor, H.C. Treatment and prognosis in cancer of the ovary. *Am. J. Obstet. Gynecol.* 74:1187–1200, 1957.

Puck, T.T. et al. Action of x-rays on mammalian cells. *J. Exp. Med.* 106:485–500, 1957.

Symmonds, R.E. Some surgical aspects of gynecologic cancer. *Cancer* 36:649–660, 1975.

Tobias, J.S., and Griffiths, C.T. Management of ovarian cancer. *N. Engl. J. Med.* 294:818–823, 1976.

Young, R.C.; Hubbard, S.P.; and DeVita, V.T. The chemotherapy of ovarian carcinoma. *Cancer Treat. Rev.* 1:99–110, 1974.

PERSPECTIVE:

The Appropriate Extent of Bulk Resection in Advanced Ovarian Cancer

Howard D. Homesley

In the past, extensive tumor bulk reduction in advanced epithelial ovarian cancer (FIGO stage III) has been advocated by many investigators. It is impossible, however, to assess the effect of bulk reduction alone on survival without recognition of other significant factors. It is generally recognized that the actual site of disease spread, amount of residual tumor, histologic grade, and volume of ascites all greatly influence therapeutic success.

The interaction of tumor resection, surgical-pathologic findings, and treatment regimens on survival of patients with advanced ovarian cancer will be discussed. A revision of FIGO stage III will be proposed that would clearly subcategorize patients according to the major determinants of survival. Findings of recent prospective randomized studies will be reviewed to place in perspective the role of tumor bulk reduction in advanced ovarian cancer in future clinical trials.

Tumor Reductive Surgery

Unfortunately, until the 1970s data pertaining to bulk reduction were primarily derived from retrospective analysis of nonrandomized series of patients treated for advanced ovarian cancer at single institutions over many years.

Aure, Hoeg, and Kolstad (1971) noted a much lower survival in patients who did not have complete removal of tumor, whereas survival was somewhat higher in stage III patients who had complete tumor removal compared to stage II patients who had tumor remaining. Similarly, Maus, MacKay, and Sellers (1968) reported a five-year survival of 5.9% for stage III, 48.4% for stage II_a, and 19.5% for stage II_b, recognizing that survival was improved and the likelihood of early recurrence was lower in patients having complete removal than for patients treated by incomplete surgical excision. Obel (1976) similarly determined that the extent of residual tumor as well as histologic grade were decisive in determining long-term survival.

Munnell (1968) reported in patients with advanced ovarian cancer (stage III) a 28% five-year survival in 36 patients who had undergone a "maximal surgical effort," a 9% five-year survival for 37 patients who had partial resection, and a 3% five-year survival for 34 patients who had biopsies only. Most of the survivors, however, had tumors of low histologic grade in which hysterectomy, bilateral salpingo-oophorectomy, and omentectomy were successful in removal of tumor bulk limited to these sites. It must be emphasized that improvement in survival occurred primarily in patients undergoing tumor resection where limited or less invasive tumor growth was completely resected when technically feasible. Omentectomy was not even performed in 200 patients from 1930 to 1943 and only in 52 of 235 patients from 1952 to 1961. Munnell, however, did conclude that, because of maximal operative procedures, there was improved survival directly related to use of more extensive surgery combined with radiation therapy in the later series of patients. Hudson and Chir (1973) advocated radical oophorectomy in which removal of the internal genitalia is combined with excision of the entire visceral and pelvic peritoneum through a retroperitoneal approach beginning at the pelvic brim. Obviously, this technique could not be applied to most patients with advanced ovarian cancer with extensive upper abdominal disease.

The retrospective analysis by Griffiths, Grogan, and Hall (1972) revealed that prolonged survival was achieved only when tumor volume was significantly reduced by surgery, particularly when localized to the pelvis, where full radiation therapy was added. Survival was directly related to the postoperative residual tumor volume, which was highly dependent upon the original volume and site of tumor. In a comprehensive statistical analysis Griffiths, in 1975, determined that the histologic grade of the tumor and the actual size of the largest residual mass were the only two factors of independent importance contributing to survival. Moreover, only when size of the largest residual mass was smaller than 1.6 cm in diameter was prolonged survival achieved. There was no correlation between the resection index (amount of tumor resected) and survival. Admittedly, the goal of the primary operation was removal of all or nearly all gross tumor, but unless at the conclusion of the procedure the tumor volume was reduced to less than 1.6 cm in diameter, survival was extremely poor.

Kjorstad, Welander, and Kolstad (1977) (table 13.1) reviewed a series of patients with advanced ovarian cancer in which preoperative irradiation was given to patients deemed inoperable prior to referral. Nearly half of these patients (41%), following 3000 rad, had tumor completely removed; however, there was only a 13% five-year survival in 36 patients who underwent complete resection who were deemed inoperable at first laparotomy. There was a

Table 13.1
Survival Rates in Relation to Treatment and
Operability

Treatment Groups	Number of Patients	Survival (%)		
		1 Year	2 Years	5 Years
Tumor totally resected prior to referral; no irradiation	154	51	32	24
Total resection of tumor after 3000 rad	36	42	27	13
Not totally resectable after 3000 rad following first laparotomy	34	28	17	5
Not totally resectable after 3000 rad deemed clinically inoperable initially	49	45	32	15

Source: Kjorstad, Welander, and Kolstad 1977.

9% postoperative mortality (13 deaths out of 145 patients) in patients undergoing resection. There was, however, a correlation found between amount of residual disease and survival. The amount of residual tumor following tumor bulk reduction in patients with advanced ovarian cancer greatly determines the success of subsequent management by radiation therapy. Delclos and Smith (1975) reported that for irradiation of carcinoma of the ovary a proportionate decrease in two- and five-year survivals was directly related to size of the largest residual tumor mass. Delclos and Quinlan (1969) reported that when radiation was used in patients with no palpable residual tumor in stage III, there was a four-year survival of 25% (5 out of 25 patients); however, when there was palpable tumor, they reported a four-year survival of only 8% (2 of 24 patients). Buchler and associates (1977) reported on patients treated by radiation therapy and by chemotherapy with subdivision of patients into favorable and unfavorable groups. The favorable group had a pelvic mass less than 8 cm or upper abdominal tumor nodules less than 2 cm. Patients with more massive disease were included in the unfavorable category. All the patients receiving radiation therapy were dead at nine months in the unfavorable category while there was longer survival in the chemotherapy group. Survival was similar between radiation therapy and chemotherapy in the favorable group. There was no analysis of the effects of histologic types, histologic grades, or ascites on survival.

Day and Smith (1975), although emphasizing that maximum reduction of tumor volume has probably been of benefit to patients with advanced ovarian cancer, did not advocate extensive operations or multiple bowel resection. They stressed that each residual lesion should be accurately recorded by notation of exact size and location with an estimate of the percentage of tumor removed and of aggregate tumor present. Accurate reporting of information gained at the time of operation was noted to be essential to evaluation of treatment by later clinical appraisal. As reported by Day and Smith, when patients had residual tumor greater than 1 cm, survival was extremely poor, with a five-year survival of 5% to 6%, compared to a 27% five-year survival for patients having no residual tumor and a 35% five-year survival for patients with 1 cm or less of residual disease (table 13.2).

Histologic Grade

Hart (1977) emphasized that a major factor in the wide variation in reported survival statistics in patients with ovarian carcinoma could be attributed largely to the inclusion of tumors of intermediate or borderline type in such reports. Unless the borderline tumor is specifically delineated, meaningful assessment of prognosis and efficacy of therapeutic modalities for ovarian carcinomas are severely hampered. Because the malignant potential of a tumor is determined by the least-differentiated portion, extensive sampling and multiple sections are essential for accurate diagnosis. As a general guideline, a block of tissue for each 1 to 2 cm of the tumor's maximal dimension must be evaluated.

Day and Smith noted a strong correlation in patients with advanced ovarian cancer between histologic grade and survival whereby survivals at one year were 80% for grade I, 30% for grade II, and 20% for grade III. The effects of grade on prognoisis held true for each histologic type, with decreased survival consistent with increased tumor grades. Low-grade tumors were more often confined to the pelvis than were high-grade tumors. The effect of grade on prognosis was not dependent upon extent of disease for serous carcinoma confined to the pelvis inasmuch as there was poor survival in

Table 13.2
Survival by Residual Disease—Stage III

Residual Tumor	Number of Patients	Survival (%)		
		1 Year	2 Years	5 Years
0	34	67	55	27
1 cm	31	55	39	35
1.1–2 cm	24	50	14	0
2.1–6 cm	95	22	13	0
> 6 cm	172	18	13	5
Unknown	32	—	—	—
Total	388			

Source: Day and Smith 1975.

high grade stage I and II patients as well as a markedly lower survival for grades II and III patients with stages III and IV disease.

Webb, Malkasian, and Gorgensen (1974) confirmed that the extent of surgical resection and tumor grade appeared to be the two major factors influencing survival, whereas the addition of radiation therapy to the treatment program did not. There was no significant difference between groups of patients having successful surgical resection after preoperatively receiving 3000 rad of therapy and those who had complete resection without preoperative irradiation.

Gallager (1975) has discussed a relationship between histologic type and prognosis as well as histologic grading of patients with cancer of the ovary, particularly emphasizing the complexities and interacting factors. He stressed that accurate histologic classification is essential before prospective treatment regimens can be expected to produce conclusive results. The problems in histologic classification relate to the common occurrence of more than one epithelial type in a single ovarian mass, where limited sampling may lead to inaccurate assessment of the basic dominant epithelial pattern. The major pathologic dilemma is to distinguish between epithelial types when tumors are poorly differentiated. In the past, the difficulty of distinguishing between poorly differentiated epithelial tumors apparently has encouraged lumping of tumors into the serous category, which would make mucinous and endometrioid tumors appear more benign than they may really be. Likewise, unresectable tumors may actually lead to deficient sampling when necrosis and hemorrhage in large masses preclude satisfactory histologic examination. Confusion can occur when metastatic neoplasms to the ovary are mistakenly determined to be primary carcinomas. As noted by Julian and associates (1974) in a review of 106 cases indexed as ovarian carcinoma at Johns Hopkins, on review only 82% (87 of 106 cases) were considered to represent primary ovarian malignancies. The other tumors were determined to be cancers secondary to gastrointestinal cancer, mixed tumors of the uterus, or lymphomas.

Malkasian, Decker, and Webb (1975), in an extensive review of 741 cases of epithelial ovarian cancer using Broder histologic grading, did determine that stage III grade I lesions had a 22% five-year survival, compared to a 3% five-year survival for grade III and IV for patients with serous cystadenocarcinomas. They concluded that a reliable evaluation of therapeutic results in ovarian carcinoma could not be achieved unless grade as well as stage were considered.

Ascites

Piver, Lele, and Barlow (1976) determined that 83% of ovarian cancer patients explored prior to referral to Roswell Park had an incision that was inadequate for evaluation of upper abdominal metastases to the diaphragm, liver, and periaortic nodes. Thorough surgical exploration is vital for accurate assessment of the extent of tumor spread. The presence of subdiaphragmatic involvement in ovarian cancer is extremely important as subdiaphragmatic spread may herald development of widespread peritoneal disease and ascites. Advanced disease within the diaphragm is likely to be associated with the presence of massive ascites. When the diaphragmatic lymphatic pathways become obstructed, the omentum likely becomes the principal route of peritoneal drainage. This may account for extensive omental involvement in patients with stage III disease.

Day and Smith noted that the amount of ascites present was directly related to survival, particularly at one year, where patients with no ascites had a 40% survival, compared to 21% for patients with ascites greater than 500 ml (table 13.3). The five-year survival for patients with massive ascites was 4% contrasting with patients with minimal (less than 500 cc) or no ascites, having five-year survivals of 17% and 15%, respectively. The one-year survival in patients with ascites greater than 500 cc was similar to the five-year survival in patients with minimal or no ascites.

Staging of Advanced Ovarian Cancer

Without doubt, the major prognostic factor in patients with ovarian cancer is the actual extent of disease, which is reflected by FIGO staging. Fortunately, staging for ovarian cancer is based on surgical-pathologic findings, unlike staging for the other gynecologic malignancies. Current FIGO staging, however, does not specify the wide variation in postoperative residual tumor bulk in patients with advanced ovarian carcinoma. There is no allowance for the amount of tumor present and the amount of tumor removed at the time of surgical exploration to reflect the true influence of surgical debulking on the further progress of the patients. It would be impractical to quantify the

Table 13.3
Survival by Ascites—Stage III

Ascites	Number of Patients	Survival (%)		
		1 Year	2 Years	5 Years
0	116	40	29	15
Minimal < (500 ml)	38	33	23	17
Large >(500 ml)	146	21	12	4
Unknown	88	—	—	—
Total	388			

Source: Day and Smith 1975.

326

amount of tumor removed, and this may not be all that important. Staging, however, should be devised to stratify patients into optimal and suboptimal categories based on the amount and site of residual disease. The other two significant prognostic factors of histologic grade and volume of ascites are ignored by current FIGO staging. Adequate surgical-pathologic staging would delineate the site and amount of residual tumor and subcategorize patients according to histologic grade and denote presence or absence of ascites (table 13.4). It makes little sense to have five subcategories for stage I, which includes less than 10% of ovarian cancer patients, and no subclassifications at all for the nearly 80% who have stage III disease.

Rubin (1975) has pointed out that ovarian cancer has been understaged and undertreated for decades because of concentration in the staging system on pelvic spread patterns. The extent of the tumor spread is the critical factor, and any attempt to analyze past reports is difficult because the lack of complete data can lead to invalid conclusions. Proper staging may include cytologic washings from the pelvis, lateral gutters, and diaphragm; inspection and biopsy of the diaphragm; pelvis and periaortic node biopsy; liver biopsy; omentectomy; and biopsies of any suspicious areas of the peritoneum of the bladder, cul-de-sac, and lateral gutters. This *requires* a vertical abdominal incision.

Young and Fisher (1978) discovered that patients prior to referral designated as stage I and II often had occult disease within the upper abdomen. Accurate staging is essential in determining the precise prognosis upon which further therapy is validly based.

Table 13.4
Proposed Staging Classification for Advanced
Ovarian Cancer Stage III

Stage III$_a$	Growth involving one or both ovaries with intraperitoneal metastasis outside the pelvis or with positive retroperitoneal nodes or both with or without histologically proved malignant extension to small bowel or omentum with no gross residual disease present following surgical resection
	Grade I: well differentiated Grade II: moderately differentiated Grade III: poorly differentiated
Stage III$_b$	Same as stage III$_a$ except residual tumor present with no single aggregate greater than 2 cm in diameter. Classify as grade I, II, or III
Stage III$_c$	Same as III$_a$ except residual tumor mass present with tumor diameter 2 cm greater. Classify as grade I, II, or III
Stage III$_d$	Stage III$_a$, III$_b$, or III$_c$ plus ascites greater than 500 cc present. Classify as grade I, II, or III

Major prognostic factors must also be incorporated into the staging classification to signify meaningful subcategories of disease within the same stage. There is such an extremely variable and wide range of tumor distribution and bulk in stage III ovarian cancer that interpretation and reporting of treatment results are confusing.

Clinical Trials

Johnson and associates (1972), in a study of stage III ovarian cancer for patients randomized to receive surgery and cyclophosphamide versus radiation therapy versus surgery, radiation therapy, and cyclophosphamide, noted a 20% survival at two years and less than 10% survival at five years with no difference between the treatment regimens. Most patients underwent total abdominal hysterectomy, bilateral salpingo-oophorectomy, and omentectomy with removal of as much tumor as feasible with residual nonpalpable tumor remaining in all patients.

In current Gynecologic Oncology Group protocols, patients with stage III ovarian cancer are subdivided into an optimal group (residual tumor 3 cm or less) and a suboptimal group (residual tumor greater than 3 cm). In reporting results of a prospective randomized study recently completed by the Gynecologic Oncology Group, Brady and associates (1979) found no difference in progression-free interval and survival in stage III patients treated by melphalan alone, radiation alone (abdominal and pelvic), melphalan followed by radiation therapy, and radiation therapy followed by melphalan (fig. 13.1). Median survival in the optimal group, however, was 15.7 months compared to 5 months for the suboptimal group (fig. 13.2). The majority of patients had grade II and III lesions, although patients with optimal disease had a higher percent (17.9%) of grade I lesions when compared to suboptimal patients (6.8%).

Patients with suboptimal stage III ovarian carcinoma prospectively randomized by the Gynecologic Oncology Group to melphalan alone versus melphalan and hexamethylmelamine versus Adriamycin and cyclophosphamide were recently determined to have similar response rates to melphalan alone compared to either of the other two combination chemotherapy regimens. Thus, in stage III suboptimal patients where tumor cannot be nearly completely excised, it remains controversial as to what chemotherapy will produce the best results.

Summary

The justification for extensive bulk reduction of advanced ovarian cancer should be improved survival, not palliation. There has not been and likely never will be a prospective randomized trial between groups of patients undergoing extensive surgical resection compared to a group having minimal

Figure 13.1

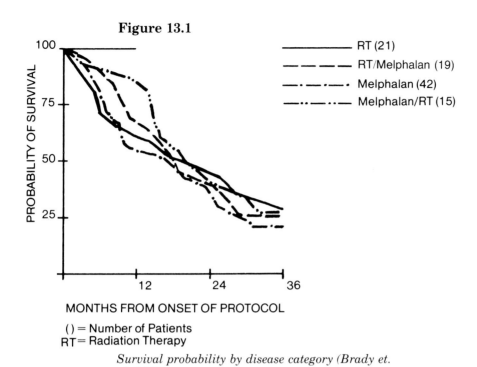

() = Number of Patients
RT = Radiation Therapy

Survival probability by disease category (Brady et. al. 1979).

diagnostic biopsies. The primary determinant survival factors in advanced epithelial ovarian cancer are amount of residual disease, histologic tumor grade, and presence of significant ascites. Histologic type may be of much less importance. FIGO staging does not adequately allow for stratification of patients according to these prognostic factors in stage III. Thus it is virtually impossible to assess the impact of tumor bulk reduction in which all significant factors are not evaluated or reported. Moreover, the response of patients with advanced ovarian cancer to various chemotherapeutic regimens or combinations of surgery, chemotherapy, and radiation therapy are uninterpretable without stratification for residual disease, histologic grade, and ascites.

Recent prospective randomized studies indicate that subsequent therapy may have less effect upon survival than whether the patient initially had optimal or suboptimal advanced ovarian cancer based on the amount of residual tumor following initial surgery. Patients with residual tumor masses greater than 2 to 3 cm should be designated as a poor prognostic or suboptimal group. In addition, histologic grade and ascites must be thoroughly evaluated in assessment of response to therapy. The practice of reduction of ovarian cancer tumor volume with preoperative radiation therapy has been largely abandoned because of poor results associated with significant operative complications. The combination of chemotherapy and surgery may prove more beneficial when more effective chemotherapy regimens have been de-

Figure 13.2

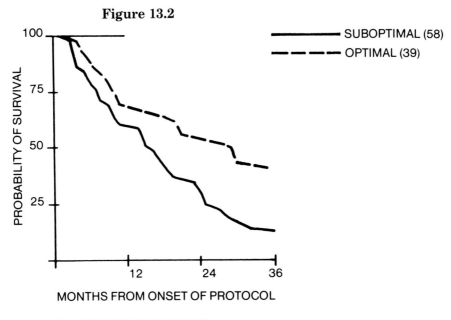

() = NUMBER OF PATIENTS

Survival probability by disease category (Brady et. al. 1979).

veloped. The appropriate extent of bulk reduction in advanced ovarian cancer should be based not upon how much tumor can be removed but how much will remain at the completion of the operation. Subsequent chemotherapy and/or radiation therapy has been relatively ineffective in arresting tumor progression in patients with poorly differentiated tumors and massive ascites associated with residual tumor masses greater than 2 to 3 cm in size.

The goal in bulk reduction in advanced ovarian cancer ideally would be removal of all tumor; however, it is apparent that unless nearly all tumor has been removed (no remaining tumor nodules should be larger than 1 cm in diameter), extensive or partial resection of large masses has not markedly improved survival. In future clinical trials, it will be extremely important to subcategorize stage III patients according to amount of residual disease related to histologic grade and presence or absence of ascites in order to substantiate the significance of each of these critical factors.

References

Aure, J.C.; Hoeg, K.; and Kolstad, P. Clinical histologic studies of ovarian carcinoma. *Obstet. Gynecol.* 37:1–9, 1971.

Brady, L.W. et al Radiotherapy, chemotherapy and combined therapy in stage III epithelial ovarian cancer. *Cancer Clin. Trials* 2:111–120, 1979.

Buchler, D.A. et al. Stage III ovarian carcinoma: treatment and results. *Radiology* 122:469–472, 1977.

Day, T.G., Jr., and Smith, J.P. Diagnosis and staging of ovarian carcinoma. *Semin. Oncol.* 2:217–222, 1975.

Delclos, L., and Quinlan, E. J. Malignant tumors of the ovary managed by postoperative megavoltage irradiation. *Radiology* 93:659–663, 1969.

Delclos, L., and Smith, J.P. *Tumors of the ovary. Textbook of radiotherapy,* ed. G. Fletcher. Philadelphia: Lea & Febiger, 1973.

Gallager, H.S. Prognostic importance of histologic type of ovarian carcinoma. *Natl. Cancer Inst. Monogr.* 42:13–14, 1975.

Griffiths, C.T. Surgical resection of tumor bulk in the primary treatment of ovarian carcinoma. *Natl. Cancer Inst. Monogr.* 42:101–104, 1975.

Griffiths, C.T.; Grogan, R.H.; and Hall, T.C. Advanced ovarian cancer, primary treatment with surgery, radiotherapy, chemotherapy. *Cancer* 29:1–7, 1972.

Hart, W.R. Ovarian epithelial tumors of borderline malignancies (carcinomas of a low malignant potential). *Hum. Pathol.* 8:541–549, 1977.

Hudson, C.N., and Chir, M. Surgical treatment of ovarian cancer. *Gynecol. Oncol.* 1:370–378, 1973.

Johnson, C.E. et al. Advanced ovarian cancer: therapy with radiation and cyclophosphamide in a randomized series. *Radiology* 114:136–141, 1972.

Julian, C.G. et al. Biologic behavior of primary ovarian malignancy. *Obstet. Gynecol.* 44:873–884, 1974.

Kjorstad, K.E.; Welander, C.; and Kolstad, P. Preoperative irradiation in stage III carcinoma of the ovaries. *Acta Obstet. Gynecol. Scand.* 56:449–452, 1977.

Malkasian, G.D., Jr.; Decker, D.G.; and Webb, M.J. Histology of epithelial tumors of the ovary. Clinical usefulness and prognostic significance of histologic classification and grading. *Semin. Oncol.* 2:191–201, 1975.

Maus, J.H.; MacKay, E.N.; and Sellers, A.H. Cancer of the ovary. *Radiat. Ther. Nucl. Med.* 102:603–607, 1968.

Munnell, E.W. The changing prognosis and treatment in cancer of the ovary. *Am. J. Obstet. Gynecol.* 100:790–805, 1968.

Obel, E.B. A comparative study of patients with cancer of the ovary who have survived more or less than 10 years. *Acta Obstet. Gynecol. Scand.* 55:429–439, 1976.

Piver, M.S.; Lele, S.; and Barlow, J.J. Preoperative and intraoperative evaluation of ovarian malignancies. *Obstet. Gynecol.* 48:312, 1976.

Rubin, P. Understanding the problem of understaging in ovarian cancer. *Semin. Oncol.* 2:236–242, 1975.

Webb, M.J.; Malkasian, G.D., Jr.; and Gorgensen, E.O. Factors influencing ovarian cancer survival after chemotherapy. *Obstet. Gynecol.* 44:564–572, 1974.

Young, R.C., and Fisher, R.I. Staging and treatment of epithelial ovarian cancer. *Can. Med. Assoc. J.* 119:249–256, 1978.

Chapter 14

The Value of a Second Look Laparotomy in Patients with Ovarian Carcinoma

PERSPECTIVE:

Thomas W. Castaldo

Ovarian carcinoma remains an enigma for the gynecologic oncologist. The overall poor results of treatment have frequently been attributed to the inability to diagnose malignant growth when it is still confined to the ovary. This is reflected in the reported incidence of stage I disease, which ranges from 19% to 43% (Burns et al. 1967; Parker, Parker, and Wilbanks 1970; Aure, Hoeg, and Kolstad 1971). Even when diagnosed at an early stage, however, cure rates at five years are less than 70% when treatment is by operation alone (Bagley et al. 1972). This may in part be related to a lack of diagnostic accuracy, as reported by Rosenoff and associates (1975a, 1975b). They reported on 49 consecutive patients referred to the National Cancer Institute with ovarian carcinoma who were subjected to pretreatment laparoscopy. All had undergone laparotomy within one month of referral. Of 16 patients believed to have disease localized to the pelvis (stage I or II) at laparotomy, 9 were found to have more advanced disease at laparoscopic examination. Since most patients have extraovarian spread at the time of diagnosis, residual disease is frequently present after operation. Consequently, radiation therapy and chemotherapy have been added in an effort to improve survival.

The use of radiotherapy following surgery has frequently been employed. In patients with stage I carcinoma of the ovary, the adjunctive use of radioisotopes to bathe the intraperitoneal surfaces has been tried. In a few reports, five-year survivals of greater than 90% have been obtained (Buchsbaum, Keetel, and Latourette 1975). Whole pelvic radiation therapy in patients with local pelvic spread has achieved 50% cure rates (Fuks 1975). But when disease has spread beyond the confines of the pelvis to involve the upper abdomen, whole abdominal radiation must be employed. Such therapy is not

335

without its morbidity and has achieved little in the way of improving the dismal salvage rate of patients with advanced disease.

Chemotherapy has in recent years been used more frequently than radiotherapy. Alkylating agents have been reported to give response rates between 30% and 60% (Bagley et al. 1972). Combination chemotherapy has been used but has not clearly demonstrated improved survival (Smith, Rutledge, and Wharton 1972; Barlow and Piver 1977). Because of the increased toxicity of combination chemotherapy, alkylating agents remain the most commonly employed drugs in the treatment of ovarian carcinoma. More recent literature on combination drug protocols has shown improved response rates (Young et al. 1978). Clinical trials with cis-platinum in combination with other agents are also encouraging (Ehrlich, Einhorn, and Morgan 1978), and combination therapy may therefore offer improved survival in the future.

Because of the frustration encountered in the treatment of advanced ovarian carcinoma, repeat laparotomy has also been suggested to be of value. It has been used predominantly as a second surgical attempt to resect residual disease, but is also used in those patients fortunate enough to have had a complete response to chemotherapy. The issue of induction of secondary malignancy is of concern in patients who remain on cytotoxic therapy for a prolonged period of time. Thus so-called second look laparotomy has been suggested by many authors in order to safely discontinue the use of these drugs when the patient has achieved clinical remission.

Much of the controversy surrounding second look laparotomy in ovarian carcinoma relates to the lack of a consistent definition. The term would seem to imply a diagnostic procedure, yet much of the available literature describes planned therapeutic operations at the time of second look. In addition, both diagnostic and therapeutic procedures have been carried out not only following completion of therapy but also in the midst of ongoing treatment. The rationale for second look operations includes (1) assessment of tumor response during therapy; (2) previous unresectable tumor masses may have had sufficient response to be resectable; (3) to discontinuing the use of cytotoxic chemotherapy when the patient is clinically free of disease and has received sufficient drug; and (4) resection of residual disease following treatment.

This chapter will review the present literature and attempt to define second look laparotomy and its value in the treatment of ovarian malignancy.

Historical Background

In 1945, Parks described three patients who had inoperable ovarian carcinoma at laparotomy. Following biopsy only, the patients received radiation therapy. All of them were subjected to repeat laparotomy with resection of the primary tumor. Although the original intent of Parks's manuscript was to document the usefulness of radiotherapy, the concept of second laparotomy in selected patients was introduced. The use of second look surgery in asymptomatic patients was first popularized by Wangensteen in 1949. Although this concept was first proposed for patients with malignant tumors of the gastrointestinal tract, women with ovarian carcinoma were also included in his second look program. Patients with ovarian carcinoma were managed as follows.

> Reoperation is carried out in patients known to be asymptomatic and without clinical evidence of cancer approximately 6 months after original excision of malignancies with gross or microscopic evidence of spread beyond the primary site. If possible, residual or recurrent tumor is removed in its entirety. Additional looks are employed, if necessary, to render the patient free of cancer. In the event that painstaking exploration and biopsies at any of the secondary operations fail to show evidence of the disease, the systematic reexploration at 6-month intervals is discontinued and further surgical effort is made only in the event of recurrence or in selected cases in which the original lesion is widespread (Wangensteen 1949).

His use of this approach in 14 patients with ovarian carcinoma resulted in the conversion of 2 patients to a tumor-free state after a positive second look. One such patient had a recurrence 10 years after her original disease and thus biologically had a low-grade cancer. She also suffered multiple postoperative fistulae from the procedure. In addition, there were two postoperative mortalities. Thus this approach did not gain widespread acceptance. The philosophy of second look procedures not prompted by recurrence or intestinal obstruction, however, has persisted.

Evaluation of Tumor Response during Therapy

The inability to diagnose ovarian carcinoma at an early stage has been referred to previously. Even more frustrating is the inability to evaluate postoperatively those patients known to have residual tumor. Disease is often not clinically evaluable by objective means. Our subjective clinical evaluation of response is frequently inaccurate, as pointed out by Smith in 1976. In a series from the M. D. Anderson Hospital and Tumor Institute, 103 patients were subjected to a second look laparotomy. All had shown complete or nearly complete clinical response to chemotherapy. Thirty-three percent of the patients were found to have either stable disease or progressive cancer when their original operative notes were compared with findings at second look. This problem has prompted some investigators to carry out periodic second look laparoscopy during chemotherapy in order objectively to assess response to cytotoxic chemotherapy.

Berek and associates (1979) have followed 57 patients in such fashion. They have done a total of 112 laparoscopies, with 12 complications, in these women and have suggested that further studies are needed. This approach may become more widely accepted as chemotherapeutic response rates improve.

Resection of Residual Tumor Masses

The most common use for the second look laparotomy has been a second surgical attempt to resect tumor masses. This has usually followed radiation therapy or a sufficiently good response to chemotherapy. Table 14.1 lists the results of these attempts in 133 patients in five published series. The largest series is that of Smith and associates (1972, 1976) from the M. D. Anderson Hospital and Tumor Institute. Eighty patients had tumor resection at the time of a second look. Twenty-nine had all gross tumor removed. Fourteen of the 80 were clinically free of disease at the time of their report. Unfortunately, follow-up is not sufficient to determine whether survival was improved by complete resection, although two-year survival figures would suggest so (77% complete resection, 48% incomplete resection). Only Tepper, in 1971, and Frick, in 1978, comment on complete resectability of the residual disease found at second look laparotomy. Nine of 17 and 7 of 19 in their respective series had total removal of all gross tumor. Thus approximately 39% of women with adequate tumor response could be expected to have resectable disease. Tepper suggests that even if cure rates are not improved, those patients having complete surgical resection survive twice as long as women having incomplete resection (39 versus 20 months). This is confirmed by Frick (38 versus 20 months). Wallach (1970, 1975), on the other hand, suggests that any tumor palpable preoperatively bodes a poor outcome. In his series of 10 patients, only 1 patient is without evidence of disease and this patient had no evidence of cancer prior to second look. Of the remaining 9 patients, 7 were dead within one year, 1 died at 44 months, and 1 is living with disease.

This group of 133 patients is obviously a select one. Selection criteria are not always clearly stated. Manka, in 1971, did not state criteria for second look. Two of his five surviving patients had tumor of low malignant potential, indicating that selection will obviously alter results. Frick, Smith, and Wallach state the total number of patients in their series and the total number of second looks. Of 1261 patients with ovarian carcinoma, 109 (8.6%) had tumor resection at the time of second look laparotomy. Since 23 patients remain without evidence of disease in these three collected series, less than 2% of women could be expected to be cured by this approach, and the figure could not be expected to exceed 5% if the approach were limited to patients with advanced stage carcinoma.

Table 14.1
Second Attempt at Surgical Resection at the
Time of Second Look

Year	Author	Number of Patients	NED*	DOD*	AWD*
1972, 1976	Smith et al.	80†	14	56	8
1971	Tepper et al.	17	3	14	0
1970, 1975	Wallach et al.	10	1	8	1
1977	Manka and Belohorsky	7	2	5	0
1978	Frick et al.	19	8	11	0
	Totals	133	28	94	9

*NED: no evidence of disease; DOD: dead of disease; AWD: alive with disease.
†Two patients died of intercurrent disease.

Discontinue the Use of Cytotoxic Chemotherapy When the Patient Is Clinically Free of Disease and Has Had Sufficient Drug

The concern of secondary malignancy induced by cytotoxic chemotherapy is troubling to anyone who prescribes these medications. It has been shown that women treated with alkylating agents for ovarian carcinoma are at increased risk for the development of acute nonlymphocytic leukemia (Reimer et al. 1977). Thirteen cases occurred among 5455 women as compared to 0.62 cases expected. All 13 had received alkylating agents. Nine also received radiotherapy. Of the four patients who had not received radiotherapy, the latency period between the start of alkylating agent therapy and the development of leukemia was 52, 84, and 90 months. (It was unknown in one patient.) Although the latency period was known, the duration of therapy was not clearly stated. The exact risk of inducing leukemia is not known; however, it is clear that such a risk is present.

In those patients who are undergoing treatment with chemotherapy and have no clinical evidence of disease, a treatment dilemma eventually arises. How long should one continue chemotherapy? What are the chances of developing leukemia as the duration of therapy increases? Clearly these are questions of the utmost importance which have uncertain answers. The logic of second look surgery to determine the presence of disease is obvious to all. This has raised additional questions, however. Is laparoscopy an acceptable means of second look? What is the best time for second look surgery? What are the chances of a relapse following the cessation of therapy after a negative second look? Are the chances of relapse related to the duration of therapy?

The use of laparoscopy as a second look procedure for the purpose of discontinuing chemotherapy was best evaluated by Rosenoff (1975a, 1975b) of the National Cancer Institute, W. G. Smith and associates (1977) of the M. D. Anderson Hospital, and Spinelli and associates (1976) of the Italian National Cancer Institute in Milan. These results are summarized in tables 14.2 and 14.3. Of 85 patients thought to be clinically free of disease, 29% were found to have cancer at the time of laparoscopy. No serious complications of the procedure were encountered. In the study from M. D. Anderson, all 11 patients with a negative laparoscopy were subjected to a laparotomy. Five of them were found to have tumor. In addition, five patients in their series were felt to have significant adhesions, which prevented adequate examination of the intraabdominal contents. Rosenoff and Spinelli did not address the question of lack of adequate visualization at laparoscopy. In the series from the National Cancer Institute, a laparotomy did not follow a negative laparoscopy i the first five patients. Three of these patients subsequently relapsed after chemotherapy was discontinued. Since that experience, laparotomy is now routine after a negative second look laparoscopy. Of the first four patients having laparotomy after a negative laparoscopy, two were found to have tumor. Spinelli reports that one patient relapsed after chemotherapy was discontinued following a negative laparoscopy. He does not, however, state how many of the 36 patients with a negative laparoscopy had cytotoxic therapy discontinued. Clearly a negative laparoscopy provides insufficient information, and chemotherapy should not be discontinued on this basis alone.

Only J. P. Smith and colleagues report a number of patients found to have no evidence of disease at second look laparotomy adequate enough to address some of the other questions. Twenty-three of the 103 patients subjected to second look laparotomy were found to be free of disease. Of these, 18 have remained without evidence of carcinoma. One has died of intercurrent disease and four have relapsed and died of recurrent cancer. All four of the patients who relapsed had only four courses of chemotherapy prior to second look. J. P. Smith and associates have suggested that patients have a minimum of 12 months of chemotherapy prior to second look procedures. This

Table 14.2
Use of Laparoscopy as a Second Look

Year	Author	Number of Patients	NED*	Disease Present	Inadequate Examination
1975	Rosenoff	18	11	7	—
1977	Smith	24	11	8	5
1976	Spinelli	47	36	11	—
	Totals	89	58	26	5

*NED: no evidence of disease.

Table 14.3
Patients Having Negative Second Look
Laparoscopy

Year	Author	Number of Patients	Findings at Laparotomy		Number of Patients Relapsing if Laparoscopy not done
			Positive	Negative	
1977	Smith	11	5	6	—
1975	Rosenoff	4	2	2	—
		5			3
	Totals	20	7	8	3

would suggest that the duration of therapy might be related to chance of relapse following cessation of chemotherapy. We eagerly await additional literature on this aspect of ovarian cancer treatment.

Discussion

As mentioned previously, the lack of a consistent definition of second look procedures has clouded the literature. In this author's opinion, repeat laparotomy with second attempts at surgical cure when palpable tumor is present is not a second look procedure. Admittedly there are occasional patients who benefit from these procedures, but no large series has ever documented this approach to be of significant value.

Repeat laparotomy in patients without evidence of cancer after an appropriate duration of chemotherapy is logical, on the other hand, and offers a planned method of management which can be applied to a defined subgroup of women. Obviously this is also a select group since they must have demonstrated a clinical response to chemotherapy. They, however, by virtue of their response, select themselves as the most likely individuals to be benefited by second look operation. Those patients found to be clinically free of disease can have cytotoxic chemotherapy discontinued. This may not completely eliminate the risk of developing leukemia, but it should decrease such a risk. The cessation of chemotherapy without the benefit of second look in patients clinically free of disease is not without risk. Sixty to 65% of patients felt to be without clinical evidence of cancer are found to have viable tumor at second look operations (Smith et al. 1972; Tepper et al. 1971; Wallach and Blinick 1970). When tumor is present at these operative procedures, 39% of patients have had all gross tumor removed. These patients have survived longer than those whose disease was not resectable. This appears to be the only place where planned reexploration and tumor resection may be of value, although it is far from proved. This approach, however, has certainly identified a subgroup of patients where aggressive new combination drug protocols may be of significant benefit. Those patients with persistent tumor can be carried on chemotherapy with the knowledge that the potential benefit far outweighs the risks of induction of secondary malignancy.

The second look procedure is far from a simple laparotomy. If one chooses to do laparoscopy, it should be understood that it is frequently a preliminary procedure. If gross residual disease not considered resectable is present, biopsies should be obtained and laparotomy may be deferred. If, however, visualization is inadequate to make such a decision, or if no disease is seen, it is mandatory to proceed with laparotomy. If resectable disease is present, it should be removed. If no gross disease is present, a thorough, complete, and systematic exploration should be carried out. This should include washings of the pelvis and colic gutters for cytologic examination. Strandlike adhesions should be excised and sent for pathologic review. Biopsy of the infundibulo-pelvic ligament stumps should be obtained. Random biopsy of the pelvic peritoneum is also suggested. If the uterus, tubes, ovaries, or omentum are present, they should be removed. The retroperitoneal space is to be opened and the periaortic nodes sampled. Diaphragmatic biopsy is also of importance. It is imperative that this procedure be carried out through an incision allowing total visualization of the entire intraabdominal contents. There is no place for a cosmetic Pfannenstiel incision at a second look laparotomy. A vertical incision offers the best opportunity to visualize the undersurfaces of the diaphragm, and often the laparoscope can be used intraoperatively to visualize this area, especially posteriorly. Only after such an operative procedure has failed to reveal residual carcinoma can chemotherapy be discontinued with confidence.

Summary

In conclusion, the following points should be restated:

1. Second operative attempts at surgical cure in the presence of palpable disease are of questionable value and should not be termed second look surgery.
2. The term second look laparotomy should be confined to systematic intra-abdominal exploration as previously described in a patient who is clinically free of disease. This operation should be performed in the hope of discontinuing cytotoxic chemotherapy and should be carried out after a minimum of one year of drug therapy.
3. If resectable disease is found at the time of a second look laparotomy, it should be removed. Chemotherapy should probably be changed but at the very least continued.
4. A negative laparoscopy is insufficient evidence to discontinue chemotherapy and must be followed by a second look laparotomy. Only after a negative laparotomy can one safely discontinue cytotoxic therapy.

References

Aure, J.C.; Hoeg, R.; and Kolstad, P. Clinical and histologic studies of ovarian carcinoma. *Obstet. Gynecol.* 37:1–9, 1971.

Bagley C.M. et al. Treatment of ovarian carcinoma: possibilities for progress. *N. Engl. J. Med.* 287:856–862, 1972.

Barlow, J.P., and Piver, M.S. Single agent versus combination chemotherapy in the treatment of ovarian cancer. *Obstet. Gynecol.* 49:609–611, 1977.

Berek, J.S.; Griffiths, T.; and Leventhal, J.M. Survival predictability, indications and improved technique of laparoscopy for second look evaluation in ovarian cancer. Presented at annual meeting of the Society of Gynecologic Oncology, January 1979.

Buchsbaum, H.J.; Keetel, W.C.; and Latourette, H.B. The use of radioisotopes as adjunct therapy of localized ovarian cancer. *Semin. Oncol.* 2:247–251, 1975.

Burns, B.C. et al. Management of ovarian carcinoma. *Am. J. Obstet. Gynecol.* 98:374–386, 1967.

Ehrlich, C.C.; Einhorn, L.H.; and Morgan, J.L. Combination chemotherapy of ovarian carcinoma with cis-diamminedicholoplatinum (CDDP), Adriamycin (ADR) and cytoxan (CTX). *Proc. Am. Assoc. Cancer Res.* 19:379, 1978.

Frick, G. el at. Relaparotomy in advanced ovarian carcinoma. *Acta Obstet. Gynecol. Scand.* 57:165, 1978.

Fuks, Z., and Bagshaw, M. The rationale for curative radiotherapy for ovarian cancer. *Int. J. Radiat. Oncol. Biol. Phys.* 1:21–32, 1975.

Manka, I., and Belohorsky, B. Chemotherapy and second look procedure in the treatment of ovarian carcinoma. *Neoplasma* 24:207–211, 1977.

Parker, R.T.; Parker, C.H.; and Wilbanks, G.D. Cancer of the ovary. *Am. J. Obstet. Gynecol.* 108:878–888, 1970.

Parks, T.J. Carcinoma of the ovary treated preoperatively with deep x-ray: report of three cases. *Am. J. Obstet. Gynecol.* 49:676–685, 1945.

Reimer, R.R. et al. Acute leukemia after alkylating agent therapy of ovarian carcinoma. *N. Engl. J. Med.* 297:177–181, 1977.

Rosenoff, S.H. et al. Use of peritoneoscopy for initial staging and post therapy evaluation of patients with ovarian carcinoma. *Natl. Cancer Inst. Monogr.* 42:81–84, 1975a.

Rosenoff, S.H. et al. Peritoneoscopy in the staging and follow-up of ovarian cancer. *Semin. Oncol.* 2:223–228, 1975b.

Smith J.P.; Delgado, G.; and Rutledge, F. Second look operation in ovarian carcinoma—post chemotherapy. *Cancer* 38:1438–1442, 1976.

Smith, J.P.; Rutledge, F.; and Wharton, J.T. Chemotherapy of ovarian cancer—new approaches to treatment. *Cancer* 30:1565–1571, 1972.

Smith, W.G.; Day, T.G.; and Smith, J.P. The use of laparoscopy to determine the results of chemotherapy for ovarian cancer. *J. Reprod. Med.* 18:257–260, 1977.

Spinelli, P. et al. Laparoscopy in staging and restaging of 95 patients with ovarian carcinoma. *Tumori* 62:493–500, 1976.

Tepper, E. et al. Second look surgery after radiation therapy for advanced stages of cancer of the ovary. *Am. J. Roentgenol.* 112:755–759, 1971.

Wallach, R.L. et al. The importance of second look surgical procedures in the staging treatment of ovarian carcinoma. *Semin. Oncol.* 2:243–246, 1975.

Wallach, R.L., and Blinick, G. The second look operation for carcinoma of the ovary. *Surg. Gynecol. Obstet.* 131:1085–1089, 1970.

Wangensteen, O.H. Cancer of the colon and rectum: with special reference to (1) earlier recognition of alimentary tract malignancy; (2) secondary delayed re-entry of the abdomen in patients exhibiting lymph node involvement; (3) subtotal primary excision of the colon; (4) operation in obstruction. *Wis. Med. J.* 48:591, 1949.

Young, R.C. et al. Advanced ovarian adenocarcinoma—a prospective clinical trial of melphalan (L-PAM) versus combination chemotherapy. *N. Engl. J. Med.* 299:1261–1266, 1978.

344

PERSPECTIVE:

The Value of a Second Look Laparotomy in Patients with Ovarian Carcinoma

Peter E. Schwartz

The clinical assessment of patients receiving chemotherapy for the treatment of ovarian cancer is hampered by a lack of sensitive serum or diagnostic radiologic examinations to determine routinely the presence of persistent disease in patients who are clinically free of cancer. Long-term therapy with cytotoxic agents may expose patients who no longer have cancer to possible life-threatening complications of chemotherapy (Reimer et al. 1977; Alexander et al. 1979). The introduction of new chemotherapeutic agents into the management of ovarian cancer also requires a way to assess the effectiveness of such agents in managing this disease. The value of second look laparotomy in patients with ovarian carcinoma is that it is the most accurate technique in assessing the patients' response to cytotoxic chemotherapy.

Second look laparotomy is employed in patients who are clinically free of disease and have completed a prescribed program of chemotherapy. Its purpose is to determine the extent of persistent disease and allow resection of such disease. Patients who are found to be free of gross and microscopic disease may have chemotherapy discontinued (Smith, Delgado, and Rutledge 1976). Reexploration for clinically obvious masses or for relief of bowel obstruction should not be considered second look surgery.

History

Second look laparotomy was originally introduced by Wangensteen as a means of diagnosing early recurrence of bowel malignancies in patients who were clinically asymptomatic (Wangensteen, Lewis, and Tongen 1951). The technique was subsequently introduced in patients with ovarian cancer at the M. D. Anderson Hospital and Tumor Institute in the early 1960s, initially employed in patients who had received melphalan chemotherapy for the management of advanced or recurrent epithelial tumors of the ovary (Rutledge and Burns 1966). Many of these patients had failed radiation therapy or had such massive tumors that even the most aggressive of radiotherapists believed the tumors would not respond to radiation therapy. The original concept was to employ second look laparotomy at a time when large fixed pelvic-abdominal masses became smaller and mobile or when tumor became clinically nondetectable. The duration of response to melphalan was unknown, and it was believed that once a response occurred, operation should be performed.

In an attempt to increase the number of patients who would be clinically and surgically free of disease, reexploration was postponed until the patient developed bone marrow depression, causing a break in the melphalan four-week schedule. Many patients were able to receive up to nine courses of melphalan before bone marrow depression occurred, but the incidence of negative second look operations was not dramatically increased. It was only when patients were required to receive 10 courses of melphalan, regardless of the time necessary to complete therapy, that the incidence of negative reoperations appeared to increase significantly (Smith, Delgado, and Rutledge 1976). Many patients clinically free of gross disease, however, had persistent microscopic disease. The melphalan schedule was then increased to 12 courses prior to reexploration and there was a dramatic increase in negative second look laparotomies, particularly in those patients with significant residual tumor left at the initial operation (Schwartz and Smith 1977). In a group of 109 patients with advanced epithelial ovarian cancers treated at the M. D. Anderson Hospital, 15% of those who received 9 or less courses of melphalan had no evidence of disease at second look surgery, whereas 28% of those who received 10 courses and 47% of those who received 12 or more courses of melphalan were free of cancer at second look surgery. The highest incidence of negative second look surgery (60%) was found in those patients who had more than 12 courses of melphalan chemotherapy (Schwartz and Smith 1977).

Technique

Exploratory laparotomy following completion of a program of chemotherapy is a carefully planned procedure. Upon entry into the peritoneal cavity via a vertical midline incision, any fluid present should be aspirated and sent for cytology and cell block analysis. In the event no free fluid is present, the pelvis and each lateral paracolic space should be irrigated with normal saline and the aspirate sent for cytology and cell block evaluation. A careful inspection of all peritoneal surfaces should be performed. Each diaphragm should be carefully palpated. A laparoscope inserted through the incision may be a useful adjunct for inspecting the diaphragm. The retroperitoneum should be palpated in search of retroperitoneal lymph node enlargement. Adhesions should be carefully inspected for possible residual disease, and the bowel and its mesentery should be inspected. The pelvis must not only be visualized, but carefully palpated, looking for persistent retroperitoneal disease.

All gross tumor found at second look laparotomy should be resected. When the tumor is found to be discrete and bulky, this goal may more readily be accomplished than in a situation where diffuse seeding is present. The greater the maximum diameter of the residual tumor left at second look surgery, the poorer the prognosis. Patients with large, bulky residual tumor left at the initial surgery are most likely to have persistent disease at second look operations. Patients with advanced or bulky cancer should be placed on a bowel preparation prior to second look laparotomy, as these patients most often have persistent disease and may require bowel resections to remove gross cancer. Patients receiving prophylactic chemotherapy, that is, those patients with early stage disease and no residual cancer at initial operation, are not routinely placed on preoperative bowel preparations.

The finding of no gross tumor at second look laparotomy cannot be interpreted to mean the patient is free of cancer. The application of modern chemotherapeutic agents, particularly in combinations containing agents each of which when used alone is active in controlling ovarian malignancies, will produce a significant number of patients who are clinically and surgically free of disease at second look operations. It is the surgeon's role to provide adequate sampling of the abdominal and pelvic peritoneum and retroperitoneum for the pathologist to determine a patient's cancer status.

Peritoneal surfaces must be sampled from the diaphragm to the cul-de-sac. Any palpable or visualized irregularity is subjected to biopsy. Sampling the diaphragm may be readily accomplished with a Kevorkian-type biopsy instrument which permits a superficial grasping of the diaphragm peritoneum. The peritoneum is tented up, a purse-string suture of 3-0 catgut suture is placed around the periphery of the tented peritoneum, the biopsy is completed, and the purse-string suture is tied. Similar biopsies are obtained along each paracolic space. Bowel serosa and mesentery are sampled at sites of adhesions, as is the omentum (if a total omentectomy was not performed at the original operation). The paraaortic fat pad is sampled—a recent report has demonstrated that this may be the only site of persistent disease at the completion of a program of chemotherapy for epithelial cancers of the ovary (Creasman, Abu-Ghazaleh, and Schmidt 1978).

The most frequent sites of persistent epithelial ovarian cancer at second look laparotomy are the omentum, residual ovaries, and pelvic peritoneum. Hysterectomy and/or oophorectomy should be performed if the uterus and/or ovaries were not removed at the initial operation. Any site where the ovary may have adhered to the pelvic sidewall should be sampled, including the area of the infundibulopelvic ligaments and round ligament stumps. Biopsies of the serosa of the sigmoid colon, cul-de-sac, and bladder peritoneum, as well as any induration in the retroperitoneal space should be performed.

A minimum of 20 separate sites should be subjected to biopsy to insure adequate sampling of peritoneal surfaces and the retroperitoneal space in those patients with no gross evidence of disease. An attempt should be made to remove all gross tumor present at second look surgery as survival is enhanced if the diameter of the largest residual tumor is less than 2 cm. The two- and five-year survival in the M. D. Anderson Hospital experience for those patients who underwent complete removal of all gross tumor was 47.5% and 27%, respectively (Schwartz and Smith 1977). Patients with residual cancer of less than 2 cm in diameter had a 29% two- and five-year survival following second look operation, but the survival when residual tumor was greater than 2 cm in diameter was only 9% for these time intervals.

Epithelial cancers of the ovary most often occur as stage III or IV disease and tend to involve both ovaries at the time of initial diagnosis. Such cancers usually occur in older women who have completed childbearing, rarely occur in the second decade of life, and infrequently occur in the third decade.

Germ cell tumors most often occur in the second and third decade of life, usually occur as stage I disease, and, until the introduction of combination chemotherapy (vincristine, actinomycin-D, cyclophosphamide), were associated with extremely poor survival (Smith and Rutledge 1975). These malignancies tend to be unilateral, and the removal of the uninvolved ovary and uterus at the initial surgery does not enhance survival (Kurman and Norris 1977). Second look laparotomy is extremely valuable in managing patients with germ cell tumors, particularly if the patient has not lost her reproductive capabilities as a consequence of the initial surgery. Those individuals found to be grossly free of disease at second look operation should undergo routine sampling of all peritoneal surfaces and of retroperitoneal lymph nodes as described above. The ovary and uterus, however, may be left in place if the patient desires to preserve reproductive function. A biopsy of the remaining ovary should be obtained.

Patients on combination chemotherapy (vincristine, actinomycin-D, cyclophosphamide) whose initial surgery for a stage I germ cell tumor was confined to a unilateral adnexectomy may continue to have ovarian function on therapy. At Yale–New Haven Hospital second look surgery has been performed in patients treated for germ cell neoplasms, and the only remarkable finding in two of these patients were 4 to 5 cm corpus luteum cysts in the remaining ovary. One was treated for an endodermal sinus tumor with focal areas of dysgerminoma, which had ruptured intraabdominally and was associated with elevated levels of serum alpha-fetoprotein prior to institution of combination chemotherapy. She is alive and free of disease three and one-half years following the diagnosis, over two years following negative second look operation, and has conceived and subsequently delivered a healthy child 20 months following the negative second look. The other patient has just undergone negative second look laparotomy following 12 monthly courses of combination chemotherapy and will have chemotherapy discontinued. These patients clearly demonstrate the value of such procedures involving germ cell tumors which in the past were associated with a high fatality rate despite presentation as early stage disease, and now may be associated with preservation of ovarian function and fertility. These patients must be evaluated by the most accurate technique to be certain no residual tumor is present before they attempt to become pregnant. Recent data from testicular tumors suggest that patients found to have clinically unsuspected persistent evidence of ovarian germ cell tumor at second look laparotomy may be successfully treated with alternative combination chemotherapy (Cis-diamminedichloroplatinum, vinblastine, bleomycin (Einhorn and Donahue 1977).

Sex cord–mesenchyme tumors, for example, granulosa cell tumors, Sertoli-Leydig tumors, appear most often as stage I disease and are adequately treated with unilateral adnexectomy in women desiring preservation of ovarian function. Advanced-stage malignancies in this histologic group have infrequently been successfully treated with chemotherapy, but in a few reported cases second look laparotomy has been valuable for determining when to discontinue therapy (Schwartz and Smith 1976).

Mixed mesodermal tumors of the ovary are extremely rare and have been considered to be insensitive to radiation therapy or chemotherapy. The combination of radiation therapy with multiagent chemotherapy has been advocated for controlling such tumors (Smith and Rutledge 1975). At Yale–New Haven Hospital combination chemotherapy (vincristine, actinomycin-D, and cyclophosphamide) has been successfully employed in inducing remissions in patients with ovarian mixed mesodermal tumors. One patient with a ruptured stage II$_b$ tumor which was predominantly a rhabdomyosarcoma was treated with this regimen for 18 months prior to a negative second look laparotomy. Chemotherapy was discontinued at that point and the patient is alive and free of disease 19 months following reexploration.

Discussion

Second look laparotomy is the most accurate technique for assessing a patient's response to chemotherapy, but it remains a highly controversial procedure. The major criticisms of this technique appear to be that (1) clinical assessment is as accurate as operative assessment, particularly in those patients with no evidence of cancer left at the initial surgery; (2) if the patient is found to have persistent cancer at second look, the patient has no hope for cure; (3) chemotherapy does not cure ovarian cancer; therefore, when a remission is induced the patient should be maintained on therapy indefinitely; and (4) laparoscopic evaluation is an acceptable alternative to an exploratory laparotomy.

The answers to these criticisms may be found in the M. D. Anderson experience (Schwartz and Smith 1977), which revealed that one-half of the group of patients treated with melphalan and found to have cancer at second look (64 patients) were clinically free of disease immediately prior to operation. Nine of 27 patients with stage I epithelial ovarian cancer had clinically unsuspected cancer at reexploration, and changing therapy in this group has led to prolonged survival.

A similar experience has recently been reported from the Mount Sinai Medical Center (New York), where 15 of 25 patients with advanced ovarian cancer treated with combination chemotherapy consisting of Adriamycin and cis-diamminedichloroplatinum were clinically free of disease but had microscopic disease (11) or gross tumor (4) at second look laparotomy (Cohen et al. 1979).

Persistent cancer found at second look laparotomy has been an ominous prognostic sign. Nevertheless, seven patients clinically free of disease immediately prior to second look were found to have persistent disease at the M. D. Anderson Hospital. Their management was changed based on the operative findings, and each has survived five or more years free of disease following second look laparotomy.

Epithelial ovarian cancers tend to present in advanced stages and have responded poorly to external beam irradiation therapy. Five-year survival for stage III disease treated in such a manner is reported in the 6% to 10% range (Kottmeier 1976). Survival rates in stage IV disease are lower. In an attempt to increase survival, many medical centers are employing chemotherapy as the primary mode of therapy for advanced ovarian cancer. Although preliminary results are extremely encouraging, five-year survival rates following completion of chemotherapy programs are not yet available. There is a paucity of data in the literature to support the concept that chemotherapy cures advanced ovarian cancer. Eight patients treated for advanced ovarian cancer at the M. D. Anderson Hospital with significant residual tumor left at the initial operation have survived five or more years following completion of a program of chemotherapy and negative second look laparotomy. Treatment was discontinued following the latter operation, and the patients appear to represent chemotherapy cures (Schwartz and Smith 1977).

Long-term therapy with alkylating agents can lead to the development of leukemia. The combination of external beam irradiation therapy and alkylating agent chemotherapy is reported to shorten the latent period before this complication is observed (Reimer et al. 1977). Most patients who develop this complication have been exposed to alkylating agents alone for more than two years. The eight M. D. Anderson patients with advanced ovarian cancer who have survived five or more years following negative second look would have needlessly been exposed to long-term complications of alkylating agents had no second look laparotomy been performed.

Laparoscopy has been advocated as the alternative to a formal laparotomy to assess the patients' response to chemotherapy (Smith, Day, and Smith 1977). Laparoscopy may obviate the need for laparotomy in those patients found to have diffuse intraperitoneal seeding of cancer following completion of a program of chemotherapy. Laparoscopically directed biopsies should confirm whether or not the seedings are malignant and the patient may then receive appropriate therapy. Patients most likely to have persistent disease upon completion of a chemotherapy program are those found to have advanced cancer and significant residual tumor left at the original procedure. Patients with no evidence of disease at laparoscopy require second look laparotomy, as laparoscopy gives an incomplete view of the peritoneal cavity and permits no evaluation of the retroperitoneal space. A recent report has demonstrated that the only site of persistent disease at second look operation may be the paraaortic lymph nodes, an area inaccessible to the laparoscope (Creasman, Abu-Ghazaleh, and Schmidt 1978). Patients found to have bulky, but possibly resectable, tumor at laparoscopy should also undergo laparotomy because the survival rates are enhanced if bulk tumor is removed at second look operations (Smith, Delgado, and Rutledge 1976).

The timing of second look laparotomy is extremely important. The available data strongly suggest that the number of courses of chemotherapy a patient receives prior to undergoing second look for epithelial cancer of the ovary correlates directly with the incidence of negative second look operations (Schwartz and Smith 1977). At Yale–New Haven Hospital patients with early stage epithelial ovarian cancers receive a single alkylating agent for 18 months prior to second look. Patients with advanced stages of epithelial ovarian cancer receive two years of chemotherapy consisting of combinations employing Adriamycin, cyclophosphamide, hexamethylmelamine, and Cis-diamminedichloroplatinum.

Adriamycin is associated with cardiac toxicity and is usually discontinued when a total dose of 540 mg/m^2 has been administered. Recent investigations employing left ventricular ejection fractions (LVEF) indicate that cardiotoxicity can be anticipated when Adriamycin therapy results in significant depression of the LVEF (Alexander et al. 1979). Patients with ovarian cancer have received Adriamycin (40 mg/m^2 IV every 4 weeks) at Yale–New Haven Hospital for as long as 24 months prior to second look using LVEF monitoring without developing cardiotoxicity. Cyclophosphamide bladder toxicity may be avoided with hydration and long-term complications of leukemia may be avoided by second look at the end of 24 months of treatment. Hexamethylmelamine neurotoxicity may be avoided by administering pyridoxine (Wharton et al. 1979). Cis-diamminedichloroplatinum nephrotoxicity may be avoided with pre- and posttreatment hydration (Hayes et al. 1977).

Germ cell tumors of the ovary have recently been demonstrated to be extremely sensitive to chemotherapy. It is unclear that patients treated for stage I disease require two years of treatment, as advocated by Smith and Rutledge in 1975. At Yale–New Haven Hospital such patients are currently treated for one year with vincristine, actinomycin-D, and cyclophosphamide. Creasman (1979) has presented data suggesting the combination of methotrexate, actinomycin-D, and chlorambucil may be used prophylactically in stage I disease for shorter intervals. Advanced stage germ cell malignancies and sex cord–mesenchyme and mixed mesodermal tumors of the ovary are treated with combination chemotherapy for 18 months at Yale–New Haven Hospital prior to second look laparotomy.

Summary

For a surgical procedure to be considered of value for ovarian cancer patients, it should influence management and result in an enhancement of survival. A second look laparotomy following completion of a program of chemotherapy accomplishes these goals. It is the most accurate way of assessing the cancer status of a patient clinically free of disease. Those patients found to have no evidence of disease by cytologic and histologic criteria may have chemotherapy discontinued and avoid the long-term, life-threatening complications of cytotoxic chemotherapy. If unsuspected cancer is found at the reexploration, removal of bulk tumor and modification of subsequent therapy enhances survival. Preliminary data suggest that advanced epithelial tumors of the ovary may be cured with alkylating agents, and more recent data suggest that combination chemotherapy may increase the number of patients potentially cured, although longer follow-up is definitely needed (Schwartz and Smith 1977; Cohen et al. 1979; Young et al. 1978). A second laparotomy is extremely valuable in assessing the response of the ovarian cancer to new chemotherapeutic agents. Preliminary data also demonstrate that patients with unsuspected persistent cancer diagnosed at a second look laparotomy may survive five or more years when treatment is changed. Germ cell tumors of the ovary are quite sensitive to combination chemotherapy and a second look laparotomy will permit discontinuation of therapy, preserving ovarian function and reproductive capabilities in patients with these rare tumors.

References

Alexander, J. et al. Serial assessment of doxorubicin cardiotoxicity with quantitative radionuclide angiocardiography. *N. Engl. J. Med.* 300:278–283, 1979.

Cohen, C.J. et al. Reoperation for patients with advanced ovarian carcinoma. Presented at the tenth annual meeting of the Society of Gynecologic Oncologists, Marco Island, Florida, January 1979.

Creasman, W.T. et al. Germ cell malignancies of the ovary. *Obstet. Gynecol.* 53:226–230, 1979.

Creasman, W.T.; Abu-Ghazaleh, S.; and Schmidt, H.J. Retroperitoneal metastatic spread of ovarian cancer. *Gynecol. Oncol.* 6:447–450, 1978.

Einhorn, L.H., and Donahue J. Cis-diamminedichloroplatinum, vinblastine, and bleomycin combination chemotherapy in disseminated testicular cancer. *Ann. Intern. Med.* 87:293–298, 1977.

Hayes, D.M. et al. High dose cis-platinumdiamminedichloride. *Cancer* 39:1372–1381, 1977.

Kottmeier, H.L., ed. *Annual report on the results of treatment in carcinoma of the uterus, vagina, and ovary,* vol. 16. Stockholm: Pogo Print, 1976.

Kurman, R.J., and Norris, H.J. Malignant germ cell tumors of the ovary. *Hum. Pathol.* 8:551–564,1977.

Reimer, R.R. et al. Acute leukemia after alkylating agent therapy for ovarian cancer. *N. Engl. J. Med.* 297:177–181, 1977.

Rutledge, F., and Burns, B. Chemotherapy for advanced ovarian cancer. *Am. J. Obstet. Gynecol.* 96:761–770, 1966.

Schwartz, P.E., and Smith, J.P. Treatment of ovarian stromal tumors. *Am. J. Obstet. Gynecol.* 125:402–408, 1976.

Schwartz, P.E., and Smith, J.P. The role of second look surgery in ovarian cancer management. Presented at the eighth annual meeting of the Felix Rutledge Society, Los Angeles, California, July 1977.

Smith, G.W.; Day, T.G.; and Smith, J.P. The use of laparoscopy to determine the results of chemotherapy for ovarian cancer. *J. Reprod. Med.* 18:257–260, 1977.

Smith, J.P.; Delgado, G.; and Rutledge, F. Second look operation in ovarian carcinoma. *Cancer* 28:1438–1442, 1976.

Smith, J.P., and Rutledge, F. Advances in chemotherapy for gynecologic cancer. *Cancer* 36:669–674, 1975.

Wangensteen, O.H.; Lewis, F.J.; and Tongen, L.A. The second-look in cancer surgery. *Lancet* 71:303–307, 1951.

Wharton, J.T. et al. Hexamethylmelamine: an evaluation of its role in the treatment of ovarian cancer. *Am. J. Obstet. Gynecol.* 133:833–841, 1979.

Young, R.C. et al. Advanced ovarian adenocarcinoma: a prospective trial of melphalan (L-PAM) versus combination chemotherapy. *N. Engl. J. Med.* 299:1261–1266, 1978.

Chapter 15

The Treatment of Ovarian Dysgerminoma

PERSPECTIVE:

Garry V. Krepart

Ovarian dysgerminoma is an uncommon malignant tumor of the ovary, germ cell in origin, accounting for approximately 2% of ovarian malignancies. The primordial germ cells, in the arrested prophase of the first meiotic division, are the presumptive stem cells for this tumor, in which no sex chromatin is found and which contain twice the DNA content of normal somatic cells (Asadourian and Taylor 1969). Dysgerminomas may arise as a pure tumor or mixed with choriocarcinomas, malignant teratomas, and embryonal carcinomas of the ovary. The prognosis of these tumors varies greatly from author to author and depends not only on treatment but also on whether these tumors are pure or are associated with other germ cell elements.

Clenot first described these germ cell tumors in 1911, however, it was not until 1931 that Myer coined the term dysgerminoma. Initially thought to be tumors of low malignant potential (Asadourian and Taylor 1969; Brody 1961), over the decades their true malignant potential has become appreciated. Survivals have increased as a result of more aggressive therapy. Treatment recommendations range from pelvic cleanout plus radiotherapy for all stages (Boyes et al. 1978), to prophylactic paraaortic, mediastinal, and supraclavicular radiotherapy in spite of negative lymphangiography (Markovits et al. 1977). Dysgerminomas are frequently unilateral and occur in a young age group desiring future childbearing function. The problem, then, lies in identifying a group of patients in whom a conservative approach is justified, without risking future recurrence.

Before treatment planning, all patients should be thoroughly evaluated. At laparotomy, all suspicious areas should undergo biopsy, including pelvic and paraaortic nodes. Pretreatment or postlaparotomy lymphangiography is needed to evaluate pelvic, paraaortic, and possibly mediastinal and supra-

355

clavicular nodes in spite of negative node biopsies. Thirty-three percent of lymphangiograms have been reported abnormal in patients presenting with dysgerminomas (Markovits et al. 1977). In unilateral tumors, the other ovary should be carefully assessed and, if normal, need not undergo biopsy or bivalving. Bilateral disease should be treated with hysterectomy and bilateral salpingo-oophorectomy. Metastatic disease must be documented as to site, and all attempts should be made maximally to reduce tumor metastases if found. Stage I_a lesions of less than 10 cm in young patients who desire to preserve their fertility may be treated by unilateral oophorectomy, provided there is no ascites and the tumor is well differentiated and a pure dysgerminoma.

Material and Methods

In a previously reported study (Krepart et al. 1978), 36 patients who were seen at the University of Texas System Cancer Center, M. D. Anderson Hospital and Tumor Institute between the years 1947 and 1974 were analyzed. Only those patients with pure dysgerminoma were included. Twenty-six patients had their initial surgery at the M. D. Anderson Hospital or were referred immediately after surgery at another hospital. The remaining 10 patients were referred with recurrent tumors. No patient was lost to follow-up.

Staging was carried out according to FIGO recommendations. Table 15.1 shows the status of patients at the time of operation and at the time of referral. Only 30% had tumor confined to one ovary when first seen at M. D. Anderson Hospital, whereas 61% had tumors confined to one ovary at the time of their initial surgery. Twenty-two percent of stage I_a tumors progressed. The average recurrence time of the 11 patients who received no postoperative irradiation and developed recurrent tumor was 17.6 months, with a mean recurrence time of 12 months (table 15.2). Stage III or IV lesions accounted for

Table 15.1
Stage of Tumor

Stage	At Operation		At Referral	
	Number of Patients	Percent	Number of Patients	Percent
I	22	61	14	39
II	2	6	2	6
III	10	28	13	36
IV	2	6	7	19

356

Table 15.2
Stage of Tumor of Patients with Recurrent
Tumor

Original Stage	Ovarian Size (cm)	Referral Stage	Time to Recurrence in Months
I_a	18	III	20
I_a	?	IV	48
I_a	15	II_b	8
I_a*	15	III	22
I_a	15	III	26
I_a	20	IV	7
I_a	23	IV	12
I_a	12.5	I_b	9
I_b	20	IV	3
II_a	25	IV	34
III	?	III	3

*Followed at the M. D. Anderson Hospital.

the majority of recurrent disease. The five stage IV patients had metastatic disease to the paraspinal area, liver, and left supraclavicular areas.

Age

Patients developing dysgerminomas are uniformly young (Asadourian and Taylor 1969; Koller and Gjonnaess 1967; Malkasian and Symmonds 1964; Pedowitz, Felmus, and Grayzel 1955; Santesson 1947; Talerman, Huyzinga, and Kvipers 1973; Thoeny et al. 1961). Patients in this series ranged in age from 7 to 33 years (fig. 15.1). Over 50% were less than 20 years old, with the average being 18 and the mean 17 years. Only 8% of patients were over 30 years of age.

Presenting Signs and Symptoms

Ovarian dysgerminomas occur in a nonspecific fashion, as outlined in table 15.3. Abdominal masses with or without pain account for over one-half of these presenting symptoms, while pain with or without a mass accounted for an equal number of complaints. Six patients, or 17% of the total group, had their dysgerminoma discovered in the antepartum, intrapartum, or post-partum periods, and this is consistent with the observations of other authors (Jackson 1967). The reason for this association is not obvious, other than per-

Figure 15.1

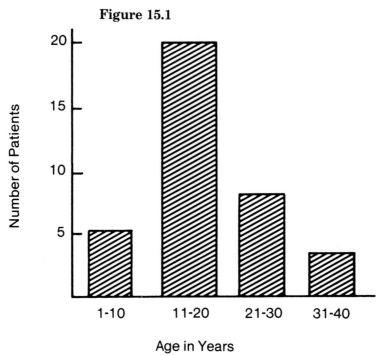

Ages of patients with dysgerminomas of the ovary.

haps the majority of these tumors are found in young women at the height of their reproductive potential. The association is not, however, noted in reviewing other germ cell tumors.

Treatment

Dysgerminomas are the gynecologic malignancies most sensitive to radiotherapy. This sensitivity results in a higher survival for ovarian dysgerminoma than for epithelial tumors of the ovary. A smaller dose is needed to eradicate dysgerminoma than is required for an equal volume of epithelial cancer. Large unresectable tumor masses often show remarkable resolution, and patients with recurrences within a previously radiated field can often be retreated.

All patients, except those with a unilateral encapsulated stage I_a lesion, should receive postoperative radiotherapy. Five patients treated with a unilateral salpingo-oophorectomy only were observed without receiving postoperative treatment. All had stage I_a dysgerminomas, with well-differentiated lesions of less than 10 cm in diameter. Subsequent pregnancy occurred in three of these patients. One patient with a 15 cm tumor who was observed

Table 15.3
Presenting Signs and Symptoms

Signs and Symptoms	Number of Patients	Percent
Abdominal mass and pain	6	17
Abdominal mass	13	36
Pain	13	36
Vaginal bleeding	1	3
At time of Caesarean section	1	3
Unknown	2	6

developed left upper quadrant metastatic disease 22 months postoperative. Subsequent treatment with radiation resulted in a cure, and she has been free of disease for over seven years. Treatment recommendations including either hysterectomy and bilateral salpingo-oophorectomy or prophylactic pelvic and nodal radiotherapy in this select group seem unjustified on the basis of current knowledge of recurrent disease.

Patients with more advanced disease should all receive postoperative radiotherapy. Table 15.2 demonstrates the stage at original laparotomy compared to the stage at referral for treatment of recurrence. Seventy-three percent of recurrences were noted in stage I_a disease as not fulfilling the criteria for conservative management.

The whole abdomen is at risk and, therefore, should be treated. In analyzing the sites of recurrent disease, abdominal metastases were present in two-thirds of the patients (table 15.4). After treatment of the abdomen, pelvic fields should be added to enhance the primary disease area. Additonal radiation should be added to biopsy proved or lymphangiogram positive paraaortic nodal areas. Prophylactic mediastinal and left supraclavicular irradiation should follow the treatment of positive paraaortic nodes. Thirty-one of 36 patients in this series received postoperative radiation. The remaining five patients were treated conservatively because of good prognosis lesions. Twenty-eight of the 31 patients received whole abdominal radiation; the remaining 3, pelvic paraaortic and/or mediastinal radiation only. Moving abdominal strip delivering a tumor dose of 2000 to 2200 rad to the entire abdomen was used in 12 patients with the remaining patients treated with open fields to a tumor dose of 2500 to 3000 rad to the entire abdomen. Additional pelvic radiation of 1500 to 2000 rad following abdominal radiation was administered to the majority of patients. Confirmed paraaortic nodal metastases were treated with 1500 rad additional radiation to the paraaortic areas in 19 patients. After three weeks of rest, these 19 patients received 2500 rad of prophylactic mediastinal and left supraclavicular radiation to complete their treatment.

359

Table 15.4
Site of Recurrence (12 Patients)

Site	Number of Patients
Abdomen	8
Pelvis	5
Paraaortic nodes	5
Supraclavicular nodes	4
Vertebral column	2
Lung	1
Liver	1

Results

Survival rates and length of survival at the time of original analysis are shown in table 15.5. The overall survival for the 36 patients is 86%. These survivals compare favorably with those in the literature, which range from 27% (Koller and Gjonnaess 1967) to over 90% (Jackson 1967; Boyes et al. 1978). Twenty-four of 26 patients receiving radiation, according to the treatment plan previously outlined, have survived (92%) and show no evidence of disease. One of these patients died of a mismatched blood transfusion and, if removed from statistics, the corrected survival would be 96%.

Seventy percent of patients referred with recurrent tumor (table 15.2) are free of disease, with the remaining patients dying of disease 16, 18, and 36 months after initial radiotherapy.

Chemotherapy

Experience with chemotherapy in dysgerminoma of the ovary is lacking. Limited remissions in this present series were obtained with cyclophosphamide and a combination of actinomycin-D, 5-fluorouracil, and cyclophosphamide as well as bleomycin and vinblastine in several patients. All eventually escaped their chemotherapy and succumbed to their disease. Others (Cohen and Goldsmith 1977) have used vincristine and bleomycin followed by vincristine and methotrexate for a prolonged response and possible cure. Unspecified alkylating agents were used for two cures in a recent series (Boyes et al. 1978). The recent success in treating testicular tumors in males with

360

Table 15.5
Survival by Stage at Referral

Stage	Number of Patients	Number Surviving	Percent	Survival in Months
I	14	14	100	36–212
II	2	2	100	102–133
III	13	10	77	36–273
IV	7	5	71	33–247
Totals	36	31	86	

vinblastine, Adriamycin, bleomycin, and Cis-diamminedichloroplatinum are encouraging and perhaps can be transposed to the treatment of ovarian dysgerminomas with success.

Conclusions

Although dysgerminomas of the ovary are rare lesions, their significance lies in their curability and their occurring most often in young women. Reproduction function may be preserved in selective cases where the tumor is a

1. stage I_a encapsulated pure dysgerminoma;
2. well-differentiated lesion;
3. tumor of less than 10 cm in diameter.

Conservative treatment with close follow-up seems, on the basis of current knowledge, altogether justified.

All other patients with dysgerminomas will need postoperative radiation. Careful intraoperative staging is imperative, as is pre- or postoperative lymphangiography. Recurrence sites demonstrate that the whole abdomen is at risk and, therefore, should be treated. Dose rates are low because of the sensitivity to radiation, and, as a result, complication rates from radiation are also low, significantly outweighing the chance of recurrence. Paraaortic metastases should be boosted and mediastinal and left supraclavicular radiation added. Over 90% of patients so treated should survive.

Chemotherapy for disease that cannot be irradiated is not, at present, well founded. Extrapolation from other germ cell tumors in both men and women seems to indicate that the active agents include alkylators, bleomycin, vinblastine, Adriamycin, and Cis-diamminedichloroplatinum. Further studies will be needed to draw any useful conclusions.

References

Asadourian, L.A., and Taylor, H.B. Dysgerminoma: an analysis of 105 cases. *Obstet. Gynecol.* 33:370–379, 1969.

Boyes, D.A. et al. Experience with dysgerminomas at the Cancer Control Agency of British Columbia. *Gynecol. Oncol.* 6:123–129, 1978.

Brody, S. Clinical aspects of dysgerminoma of the ovary. *Acta Radiol.* 56:209–230, 1961.

Cohen, S.M., and Goldsmith, M.A. Prolonged chemotherapeutic remission of metastatic ovarian dysgerminoma: report of a case. *Gynecol. Oncol.* 5:299–304, 1977.

Jackson, S.M. Ovarian dysgerminoma. *Br. J. Radiol.* 40:459–462, 1967.

Koller, O., and Gjonnaess, H. Dysgerminoma of the ovary—clinical report of 20 cases. *Acta Obstet. Gynecol. Scand.* 43:268–278, 1967.

Krepart, G.V. et al. The treatment for dysgerminoma of the ovary. *Cancer* 41:986–990, 1978.

Malkasian, G., and Symmonds, R.E. Treatment of the unilateral encapsulated ovarian dysgerminoma. *Am. J. Obstet. Gynecol.* 90:379–382, 1964.

Markovits, P. et al. Lymphography in the staging, treatment planning, and surveillance of ovarian dysgerminomas. *Am. J. Roentgenol.* 128:835–838, 1977.

Mueller, C.W.; Topkins, P.; and Lapp, W.A. Dysgerminoma of the ovary, an analysis of 427 cases. *Am. J. Obstet. Gynecol.* 60:153–159, 1950.

Myer, R. The pathology of some special ovarian tumors and their relationship to sex characteristics. *Am. J. Obstet. Gynecol.* 22:697–710, 1931.

Pedowitz, P.; Felmus, L.B.; and Grayzel, D.M. Dysgerminoma of the ovary—prognosis and treatment. *Am. J. Obstet. Gynecol.* 70:1284–1297, 1955.

Santesson, L. Clinical and pathological survey of the ovarian tumors treated at Radiumhemmet: dysgerminomas. *Acta Radiol.* 28:644–668, 1947.

Talerman, A.; Huyzinga, W.T.; and Kvipers, T. Dysgerminoma: clinical pathologic study of 22 cases. *Obstet. Gynecol.* 41:147, 1973.

Thoeny, R.H. et al. A study of ovarian dysgerminoma with emphasis on the role of radiotherapy. *Surg. Gynecol. Obstet.* 113:692–698, 1961.

PART VI

GESTATIONAL TROPHOBLASTIC DISEASE

Although relatively uncommon, gestational trophoblastic disease (GTD) deserves attention out of proportion to its incidence because of several unique features. First among these is the consistent elaboration by these tumors of human chorionic gonadotropin (HCG) into the plasma and its subsequent excretion in the urine. Chorionic gonadotropin is always found in the presence of GTD, and the clinical course of the disease as well as the response to therapy correlate with the measured level of HCG.

The elaboration of HCG by the trophoblast assumes clinical importance in the management of patients with GTD because assays are available which provide an accurate measurement of minute amounts of gonadotropin. Since 1943, a bioassay technique using a kaolin acetone extract of urine has allowed HCG to be quantitated at levels which can be accounted for on the basis of circulating pituitary FSH and LH. Radioimmunoassay has been developed using antisera generated against the beta subunit of HCG. High LH levels do not interfere with the specificity of this radioimmunoassay, and it appears ideal for monitoring serum HCG levels in patients undergoing chemotherapy as well as for the follow-up of patients after termination of molar pregnancies.

Dr. Jones reviews the chemistry and assays of HCG as they relate to all trophoblastic and gonadotropin producing tumors. Drs. Morrow, O'Brien, and Schlaerth indicate the bases for error using current assay techniques and suggest future refinements which will allow detection of even more minute quantities of circulating chorionic gonadotropin.

Chapter 16

Gestational Trophoblastic Disease: Is Human Chorionic Gonadotropin the Ideal Tumor Marker?

PERSPECTIVE:

Walter B. Jones

The development of highly sensitive techniques such as the radioimmuno-assay has made it possible to identify polypeptides and other tumor specific proteins in the blood and urine of individuals with a wide variety of neo-plasms. The term ectopic is applied to these findings when the parent tissue of the neoplasm is not ordinarily associated with such secretion. It is now well known that measurement of ectopic proteins can be useful in following the clinical course of cancer patients and thus serve as tumor markers. In some cases the persistence or recurrence of tumor after treatment can be de-termined by an elevation in specific tumor markers. Moreover, it has become apparent that aberrant hormone production may precede clinical recognition of tumor and thereby provide an early diagnosis of malignancy. Over the last decade the principle of radioimmunoassay has been applied to the study of almost all known polypeptide and steroid hormones (Ross 1977; Buster and Abraham 1975). The results of these studies have not only documented the increasing usefulness of tumor markers in current clinical diagnosis and management of malignancy but have afforded new insight into the process of normal and neoplastic protein biosynthesis (Franchimont et al. 1972; Shane and Naftolin 1975).

Fetoprotein tumor markers, carcinoembryonic antigen (CEA), and alpha feto-protein (AFP) were previously thought to be restricted to embryonic tis-sues or associated with specific neoplasms. It is now known that these mark-ers are present in the serum of normal persons as well as those with tumor, although levels are significantly higher in patients with tumors ectopically secreting the marker (Weintraub and Rosen 1973). Because of this, these pro-teins are sometimes referred to as quantitative markers (Rosen and Wein-traub 1974). The value of such markers can be seen in studies of CEA in pa-tients with colon cancer. Wanebo and co-workers (1978), for example, found the level of CEA to be of predictive value beyond that customarily provided by pathologic staging systems and suggested that preoperative levels could be used to divide patients into high- and low-risk categories. It is of interest that the highest levels of CEA are found in patients with colorectal cancer when compared to other gastrointestinal malignancies, yet a significant number of patients with colorectal cancer have normal levels of CEA (Beatty et al. 1979). Similar studies have been reported in which AFP served as the tumor marker (Waldmann and McIntire 1974). Qualitative tumor markers such as placental alkaline phosphatase, placental lactogen, and chorionic gonadotropin (HCG) and its beta subunit were similarly thought to be normally absent in the serum of men or nonpregnant women; their detection in these individuals therefore was considered diagnostic of the presence of neoplasm (Weintraub and Rosen 1973). Recent evidence suggests that these markers also exist in the serum and tissues of some normal persons as well as patients with various benign and malignant conditions. Human chorionic gonadotropin has received the most attention of this group of markers, although recent interest has also been focused on the aberrant isolated production of its subunits. After a brief review of the chemistry and procedures used to assay HCG and its subunits, their role as tumor markers will be considered.

Chemistry and Assay of HCG

Human chorionic gonadotropin is similar to other glycoproteins such as thyroid stimulating hormone (TSH), follicular stimulating hormone (FSH), and human luteinizing hormone (HLH) in that they are all composed of noncovalently linked subunits designated alpha and beta (Morgan and Canfield 1971). The alpha subunits are homologous with respect to chemical structure and appear to be interchangeable with one another. The beta subunits, although similar, have distinctive amino acid sequences and confer the unique biologic and immunologic activity of the hormone (Bahl et al. 1972). For example, the cross reaction between HCG and HLH in all biologic and nonspecific radioimmunoassays can be attributed to the fact that 80% of the first 115 amino acid terminal residues of the HCG-beta is identical to those of HLH-beta. The HCG-beta, however, has an additional 30 amino acid residues which are distinctive. The preparation and purification of native HCG and its subunits have made possible the development of specific and sensitive radioimmunoassays capable of measuring minute quantities of these proteins (Vaitukaitis, Braunstein, and Ross 1972). Extracts of tissues, serum, and urine, when subjected to fractionation by gel filtration, can be assayed so as to detect the presence of individual subunits as well as the intact hormone. The recent use of concanavalin-A to extract HCG from serum or urine prior to assay and the preparation of antisera generated against the 23 carboxy terminal amino acids of HCG-beta has resulted in assays of greater sensitivity and specificity than were previously available (Schreiber et al. 1976; Ayala et al. 1978).

Trophoblastic Neoplasms

Studies using an assay specific for HCG and its beta subunit in serum and plasma of patients with gestational trophoblastic neoplasms have become prototypes of follow-up practices in patients with hormonally active tumors. Human chorionic gonadotropin appears to be an ideal tumor marker in patients with gestational trophoblastic disease because it is invariably produced when viable tumor is present, can furnish an early diagnosis of malignancy, and can be used to monitor therapy and provide a diagnosis of remission. The value of this marker can be seen in the follow-up of patients after evacuation of a hydatidiform mole. Incomplete involution of the uterus and vaginal bleeding may be signs of persistent trophoblastic disease but measurement of HCG has been shown to be the most reliable method of identifying patients who have developed malignant sequelae (Delphs 1957). In this regard, HCG fulfills an arbitrary criterion of an ideal tumor marker in that a diagnosis of malignancy can be made prior to clinical or roentgenologic evidence of disease weeks or months in advance. Rushworth, Orr, and Bagshawe (1968) directed attention to the diagnostic value of HCG in patients with asymptomatic brain metastases. In their studies patients with tumors in this location could be identified by a higher concentration of HCG in the CSF relative to plasma than those who did not. Evidence from tissue culture, heterotransplants, and clinical studies indicates that the amount of HCG correlates well with the volume of viable trophoblastic tissue present (Kohler and Bridson 1971; Ross 1967; Pattillo et al. 1968; Ross et al. 1966). This quantitative relationship between tumor volume and HCG titer becomes important in patients with metastatic gestational trophoblastic disease because high initial HCG titers in these cases is associated with decreased survival rates (Ross et al. 1965). As a result of this, patients have been assigned to risk or therapeutic categories in which appropriate treatment is planned in part on the basis of the HCG titer (Jones 1975; Goldstein 1972; Hammond and Parker 1970). The measurement of HCG has also been shown to be a striking monitor of therapeutic effectiveness in patients undergoing chemotherapy. It is common clinical practice to alter chemotherapeutic agents or schedules in patients who evidence resistance by a plateau or elevation in HCG titer. The marker in this instance provides direct evidence of response to therapy, an observation that may antedate by weeks the recognition of disease progression by the usual clinical diagnostic measures. Perhaps the major value of HCG testing to physicians caring for these patients is its role in determining remission following treatment. While minimal levels of persisting marker indicate minimal remaining viable tumor and the need for further chemotherapy, the complete disappearance of HCG from the serum can provide a provisional diagnosis of remission. This becomes important because chemotherapy can safely be withheld in most patients when there is no hormonal evidence of remaining tumor (Jones, Lewis, and Lehr 1970). Radioimmunoassays in which extracts of urinary concentrates are analyzed for HCG

369

have made it possible to ascertain with even greater accuracy those patients who have achieved complete and sustained remission.

In summary, HCG appears to be an ideal tumor marker in patients with gestational trophoblastic disease. This opinion is based on the following observations:

1. A consistent production of marker by the tumor exists.
2. The detection of marker can provide a preclinical diagnosis of malignancy.
3. A quantitative relationship exists between marker and tumor volume.
4. The marker is an accurate monitor of response to treatment.
5. The disappearance of marker indicates remission of disease.

The presence of HCG in the serum of patients with gestational trophoblastic disease has been called a tumor specific index by Bagshawe. Perhaps there is not a more ideal tumor marker in all of clinical medicine.

Human chorionic gonadotropin is also a sensitive biologic marker in patients with trophoblastic tumors of nongestational origin such as those originating from the germ cells of the gonads or other primordial cells. Testicular tumors are by far the most commonly encountered of these neoplasms and are the subject of recent investigations using HCG and other tumor markers to monitor response to therapy. Current data indicate that 40% to 60% of patients with nonseminomatous germ cell tumors of the testicle will have a positive serum beta subunit radioimmunoassay (RIA) (Barzell and Whitmore 1979). Less commonly found is an association of HCG with seminoma (7% to 10%), although a higher frequency has been reported when assays of greater sensitivity are employed (Braunstein et al. 1973). It is of particular interest, however, that not all germ cell tumors associated with a positive test for HCG contain recognizable trophoblastic elements (Goldstein et al. 1974). The prognostic value of the marker in patients with nonseminomatous testicular tumors can be seen in the recent report by Barzell and Whitmore. In their study 74% of patients with a positive beta subunit assay had positive retroperitoneal lymph nodes on exploration. Similarly, Newlands and co-workers (1976) found that persistently elevated levels in serum after orchiectomy invariably indicated retroperitoneal metastases. Although HCG is occasionally the only positive marker detected in these cases, it is more commonly found in association with elevations of AFP or CEA, and this may occur at any time during the course of the disease. Initial and sequential measurement of these markers has been shown to reduce clinical staging errors significantly. According to Javadpour, when HCG and AFP are used together, they are the best markers available in diagnosis, detection of early recurrence, accurate staging, and reflecting the adequacy of treatment. Unlike the case for patients with gestational trophoblastic neoplasms, however, HCG may be absent from the serum and urine in a significant number of patients with germ cell tumors of the gonads. Also, in some cases with positive tests for HCG, treatment may alter hormone synthesis without an effect on tumor growth, perhaps reflecting the lack of response of heterologous elements present.

Nontrophoblastic Neoplasms

The specific radioimmunoassay based on the beta subunit of HCG, while providing the first practical method of differentiating between low levels of HCG and normal levels of HLH in patients with trophoblastic neoplasms, made it possible at the same time to survey large numbers of patients with nontrophoblastic tumors for the ectopic production of HCG. Braunstein and associates (1973) determined that approximately 10% of patients with a wide variety of tumors had positive responses using this assay with high levels found in carcinoma of the stomach, liver, pancreas, breast, and multiple myeloma. They also provided evidence that the ectopic hormone in many serum samples was in fact HCG rather than its subunits, although in some sera HCG-beta may have also been measured. Subsequent studies have confirmed the finding of ectopic HCG secretion in the serum of numerous cancer patients and more recently a material cross-reacting with the anti–B-chain antibody has been identified in the malignant cells of some of these tumors (McManus, Naughton, and Martinez-Hernandez 1976). Because of such findings it has been suggested that the presence of HCG in the blood of a man or a nonpregnant woman implied the presence of a tumor provided that a specific assay is used. Moreover, the unexpected production of HCG by such heterogeneous tumors indicated a possible role for HCG as a nonspecific marker to be used in screening for neoplasms. In the same context, Weintraub and Rosen, using radioimmunoassays permitting the differentiation of reactions with glycoproteins and their subunits, reported a case of pancreatic adenosquamous carcinoma in which the isolated ectopic production of HCG-beta was found in the serum. Based on the absence of HCG-beta in control sera it was suggested that the isolated production of this subunit may serve as yet another specific marker of neoplasms in men and nonpregnant women. Unfortunately, it appears that neither HCG nor HCG-beta is a unique secretory product of trophoblastic tumors or malignant neoplasms in general. Dosogne-Guerin and associates (1978), as an example, found significant plasma concentrations of HCG-beta as frequently in patients with benign diseases as in patients with malignant tumors (16% vs 16%). Remarkably a material reacting like HCG-beta was also found in the plasma of many normal control patients, a group composed of premenopausal and postmenopausal women, as well as men. A possible explanation for these observations may be found in recent reports documenting the presence of HCG in normal tissues. On examination of extracts of pooled normal human pituitary tissue from men and nonpregnant women, Chen and associates (1976) were able to identify substances with immunologic and physical characteristics of HCG. Similar substances have been found in extracts from normal human testes and sperm, and in the latter instance biologic potency could also be demonstrated (Braunstein, Rasor, and Wade 1975; Asch et al. 1978; Chowdhury and Steinberger 1979). Finally, Braunstein and coworkers (1978) provided evidence for the widespread distribution of a substance resembling HCG in a variety of normal human tissues. That substances biologically and antigenically similar to HCG may be more ubiquitous in nature than previously appreciated is suggested by the finding of a material similar to HCG in extracts from cultures of several microorganisms (Livingston 1974; Cohen and Strampp 1976).

As indicated previously the alpha subunit is common to all glycoproteins and thus a component of normally circulating hormones. Where normal levels have been established, however, excess free alpha has been attributed to ectopic secretion. The percentage of excessive alpha subunit concentration in patients with benign and malignant neoplasms appears to be virtually the same (17% vs 21%) (Dosogne-Guerin 1978), an incidence not unlike that found for the beta subunit. Because of the presence of subunits in the plasma of many patients with benign diseases, their measurement is thought to be of little value as a screening procedure. It should be noted, however, that very high levels of the subunits tend to be associated with the presence of malignancy, and in the occasional case where quantitative measurements have been made serum values were concordant with the clinical course of the disease (Rosen and Weintraub 1974). Free alpha and free beta subunits, when found in serum, urine, or tissue extracts in patients with gestational trophoblastic disease, have been shown to be an expression of more severe malignancy (Vaitukaitis and Ebersole 1976; Vaitukaitis 1973). Such findings suggest that follow-up of these patients requires assays responsive to the subunits as well as the intact hormone.

In summary, HCG and its subunits can normally be found in the plasma, urine, and tissues of some individuals and in the plasma of patients with nontrophoblastic tumors with ectopic HCG secretion. For these reasons, measurement of HCG is of limited usefulness as a screening procedure for occult neoplasia and when present does not identify the tumor type or site. This is in contrast to the value of HCG as a tumor marker in patients with gestational trophoblastic neoplasms. Because of the unique production of HCG whenever viable tumor is present in these cases, measurement of HCG can not only establish a diagnosis of occult malignancy, but it also provides a sensitive monitor of therapeutic response and a reliable diagnosis of remission.

References

Asch, R.H. et al. Characterization of a human chorionic gonadotropin-like material in human sperm. *Fertil. Steril. Suppl.* 30:755–756, 1978.

Ayala, A.R. et al. Highly sensitive radioimmunoassay for chorionic gonado-tropin in human urine. *J. Clin. Endocrinol. Metab.* 47:767–773, 1978.

Bahl, O.P. et al. Human chorionic gonadotropin: amino and sequence of the alpha and beta subunits. *Biochem. Biophys. Res. Commun.* 48:416–422, 1972.

Barzell, W.E., and Whitmore, W.F. Clinical significance of biologic markers: Memorial Hospital experience. *Semin. Oncol.* 6:48–52, 1979.

Beatty, J.D. et al. Clinical value of carcinoembryonic antigen. *Arch. Surg.* 114:563–567, 1979.

Braunstein, G.D. et al. Ectopic production of human chorionic gonadotropin by neoplasms. *Ann. Intern. Med.* 78:39–45, 1973.

Braunstein, G.D. et al. Widespread distribution of a chorionic gonadotropin-like substance in normal human tissues (abstr. 44). In program and abstracts of the 60th annual meeting of the American Endocrine Society, Miami, June 1978.

Braunstein, G.D.; Rasor, J.; and Wade, M.E. Presence in normal human testes of a chorionic-gonadotropin-like substance distinct from human lu-teinizing hormone. *N. Engl. J. Med.* 293:1339–1342, 1975.

Buster, J.E., and Abraham, G.E. The application of steroid hormone radioimmunoassays to clinical obstetrics. *Obstet. Gynecol.* 46:489–499, 1975.

Chen, H.C. et al. Evidence for a gonadotrophin from non-pregnant subjects that has physical, immunological and biological similarities to HCG. *Proc. Natl. Acad. Sci. USA* 73:2885, 1976.

Chowdhury, M., and Steinberger, E. Effect of age and estrogen therapy on the immunoreactive human chorionic gonadotropin content of testes. *Fertil. Steril.* 31:328–330, 1979.

Cohen, H., and Strampp, A. Bacterial synthesis of substances similar to human chorionic gonadotropins. *Proc. Soc. Exp. Biol. Med.* 152:408–410, 1976.

Delphs, E. Quantitative chorionic gonadotropin. Prognostic value in hydatidiform mole and chorionepithelioma. *Obstet. Gynecol.* 9:1–24, 1957.

Dosogne-Guerin, M.; Stolarczyk, A.; and Borokowski, A. Prospective study of alpha and beta subunits of human chorionic gonadotropin in the blood of patients with various benign and malignant conditions. *Eur. J. Cancer* 14:525–532, 1978.

Franchimont, P. et al. Polymorphism of protein and polypeptide hormones. *Clin. Endocrinol.* 1:315–336, 1972.

Goldstein, D.P. The chemotherapy of gestational trophoblastic disease. *JAMA* 220:209–213, 1972.

Goldstein, D.P.; Kosasa, T.S.; and Skarim, A.T. The clinical application of a specific radioimmunoassay for human chorionic gonadotropin in trophoblastic and non-trophoblastic tumors. *Surg. Gynecol. Obstet.* 138:747–751, 1974.

Hammond, C.B., and Parker, R.T. Diagnosis and treatment of trophoblastic disease—a report from the southeastern regional center. *Obstet. Gynecol.* 35:132–143, 1970.

Javadpour, N. The value of biologic markers in diagnosis and treatment of testicular cancer. *Semin. Oncol.* 6:37–47, 1979.

Jones, W.B. Treatment of chorionic tumors. *Clin. Obstet. Gynecol.* 18:247–265, 1975.

Jones, W.B.; Lewis, J.L., Jr.; and Lehr, M. Monitor of chemotherapy in gestational trophoblastic neoplasm by radioimmunoassay of the B-subunit of human chorionic gonadotropin. *Am. J. Obstet. Gynecol.* 36:37–43, 1970.

Kohler, P.O., and Bridson, W.E. Isolation of hormone-producing clonal lines of human choriocarcinoma. *J. Clin. Endocrinol. Metab.,* 32:683–687, 1971.

Livingston, V.W., and Livingston, A.M. Some cultural, immunological and biochemical properties of progenitor cryptocides. *Trans. N.Y. Acad. Sci.* 36:569–582, 1974.

McManus, L.M.; Naughton, M.A.; and Martinez-Hernandez, A. Human chorionic gonadotropin in human neoplastic cells. *Cancer Res.* 36:3476–3481, 1976.

Morgan, F.J., and Canfield, R.E. Nature of the subunits of human chorionic gonadotropin. *Endocrinol.* 88:1045–1053, 1971.

374

Newlands, E.S. et al. Serum alpha-fetoprotein and H.C.G. in patients with testicular tumours. *Lancet* 2:744–745, 1976.

Pattillo, R.A. et al. Human hormone production in vitro. *Science* 159:1467–1469, 1968.

Rosen, S.W., and Weintraub, B.D. Ectopic production of the isolated alpha subunit of the glycoprotein hormones. *N. Engl. J. Med.* 290:1441–1447, 1974.

Ross, G.T. In C.J. Lund and J.W. Choate, eds. Transcript of Fourth Rochester Trophoblast Conference, University of Rochester, 1967.

Ross, G.T. Clinical relevance of research on the structure of human chorionic gonadotropin. *Am. J. Obstet. Gynecol.* 129:795–808, 1977.

Ross, G.T. et al. Sequential use of methotrexate and antinomycin-D in the treatment of metastatic choriocarcinoma and relative trophoblastic disease in women. *Am. J. Obstet. Gynecol.* 93:223–229, 1965.

Ross, G.T. et al. Chemotherapy of metastatic and non-metastatic gestational trophoblastic neoplasms. *Tex. Rep. Biol. Med.* 24:326–338, 1966.

Rushworth, A.G.J.; Orr, A.H.; and Bagshawe, K.D. The concentration of HCG in the plasma and spinal fluid of patients with trophoblastic tumours in the central nervous system. *Br. J. Cancer* 22:253–257, 1968.

Schreiber, J.R. et al. Limitation of the specific serum radioimmunoassay for human chorionic gonadotropin in the management of trophoblastic neoplasms. *Am. J. Obstet. Gynecol.* 125:705–707, 1976.

Shane, J.M., and Naftolin, F. Aberrant hormone activity by tumors of gynecologic importance. *Am. J. Obstet. Gynecol.* 121:133–147, 1975.

Vaitukaitis, J.L. Immunologic and physical characterization of human chorionic gonadotropin (HCG) secreted by tumors. *J. Clin. Endocrinol. Metab.* 37:505–514, 1973.

Vaitukaitis, J.L.; Braunstein, G.D.; and Ross, G.T. A radioimmunoassay which specifically measures human chorionic gonadotropin in the presence of human luteinizing hormone. *Am. J. Obstet. Gynecol.* 113:751–758, 1972.

Vaitukaitis, J.L., and Ebersole, E.R. Evidence for altered synthesis of human chorionic gonadotropin in gestational trophoblastic tumors. *J. Clin. Endocrinol. Metab.* 42:1048–1055, 1976.

Waldmann, T.A., and McIntire, K.R. The use of a radioimmunoassay for alpha-beta protein in the diagnosis of malignancy. *Cancer* 34:1510–1515, 1974.

Wanebo, H.J. et al. Preoperative carcinoembryonic antigen level as a prognostic indicator in colorectal cancer. *N. Engl. J. Med.* 299:448–451, 1978.

Weintraub, B.D., and Rosen, S.W. Competitive radioassays and "specific" tumor markers. *Metabolism* 22:1119–1127, 1973a.

Weintraub, B.D., and Rosen, S.W. Ectopic production of the isolated beta subunit of human chorionic gonadotropin. *J. Clin. Invest.* 52:3135–3142, 1973b.

PERSPECTIVE:

Gestational Trophoblastic Disease: Is Human Chorionic Gonadotropin the Ideal Tumor Marker?

C. Paul Morrow,
Timothy J. O'Brien, and
John B. Schlaerth

The elaboration of chorionic gonadotrophin in relatively large quantities is such a constant feature of normal and neoplastic trophoblast that HCG is generally considered to be the prototype for all tumor markers. It is not this fact alone, however, which has bestowed upon HCG this mark of distinction, but rather a remarkable set of circumstances which may be related only indirectly: (1) the trophoblastic tumors, invasive mole, and choriocarcinoma are frequently curable even in the metastatic state by chemotherapy alone; (2) HCG is a biologically potent hormone and an antigenically potent protein, properties which have permitted it to be identified and quantified in very small concentrations.

Despite these unprecedented properties, HCG testing continues to be a subject of active research (Ross 1977). New markers for the trophoblastic tumors might also be desirable because of certain shortcomings of the HCG system: (1) neither qualitative nor quantitative HCG testing can distinguish among malignant, benign, normal, or nontrophoblastic sources of the hormone; (2) despite refinements in the methods for quantifying HCG, its similarity to LH on the molecular and immunologic levels can still be a source of error in HCG measurement; (3) the absence of HCG as determined by currently available methods is not absolute evidence that no viable (clonogenic) trophoblastic cells remain; at least some normal, nonpregnant women have low but detectable levels of HCG or HCG-like substances in their serum or urine (Chen et al. 1976; Borkowski and Muquardt 1979). The nature of HCG, the sensitivity and specificity of tests for its reliability as a trophoblastic marker, and potentially useful alternate or adjuvant markers are reviewed in this essay.

Supported by the Wright Foundation grant no. 55 and U. S. Public Health Service grants CA-20749 and CA-20501 from the National Institutes of Health.

376

Chemical and Immunologic Properties

Human chorionic gonadotropin is a glycoprotein hormone with a molecular weight of about 34,000 daltons (Frieden 1976). It is composed of two subunits, designated α and β, which are noncovalently linked. The subunits of HCG have been isolated, purified, and characterized (Morgan and Canfield 1971). Alpha is the smaller subunit and, except for the carbohydrate components, is nearly identical to the α subunits of the glycoprotein hormones FSH, LH, and TSH. Each contains 89 to 92 amino acid residues. It is the β subunit which gives these hormones immunologic as well as biologic specificity. β-HCG differs from LH primarily by the addition of a 30 amino acid carboxyl terminal sequence (Carlsen, Bahl, and Swaminathan 1973).

These glycoprotein hormones contain complex side chains of carbohydrates covalently bound to the polypeptides. The carbohydrate chains are composed of sialic acid, glucosamine, N-acetylglucosamine, galactose, mannose, and fucose. Removal of the sialic acid residues leads to a marked reduction of the plasma half-life and biologic (in vivo) potency of the hormone. The loss of monosaccharides from the carbohydrate side chains may also reduce the biologic activity of HCG (Tsuruhara et al. 1972). Despite the difference in the carbohydrate side chains, the antigenic determinants of the α subunits of HCG, LH, FSH, and TSH are nearly identical as measured by their reactivity to antisera; however, their potency as antigens varies. The β-subunits, on the other hand, reflecting their different polypeptide structure, induce more specific antibodies. According to Ross anti-alpha HCG sera is capable of neutralizing the biologic activities of HCG, LH, FSH, and TSH; in contrast the anti-beta HCG sera neutralizes HCG activity only. The antigenic specificity of beta HCG is due primarily to the 30 amino acid carboxyl terminal group, which has been sequenced and synthesized (Carlson, Bahl, and Swaminathan 1973). Although antisera raised against the carboxyl terminal sequence is more specific for HCG than anti-β sera, the isolated sequence is a less potent antigen, and consequently its antisera has less affinity for HCG than anti-β sera. The resultant loss of sensitivity in the radioimmunoassay (RIA) effectively neutralizes the advantage conferred on it by virtue of its greater specificity.

Metabolism

Injected HCG disappears from the blood of human subjects much more slowly than other glycoprotein hormones, providing it with a certain biologic advantage. Rizkallah and associates (1969) found the metabolic clearance rate of HCG in normal women following the intramuscular or intravenous injection of 10,000 IU of HCG to be 3.86 plus or minus 0.5 L/day (2.7 ml/min). The plasma HCG extinction curve had an initial fast exponential component with a half-life of 5.6 hours and slow component with a half-life of 23.9 hours. The volume of space into which the HCG distributed was calculated to be 1.75 to

2.83 L, a space compatible with the expected plasma volume of the subjects. Others have found similar values (Yen et al. 1968; Midgley and Jaffee 1968). The biexponential curve, usually interpreted as representing a two "pool" model, is also consistent with a multipool model. Since the half-life is strongly influenced by the degree of sialylation (Morell et al. 1971), one explanation for the observed extinction curve is that the multiple "pools" consist of HCG in various stages of desialylation, and this facilitates removal of HCG from the serum. Since only 6% to 12% of endogenous HCG is excreted in the urine (Johnson et al. 1950; Wide et al. 1968), metabolic clearance appears to be predominantly hepatic. The experiments of Tsuruhara and associates seem to confirm this notion. Comparing intact and desialylated HCG 15 minutes after injection into rats they found 8% uptake in the liver and 6% in the kidneys for the sialylated HCG versus 50% and 5% for the asialo form.

Measurement of HCG

The utility of HCG as a marker for trophoblastic tumors is essentially dependent upon the specificity and sensitivity with which it can be measured. The mouse or rat uterine weight assay and the rat ventral prostate assay exploit the biologic potency of HCG and its relatively specific bioactivity. Endogenous pituitary gonadotropins must be taken into account, however, since their biologic effects are similar to those of HCG. The sensitivity of these bioassays can be increased by concentrating the urine, or by injecting relatively large volumes of urine or serum into the small laboratory animals. Despite the success of the bioassays, they are cumbersome, expensive, and consequently have never been widely available. Biologic and immunologic activity are not necessarily parallel, and in at least one report the mouse uterine weight assay for HCG seemed to be more sensitive than a radioimmunoassay using an antisera to β-HCG (Wide et al. 1968; Schreiber et al. 1976).

The development of the radioimmunoassay (RIA) methodology was quickly adapted to the measurement of serum HCG. Unfortunately, anti-HCG sera also measures LH, a serious limitation since the ultimate criterion of any tumor marker assay is a specificity which matches its sensitivity. In 1972 Vaitukaitis and associates reported an RIA more specific for HCG using an antisera raised against the purified free beta subunit, which has different antigenic determinants than the beta subunits of the other tropic hormones. Its superiority to previous methods of monitoring trophoblastic disease patients has been the subject of numerous clinical studies (Jones, Lewis, and Lehr 1975; Pastorfide, Goldstein, and Kosasa 1974; Morrow et al. 1977; Khoo 1977).

The most recent development in HCG testing, the radioreceptor assay (RRA), uses receptor membranes of bovine corpora lutea which make it more specific and sensitive than other methods of pregnancy testing. It does not, however, distinguish HCG from LH (Kletzky et al. 1978). Furthermore, it is less sensitive than the β-HCG RIA and for these reasons is not suited to the measurement of HCG in patients with titers less than 5 to 10 mIU/ml of serum.

Limitations of the RIA for HCG

Sensitivity

The lowest concentration of HCG which can be reliably measured in the serum by currently available RIA methodology is 0.5 to 1.0 mIU/ml (0.2 to 0.4 ng/ml). Present data indicate that about 10,000 trophoblastic cells produce 8 to 40 mIU HCG per hour (Pattillo and Gey 1968; Lewis, Davis, and Ross 1969; Kohler and Bridson 1971; Braunstein et al. 1973; Knecht and Hertz 1978). Calculations of the T½ for the slow component of the HCG clearance curve range from 20 to 40 hours (Rizkallah, Gurpide, and Vande Wiele 1969; Yen et al. 1968; Midgley and Jaffe 1968). Assuming that the HCG is distributed in a plasma volume of 1500 to 3000 ml, 10^4 cells would produce in a steady state a serum HCG level of 0.03 to 0.5 mIU/ml (0.01 to 0.2 ng/ml) which is below the sensitivity of the assay. Thus the current RIA methodology limits our ability to detect fewer than 10,000 to 100,000 cells when all assay specifications are optimal. Ideally, the assay should detect the smallest number of cells capable of regrowing the tumor, in order to avoid premature termination of treatment. At the absolute minimum this would be one cell, but it is very doubtful that the last surviving cell must be killed by chemotherapy. (This also ignores the fact that choriocarcinoma consists of two cell types, the more differentiated of which, the syntrophoblastic cell, produces HCG, but is incapable of replicating.)

This deficiency in our testing methodology can be overcome, at least in part, by continuing treatment after the serum level of HCG drops below the sensitivity of the method. The duration of treatment post titer remission might be based on the presumed number of residual cells and the fractional kill calculated from the HCG titer curve during chemotherapy. For example, if the number of residual cells is estimated to be 50,000 and the fractional kill is 90% (one log drop in the nadir serum HCG after each course of drug therapy), then five more courses of chemotherapy might be necessary. While great success has been achieved by the traditional method of stopping chemotherapy as soon as titer remission is achieved, or one or two treatments later, relapses do occur, underscoring the need for continued treatment or a more sensitive assay (fig. 16.1).

Because the sensitivity of a given radioimmune assay is determined ultimately by the association constant of the antibody for the antigen, selection of specific antibodies may be capable of increasing the sensitivity of the assay from, say, 1.0 to 0.5 mIU/ml. To increase the current level of sensitivity by 10-fold or more, however, a different methodology is necessary. One approach

379

to this problem is to develop a trap system for the tumor marker. The trap could consist of a solid phase, immobilized antibody through which a body fluid such as whole blood, serum, urine, or saliva is passed. The resulting concentrated marker protein would then be assayed by any of the available methods (RIA, elisa, bioassay). We are working on such a trap system in our laboratory at the present time. Nevertheless, improvements in disease mon-

Figure 16.1

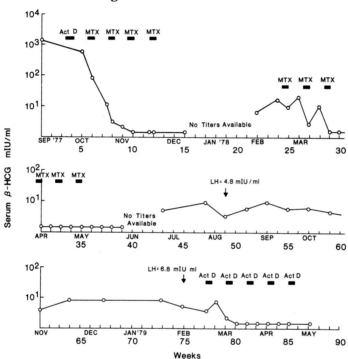

Twenty-six-year-old patient, gravida 1, para 0. Molar pregnancy evacuated in May 1977. Chest x-ray prior to chemotherapy revealed pulmonary metastases. She received one full course of methotrexate (MTX) after achieving titer remission (< 1.5 mIU/ml). Her titer rose to 10 mIU/ml and chemotherapy was again administered. This time she received three full courses of MTX after titer remission. Again her HCG titer became elevated and ranged from 5–10 mIU/ml for nine months. During this time she was on oral contraceptives. Her serum LH was measured twice to be certain it was not contributing to the persistently low HCG value. For her third round of treatment, actinomycin-D (Act-D) was employed. Titer remission was again readily achieved. The plan is to continue her treatments for six months postremission.

itoring by increasing the HCG assay sensitivity are clearly limited by the existence of low levels of HCG-like substances in the serum of normal subjects.

Specificity

Even the best antisera raised against the purified β-subunit will exhibit some measurable cross-reactivity with LH if the concentration of LH is sufficient. For example, a reasonably good antisera might have as much as 5% cross-reaction with LH. At 20 mIU/ml the LH would then contribute 1.0 mIU/ml to the HCG assay. If the assay sensitivity is 1.0 mIU/ml then a slightly elevated value of between 1.0 and 2.0 mIU/ml might result when the actual concentration of HCG is less than 1.0. Preovulatory peaks of 40 to 200 mIU/ml might spuriously raise the HCG value by 2 to 10 mIU/ml. It is not helpful to deal with this problem by calling 10 mIU/ml the upper limit of "normal" and designating it as the zero value. Since many "specific" antibeta sera will cross-react to some extent with LH in the physiologic range, estrogen-progestin contraceptive steroids should be given to patients with trophoblastic disease to suppress the serum LH and nullify this potential source of error. The occasional castrated or postmenopausal patient with tro-

Figure 16.2

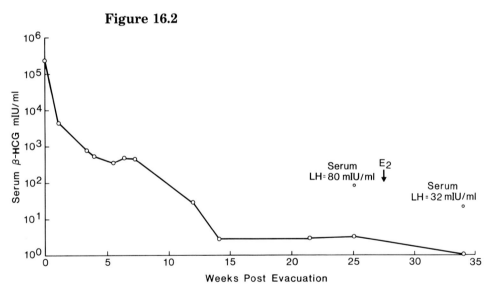

Weeks Post Evacuation

Forty-four-year-old patient had total abdominal hysterectomy and bilateral salpingo-oophorectomy 10 weeks post molar pregnancy because of a titer plateau. There was no evidence of metastases. Her serum β-HCG titer fell within 4 weeks to a level of 2–3 mIU/ml and then persisted at that level for 10–12 weeks. Serum LH at 15 weeks postoophorectomy was 80 mIU/ml. She was placed on oral estrogen therapy (E₂) and her serum β-HCG fell to less than 1.0 mIU/ml.

381

Figure 16.3

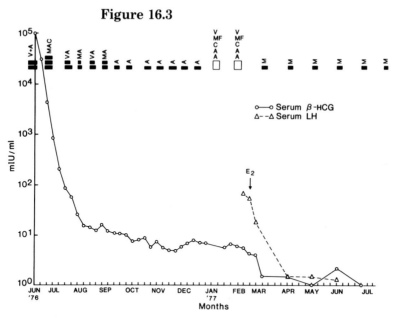

*Fifty-year-old patient presented with postabortal
choriocarcinoma metastatic to the lung and brain.
She received whole brain radiation and chemotherapy (V = velban, A = actinomycin-D,
C = cytoxan, M = methotrexate; VMFCCA =
Bagshaw's combination drug regimen). From
August 1976 to mid-November 1976 her serum
β-HCG titer fell from 20 to 6 mIU/ml. After there
was no response to VMFCCA the serum LH was
determined to be 68.1 mIU/ml. The serum β-HCG
simultaneously fell to less than 1.0 mIU/ml. She
remains in remission as of April 1979. Treatment
with single-agent chemotherapy was continued for
six months post titer remission.*

phoblastic disease presents a similar problem. Her tonic level of LH may be
as high as the preovulatory spike of the cycling patient. Even if she is taking
the conjugated estrogens usually prescribed for these women, the LH will not
be suppressed to insignificant levels (Utian et al. 1978). If these factors are
not appreciated, treatment may be discontinued prematurely (normal HCG
value arbitrarily set too high) or it may be continued (even intensified) in the
presence of a persistently low "HCG titer" due to cross-reaction with relatively high levels of LH rather than persistent disease (figs. 16.2 and 16.3).

Elimination or reduction of the cross-reactivity with LH would enhance
the reliability of the present RIA for HCG. Improved specificity has been at-
tained by developing antisera to the unique carboxyl terminal amino acid sequence of β-HCG, but unfortunately, since this antisera has less affinity for
the HCG molecule, this assay is less sensitive. Fractionation of antisera to

Figure 16.4

ANTIBODY DILUTIONS AFTER ISOELECTRIC FOCUSING

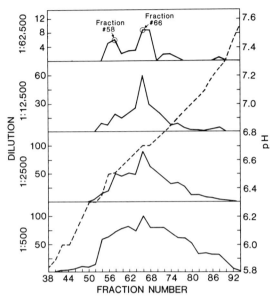

Fractionation of 100 μl of antiserum to β-HCG is accomplished by isoelectric focusing over a pH gradient (-----) of 5–8 (O'Brien et al. 1980a). Individual fractions are then titered and evaluated for sensitivity and specificity in the RIA assay.

β-HCG into individual antibody groups can be accomplished by isoelectric focusing of the whole serum. Because the primary structure of the antigenic binding site is unique for each antigenic determinant, a specific isoelectric character is associated with individual antibodies. Therefore, isoelectric fractionation over a suitable pH gradient (5 to 8) allows individual antibody groups (i.e., closely related isoelectric groups) to be selected. Fractionation of a typical antiserum to HCG prepared in our laboratory is shown in figure 16.4. Titering of individual fractions shows marked variations for different isoelectric groups. By comparing the cross-reactivity of the whole antiserum (fig. 16.5) to individual fractions, certain fractions can be selected which have almost no LH cross-reactivity (fig. 16.6, fraction 58) while maintaining good sensitivity (1.2 mIU/ml at 90% binding). Other fractions also have good sensitivity (fig. 16.7, fraction 66), but with measurable cross-reactivity for LH (3.5%). Thus LH cross-reactivity can be eliminated or reduced significantly without loss of sensitivity by isoelectric fractionation. A potential limitation of this approach is its failure to produce sufficient antibody for large numbers of radioimmune assays. If the isoelectric point can be correlated with specific antigenic determinants (and there is no evidence yet for this) then antisera from different rabbits could be processed to obtain a larger volume of homogenous antibody preparations.

Figure 16.5

CHARACTERISTICS OF WHOLE ANTISERA
PRIOR TO ISOELECTRIC FOCUSING

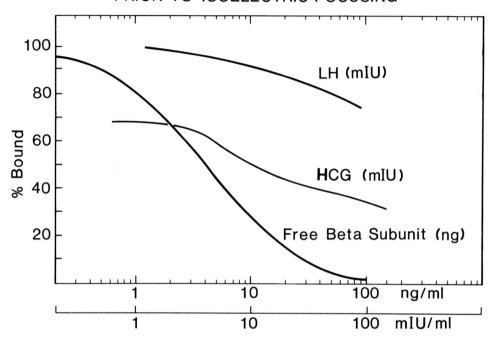

A standard curve for free β-subunit of HCG is used to compare the affinity and cross-reactivity of antiserum fraction No. 6 for HCG (whole molecule) and LH.

Alternate Assays to HCG

Free Alpha Subunit

A potential candidate as an alternate tumor marker to HCG is the free alpha subunit of the HCG molecule. This consideration is based on the evidence demonstrating the independent control of the alpha subunit gene from that of the beta subunit gene. In normal placenta the rate of synthesis of messenger RNA for the alpha subunit and subsequent protein synthesis exceeds that of the β-subunit by 6- to 10-fold (Vaitukaitis et al. 1976). Its potential as a marker for malignancy would be strengthened further if the independent regulation of the two individual subunits were such that elaboration of the alpha subunit occurred prior to beta subunit expression during the differentiation of cytotrophoblast to syntrophoblast. Such a sequence, of course, would provide a capacity to measure with greater sensitivity the presence of clonogenic cytotrophoblast and would therefore be a more meaningful eval-

Figure 16.6

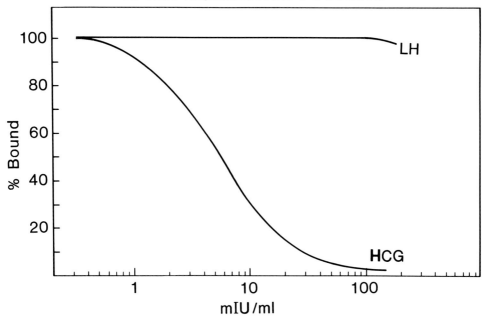

FRACTION 58
CROSS REACTIVITY OF LH WITH HCG
AFTER ISOELECTRIC FOCUSING

*Sensitivity and cross-reactivity of fraction No. 58 is
demonstrated by comparing the standard curve for
HCG (whole molecule) with LH displacement in
the RIA for HCG.*

uation of disease activity during treatment and follow-up. Difficulties which
might preclude an alpha subunit assay's becoming a more ideal tumor monitor than HCG are (1) less sensitivity than the β-HCG assay; (2) cross-
reactivity with the whole HCG molecule; (3) free subunit production by the
pituitary or other nontumor sources; and (4) lack of subunit production by
the trophoblastic cells. Both the sensitivity and the cross-reactivity problems
appear solvable, as several good antialpha sera have been developed in our
laboratory with excellent sensitivity and low cross-reactivity for HCG, LH,
and the β-subunit. (We are grateful to Drs. Robert Canfield and Griff Ross
for supplying us with purified α- and β-subunits CR119–2.) The behavior of
one such antisera is shown in figure 16.8. With this assay we have found in
preliminary studies that the serum-free alpha HCG levels range from
2.5–6 ng/ml in normal, cycling women. The free alpha concentrations in nine
women with choriocarcinoma were consistently lower than the serum HCG
until the latter dropped to normal levels (fig. 16.9). Thereafter free alpha,
presumably of pituitary origin, persisted at a low but measurable level. It is
notable that the free alpha levels in these women who were suppressed with

Figure 16.7

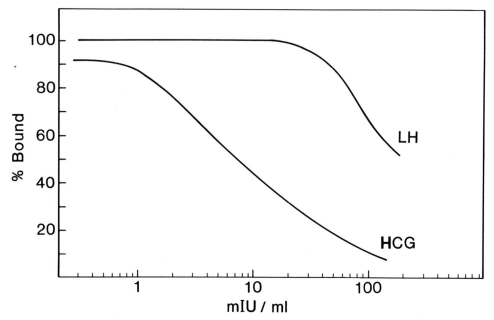

FRACTION 66
CROSS REACTIVITY OF LH WITH HCG
AFTER ISOELECTRIC FOCUSING

Analysis of fraction No. 66 compares LH cross-reactivity with an HCG standard curve for this isoelectric group of antibodies.

oral contraceptives are significantly lower than in the cycling women.

Vaitukaitis and Ebersole (1976) have examined tissue extracts, sera, and urine from women with molar pregnancies and choriocarcinoma. None of the plasm and urine samples from 18 women responding to chemotherapy contained free alpha (or beta) subunits, but the urine of one patient dying of resistant choriocarcinoma contained more free alpha than intact HCG. Other investigators have reported generally discordant findings (Dawood et al. 1977; Ashitaka et al. 1977; Rutanen 1978). The evaluation of this tumor marker is still incomplete.

Free Beta Subunit

This species is also being studied as a potential marker for chorionic tumors. It has two properties which are advantageous by comparison to the free alpha subunit. First, the slow phase serum half-life of the free beta subunit is three times that of the free alpha molecule (Wehmann and Nisula 1979); second, since the beta HCG subunit is not produced by the pituitary, its measure-

Figure 16.8

CHARACTERISTICS OF ANTISERUM
FOR FREE ALPHA SUBUNIT OF HCG

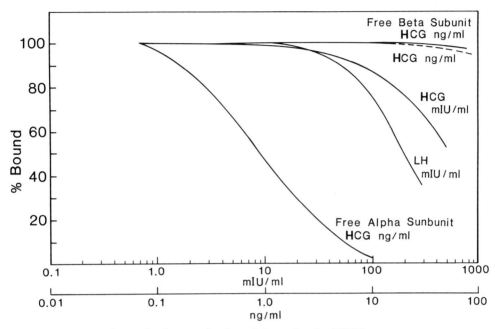

A standard curve for free alpha subunit of HCG
with antialpha antiserum fraction No. 2 is used to
compare cross-reactivity of free β-subunit of HCG,
whole molecule HCG, and LH.

ment has the potential for being not only more sensitive, but also more specific. To date, however, free beta HCG subunit has been found less often than the alpha subunit in measureable quantities in the body fluids of trophoblastic disease patients. (Vaitukaitis and Ebersole 1976; Dawood et al. 1977; Ashitaka et al. 1977).

Pregnancy Specific β_1-glycoprotein

Another oncoplacental protein which has recently received attention is the β_1-placental specific glycoprotein (SP$_1$, PAPP-C) (Horne and Towler 1978). Unlike the gonadotropins, this glycoprotein is composed of a single peptide chain. It has a molecular weight of 90,000 daltons and a carbohydrate content of 29%. In common with HCG, it is synthesized and secreted by the syntrophoblastic cell. The exact timing for the synthesis of this molecule during differentiation of the cytotrophoblast to syntrophoblast is unclear, but as with the case of HCG and the free alpha subunit, the measurement of SP$_1$ could prove to be useful in monitoring trophoblastic disease. Because of its

Figure 16.9

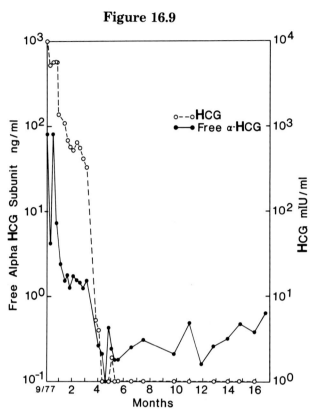

Analyses of serum concentrations of HCG and free alpha subunit are compared during chemotherapeutic follow-up in a patient with choriocarcinoma. Free alpha subunit values were corrected for a 0.4% cross-reactivity of HCG (whole molecule).

unique character (at least as far as is known) it does not suffer from the problems of (1) sharing a subunit with the other gonadotropins as HCG does with LH, FSH, and TSH or (2) sharing antigenic cross-reactivity with these hormones as β-HCG does with β-LH. It would seem, therefore, that an SP_1 assay might not have the cross-reactivity problems of the HCG assay.

Although the SP_1 assay is still under development it has reached a potentially useful status with good sensitivity and without obvious problems of cross-reactivity (O'Brien et al. 1980a, 1980b). This assay mimics the HCG assay very well in terms of monitoring therapy of choriocarcinoma patients, as shown in figure 16.10. When a conversion factor of 2.5 mIU to 1.0 ng is used to express HCG in ng/ml, the quantity of HCG in the patients' serum still exceeds that of SP_1 in most cases. While this excess of HCG is the general rule, it is usually not great (often around 2-fold), and at times the SP_1 titer exceeds that of HCG, as shown in figure 16.11. The replacement of the HCG

Figure 16.10

COMPARISON OF HCG AND SP₁
IN CHORIOCARCINOMA MONITORING

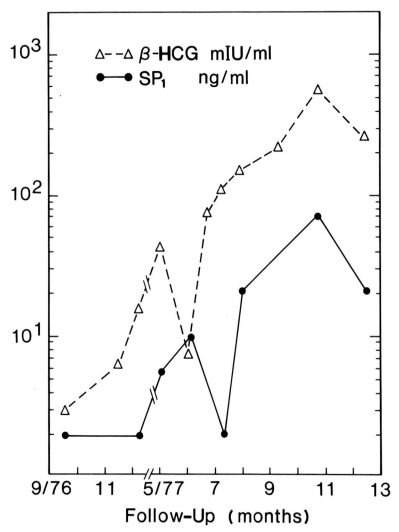

Serum concentrations of HCG and SP₁ are
compared during follow-up period of
choriocarcinoma patient who refused treatment.
SP₁ analyses were carried out at the City of Hope
National Medical Center in collaboration with Dr.
Eva Engvall.

Figure 16.11

COMPARISON OF HCG AND SP₁
IN CHORIOCARCINOMA MONITORING

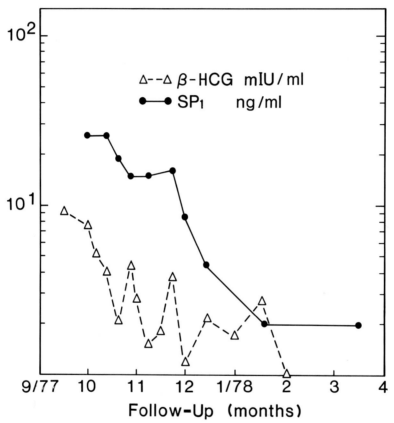

Serum concentrations of HCG and SP₁ were
analyzed as above in the follow-up monitoring of
this choriocarcinoma patient.

assay by an SP₁ assay for trophoblastic disease appraisal is not likely to occur. It is noteworthy, however, that this assay might avoid some of the pre
sent drawbacks of the HCG assay, for example, misinterpretation of low titer
values due to cross-reactivity with LH. Therefore, in the long run it may be
proved to be valuable to the clinician. Further evaluation of the SP₁ assay is
needed to establish its sensitivity at threshold values of HCG and to assess
the frequency with which nontrophoblastic tumors produce measureable
quantities of SP₁.

Miscellaneous Markers

Several other oncoplacental proteins have been described in the past several years which have attracted some interest as potential tumor markers. Best known, perhaps, is placental lactogen (HPL) (Goldstein 1971). Others are alkaline phosphatase (Goldstein 1965), oxytocinase (Babuna et al. 1970), and placental protein 5 (Bohn 1972). Carcinoembryonic antigen and alpha fetoprotein, oncofetal proteins intensively studied in patients with liver, gut, and gonadal tumors, are usually not found in the sera of women with trophoblastic disease (DiSaia et al. 1975; Ishiguro 1975).

Summary

In answer to the question of how HCG measures up to the ideal as a tumor marker, emphasis must be placed first on its unprecedented success which has made it a powerful and indispensable tool in the diagnosis and management of chorionic tumors. Nevertheless, we believe improvements are possible in the areas of specificity and sensitivity of the assay. A few patients will relapse after titer remission, a clinical fact which seems to confirm the calculations that the most sensitive HCG assays available can detect no fewer than 10^4 to 10^5 trophoblastic cells. The specificity requirements at the lower limits of sensitivity need to be improved, since even low levels of cross-reaction with similar molecules (e.g., LH) can produce spurious values. Theoretically, SP_1 has the potential to be more useful as a tumor marker than HCG at very low tumor volumes because it appears to be a unique antigen and therefore may not have the problem of cross-reactivity. Even if this proves to be an exploitable feature, the SP_1 assay cannot be expected to improve the sensitivity of testing for trophoblastic cells by more than two-fold. A more dramatic increase in sensitivity must be accomplished by concentrating the marker protein once the serum (or urine) levels drop below the sensitivity of our testing method. We are approaching this problem by immunologically trapping the marker on a solid phase support system prior to performing the assay. The application of this model system to tumor monitoring in general awaits development of the system and identification of tumor markers elaborated by specific malignancies.

References

Ashitaka, Y. et al. Alpha-subunit of human chorionic gonadotropin in fluid of molar vesicles. *Endocrinol. Jpn.* 24:115–119, 1977.

Babuna, C. et al. An enzymatic method for diagnosis of hydatidiform mole. *Obstet. Gynecol.* 35:852–856, 1970.

Bohn, H.N. Nochweis und charakterisierung von schwangerschaftsproteinen in der menschlichen plazenta, sowie ihre quantitative immunologische bestimmung in serum schwangererfrauen. *Arch. Gynaekol.* 212:165–175, 1972.

Borkowski, A., and Muquardt, C. Human chorionic gonadotropin in the plasma of normal, nonpregnant subjects. *N. Engl. J. Med.* 301:298–302, 1979.

Braunstein, G.D. et al. Secretory rates of human chorionic gonadotropin by normal trophoblast. *Am. J. Obstet. Gynecol.* 115:447–450, 1973.

Carlsen, R.B.; Bahl, O.P.; and Swaminathan, N. Human chorionic gonadotropin. *J. Biol. Chem.* 248:6810–6825, 1973.

Chen, H.C. et al. Evidence for a gonadotropin from nonpregnant subjects that has physical, immunological, and biological similarities to human chorionic gonadotropin. *Proc. Natl. Acad. Sci.* 73:2885–2889, 1976.

Dawood, M.Y.; Saxena, B.B.; and Landesman, R. Human chorionic gonadotropin and its subunits in hydatidiform mole and choriocarcinoma. *Obstet. Gynecol.* 50:172–181, 1977.

DiSaia, P.J. et al. Carcinoembryonic antigen in patients with gynecologic malignancies. *Am. J. Obstet. Gynecol.* 121:159–163, 1975.

Frieden, E.H. *Chemical endocrinology.* New York: Academic Press, 1976.

Goldstein, D.P. Neutrophil alkaline phosphatase activity in patients with choriocarcinoma and related trophoblastic tumors, undelivered hydatid mole, and in normal pregnancy. *Am. J. Obstet. Gynecol.* 92:1014–1017, 1965.

Goldstein, D.P. Serum placental lactogen activity in patients with molar pregnancy and trophoblastic tumors—a reliable index of malignancy. *Am. J. Obstet. Gynecol.* 110:583–587, 1971.

Horne, C.H.W., and Towler, C.M. Pregnancy-specific β_1-glycoprotein: a review. *Obstet. Gynecol. Surv.* 33:761–768, 1978.

Ishiguro, T. Serum α-fetoprotein in hydatidiform mole, choriocarcinoma, and twin pregnancy. *Am. J. Obstet. Gynecol.* 121:539–541, 1975.

Johnson, C.E.; Albert, A.; and Wilson, R.B. Renal and extrarenal disposal of chorionic gonadotropin in the immediate postpartum period. *J. Clin. Endocrinol.* 10:371–380, 1950.

Jones, W.B.; Lewis, J.L., Jr.; and Lehr, M. Monitor of chemotherapy in gestational trophoblastic neoplasm by radioimmunoassay of the β-subunit of human chorionic gonadotropin. *Am. J. Obstet. Gynecol.* 121:669–673, 1975.

Khoo, S.K. Measurement of the beta-subunit of chorionic gonadotrophin in uncomplicated, complicated, and molar pregnancies. *Aust. N.Z. J. Obstet. Gynaecol.* 17:137, 1977.

Kletzky, O.A. et al. A comparative study between radioreceptor assay and radioimmunoassay for HCG in patients with trophoblastic disease. *Obstet. Gynecol.* 52:328–331, 1978.

Knecht, M., and Hertz, R. Relationship between plasma levels of human chorionic gonadotropin and tumor growth during chemotherapy for human choriocarcinoma maintained in the hamster cheek pouch. *Cancer Treat. Rep.* 62:2101–2108, 1978.

Kohler, P.O., and Bridson, W.E. Isolation of hormone-producing clonal lines of human choriocarcinoma. *J. Clin. Endocrinol. Metab.* 32:683–687, 1971.

Lewis, J.L.; Davis, R.C.; and Ross, G.T. Hormonal, immunologic, and chemotherapeutic studies of transplantable human choriocarcinoma. *Am. J. Obstet. Gynecol.* 104:472–478, 1969.

Midgley, A.R., Jr., and Jaffe, R.B. Regulation of human gonadotropins: II. Disappearance of human chorionic gonadotropin following delivery. *J. Clin. Endocrinol. Metab.* 28:1712–1718, 1968.

Morell, A.G.; Gregoriadis, G.; and Scheinberg, I.H. The role of sialic acid in determining the survival of glycoproteins in the circulation. *J. Biol. Chem.* 246:1461–1467, 1971.

Morgan, F.J., and Canfield, R.E. Nature of the subunits of human chorionic gonadotropin. *Endocrinol.* 88:1045–1053, 1971.

Morrow, C.P. et al. Clinical and laboratory correlates of molar pregnancy and trophoblastic disease. *Am. J. Obstet. Gynecol.* 128:424–430, 1977.

O'Brien, T.J. et al. Antibody fractionation for improved sensitivity and specificity of HCG antisera. *Clin. Chemo.* 26:1920–1921, 1980a.

O'Brien, T.J. et al. Trophoblastic disease monitoring: evaluation of pregnancy specific β_1-glycoprotein. *Am. J. Obstet. Gynecol.* 138:313–320, 1980b.

Pastorfide, G.B.; Goldstein, D.P.; and Kosasa, T.S. The use of a radioimmunoassay specific for human chorionic gonadotropin in patients with molar pregnancy and gestational trophoblastic disease. *Am. J. Obstet. Gynecol.* 120:1025–1028, 1974.

Pattillo, R.A., and Gey, G.O. The establishment of a cell line of human hormone-synthesizing trophoblastic cells in vitro. *Cancer Res.* 28:1231–1236, 1968.

Rizkallah, T.; Gurpide, E.; and Vande Wiele, R.L. Metabolism of HCG in man. *J. Clin. Endocrinol. Metab.* 29:92–100, 1969.

Ross, G.T. Clinical relevance of research on the structure of human chorionic gonadotropin. *Am. J. Obstet. Gynecol.* 129:795–808, 1977.

Rutanen, E.M. The circulating alpha subunit of human chorionic gonadotrophin in gynaecologic tumours. *Int. J. Cancer* 22:413–421, 1978.

Schreiber, J.R. et al. Limitation of the specific serum radioimmunoassay for human chorionic gonadotropin in the management of trophoblastic neoplasms. *Am. J. Obstet. Gynecol.* 125:705–707, 1976.

Tsuruhara, T. et al. Biological properties of HCG after removal of terminal sialic acid and galactose residues. *Endocrinol.* 91:296–301, 1972.

Utian, W.H. et al. Effect of premenopausal castration and incremental dosages of conjugated equine estrogens on plasma follicle-stimulating hormone, luteinizing hormone, and estradiol. *Am. J. Obstet. Gynecol.* 132:297–302, 1978.

Vaitukaitis, J.L. et al. Gonadotropins and their subunits: basic and clinical studies. *Recent Prog. Horm. Res.* 32:289–331, 1976.

Vaitukaitis, J.L.; Braunstein, G.D.; and Ross, G.T. A radioimmunoassay which specifically measures human chorionic gonadotropin in the presence of human luteinizing hormone. *Am. J. Obstet. Gyecol.* 113:751–758, 1972.

Vaitukaitis, J.L., and Ebersole, E.R. Evidence for altered synthesis of human chorionic gonadotropin in gestational trophoblastic tumors. *J. Clin. Endocrinol. Metab.* 42:1048–1055, 1976.

Wehmann, R.E., and Nisula, B.C. Metabolic clearance rates of the subunits of human chorionic gonadotropin in man. *J. Clin. Endocrinol. Metab.* 48:753–754, 1979.

Wide, L. et al. Metabolic clearance of human chorionic gonadotropin administered to non pregnant women. *Acta Endocrinol.* 59:579–594, 1968.

Yen, S.S.C. et al. Disappearance rates of endogenous luteinizing hormone and chorionic gonadotropin in man. *J. Clin. Endocrinol. Metab.* 28:1763–1767, 1968.

PART VII

TUMOR IMMUNOLOGY

A clearly defined need exists for effective new systemic approaches to the treatment of female reproductive tract tumors. In addition, any tool that increases our ability to diagnose malignant disease at an earlier stage would enhance the effectiveness of established treatment methods. Drs. Pattillo and Smith discuss the current status of immunologic testing as it applies to the patient with genital tract tumors. Dr. Pattillo reviews the techniques currently available and their implications in the light of accepted immunobiologic concepts. Dr. Smith attempts to identify problem areas in the interpretation of available data and discusses the immune system in its role as a protector against the development and continued growth of neoplastic diseases.

Chapter 17

The Importance of an Immunologic Assessment of the Gynecologic Cancer Patient

PERSPECTIVE:

Roland A. Pattillo

Background

Strong support for the role of the immune system in host resistance comes from reported observations that surgical intensive care unit patients who remain anergic have a mortality rate over 75%, compared to less than 10% in patients whose anergy is reversed through hyperalimentation (Pietsch, Meakins, and McClean 1977). Delayed hypersensitivity skin tests including mumps, candida, PPD, streptokinase-streptodornase, and tricophytin are used to evaluate immunological recall antigens; hyperalimentation is administered to correct negative nitrogen balance and malnutrition characteristic of patients with chronic illnesses, multiple trauma, and systemic disease. Death in these immunologically anergic patients is most frequently caused by sepsis and deteriorated host resistance. It was reported by Seltzer that by asking the simple question, Have you involuntarily lost 10 pounds or more in the last six months? and by ordering two laboratory tests, a serum albumin and absolute lymphocyte count, one can identify patients whose deficient nutritional state will predict lowered host resistance. In patients with serum albumin values of less than 3.5 gm/L plus absolute lymphocytes under 1500 cu mm, 4 times the morbidity and 20 times the mortality were observed compared to rates for patients testing normally for these parameters (Seltzer 1979). Nutritional improvement by hyperalimentation is associated with correction of the absolute lymphopenia, the state of lymphocyte depletion of less than 1500 lymphs/cu mm, often associated with decreased immunological competence.

The primary role of immune surveillance and immune resistance is to detect and resist foreign antigens. In addition to delayed hypersensitivity recall skin test antigens, quantitative assessment of T and B lymphocytes func-

Figure 17.1

LYMPHOCYTE-MITOGEN STIMULATION

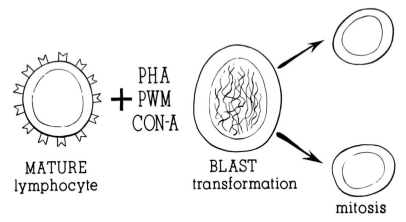

MATURE
lymphocyte

PHA
PWM
CON-A

BLAST
transformation

mitosis

Mitogen assay of lymphocyte reactivity. (Pattillo 1976. Reprinted with permission.)

Figure 17.2

MIXED LYMPHOCYTE CULTURE
(MLC) LD-A

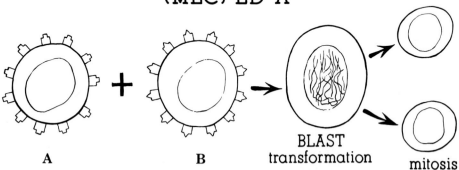

A

B

BLAST
transformation

mitosis

Lymphocytes from two individuals, A and B, undergo blast transformation and mitosis when stimulated by the differing antigens on their cell surfaces. These are lymphocyte definable antigens (LD-A) and comprise the major components of the histocompatibility system.

400

tion in the peripheral blood can be measured in the laboratory by mitogens (plant extracts which cause lymphocytes in the peripheral blood to transform, i.e., undergo blast transformation and divide) (fig. 17.1). This stimulation is similar to that observed in mixed lymphocyte cultures (MLC) by differing antigens on the surface of two different lymphocyte donors (fig. 17.2). This is the basis of the conventional MLC used to determine histocompatibility between kidney transplant pairs. The plant mitogen is recognized as a foreign antigen and the degree of response of the lymphocytes being tested reflects their immunocompetence to respond to other antigens, including tumor antigens. The mitogens used in those tests include PHA (phytohemagglutinin), conconavalin-A (con-A) and pokeweed mitogen (PWM). The response of normally mature lymphocytes in the peripheral blood to incubations with PHA is sequentially to undergo "blast transformation," synthesize DNA, and enter mitosis. This event can be quantitated and compared with normal controls by

Figure 17.3

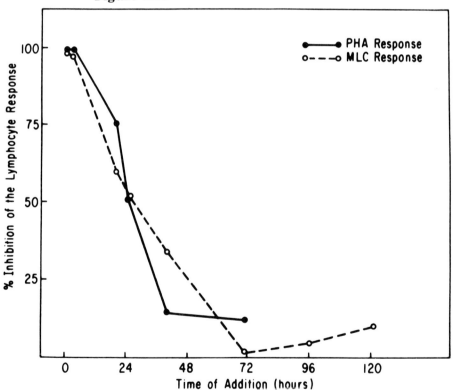

Ovarian cancer ascitic fluid contains immunosuppressive factors which completely inhibit the PHA response of normal lymphocytes. (Hess, Gall, and Dawson 1979. Reprinted with permission.)

Figure 17.4

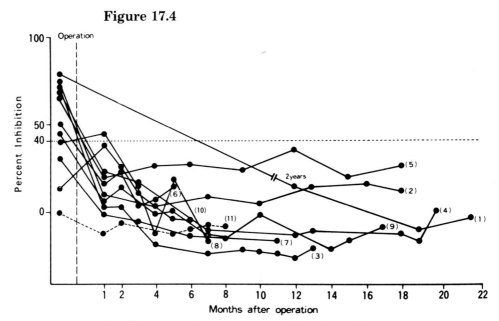

Serially measured immunosuppressive effect of the serum of patients without recurrence. (Ueda, Toyokawa, and Nakamori 1979. Reprinted with permission.)

Figure 17.5

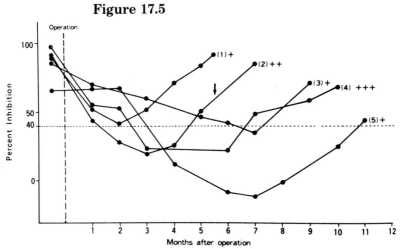

Serially measured immunosuppressive effect of the serum of patients who succumbed to advanced ovarian cancer. (Ueda, Toyokawa, and Nakamori 1979. Reprinted with permission.)

Table 17.1
Determination of Immunological Competence

1) Ficol density separation of lymphocytes.
2) Incubate stimulator c̄ 10^5 lymphs for 3 days.
3) Pulse lymphocytes c̄ ^{3}H thymidine.
4) ^{3}H DNA PPT, scintillation counting.

measuring counts per minute (CPM) of tritiated thymidine incorporated into DNA (table 17.1).

The effect of ascitic fluid from ovarian cancer patients on depressing this PHA response has been demonstrated by Hess, Gall, and Dawson (1979), as shown in figure 17.3. Serum from ovarian cancer patients likewise contains depressant factors preventing the normal PHA lymphocyte stimulation, as demonstrated in recent reports by Ueda and associates (1979), who found that serum immunosuppressive factors rose sharply in ovarian cancer patients who expired from advancing disease from 5 to 10 months after operation. Decreasing immunosuppression was observed, however, in those patients who survived. Inhibition of PHA stimulation by the serum of these patients accurately predicted prognosis, as shown in figures 17.4 and 17.5. Using the PHA evaluation of T lymphocytes, varying degrees of immunosuppression can be detected in the serum and lymphocytes from cervical cancer patients (Pattillo 1976).

Progressive decrease in immunocompetency, measured by PHA response in recurrent cervical cancer, as reported by the author, is shown in figure 17.6. Complete anergy by skin tests and in-vitro lymphocyte depressions preceded this patient's death from cervical cancer.

Specific recognition of tumor antigens by lymphocytes and by antibody constitutes the basis of the cell mediated immunity (CMI) and antibody mediated immunity (AMI), respectively—the clinical laboratory tests used to evaluate the gynecologic cancer patient. But, "blocking factors" found by these laboratory tests in the serum of cancer patients inhibit immune defense mechanisms and prevent the host from cytolytically destroying the offending cancer cell. Blocking factors can be represented by antigen, by antibody, or by antigen-antibody complex (fig. 17.7). To appreciate the present components of immunological assessments, a review of tumor immunology is necessary.

Tumor Immunology Development

Tumor immunology, in modern times, has an extremely brief history. It was not until the late 1950s that the availability of highly inbred strains of mice made possible the detection of tumor specific antigens. These strains of mice were so closely inbred that those of the same strain were genetically identical

Figure 17.6

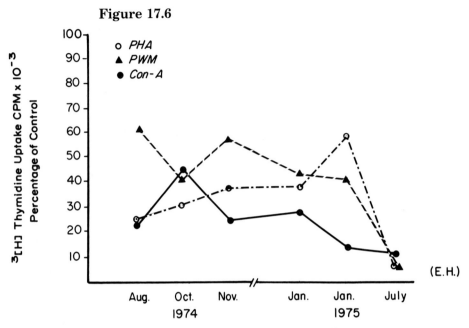

Terminal suppression of mitogen response of lymphocytes in cervical cancer patient. (Pattillo 1976. Reprinted with permission.)

Figure 17.7

BLOCKING OF TUMOR CELL LYSIS

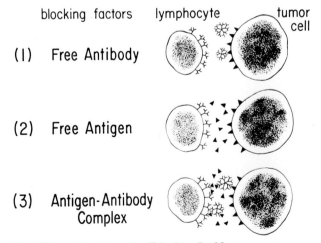

Possible mechanisms for "blocking" of host resistance. (Pattillo 1976. Reprinted with permission.)

(syngeneic), and therefore had antigenetically identical tissues. It is well known that in identical twins, normal tissues transplanted from one to another will grow permanently without eliciting an immunologic rejection reaction. If, in such genetically and antigenetically identical animals, a tumor arises or is induced by a known carcinogen and cannot be transplanted to another member of the strain because of immunologic resistance, it can then be logically concluded that the tumor contains new antigens not present in the host. In these early syngeneic mice experiments, using Methylcholanthrene induced sarcomas, Foley (1953), Prehn and Main (1957), and Klein and associates (1960) were able to demonstrate that these new antigens were intrinsic to the tumor cells, that is, they were not secondary to contaminating extraneous organisms and were therefore tumor-associated antigens. Similarly, it was shown that the genomes of DNA and RNA oncogenic viruses which induce tumors in experimental animals and which can infect man, such as the Epstein-Barr virus (EBV), simian virus 40 (SV40), and adenoviruses, direct the synthesis of tumor associated neoantigens that are distinct from the antigens of the virus particle. It can be seen, therefore, that the basic questions of the existence of tumor associated antigens and the response of tumor bearing hosts to such antigens have been well demonstrated in experimental animals. The question of immunologic mechanisms, the presence of tumor associated antigens in gynecologic tumor patients, and immunologic competence to detect and resist these antigens, therefore, needs further exploration. We will start with the evidence for demonstration of tumor associated antigens in some selected gynecologic cancers.

Demonstration of Tumor Associated Antigens in Human Gynecologic Malignancies

Demonstration of tumor associated antigens in cervical cancer was reported by Gall using microimmunodiffusion and immunoelectrophoresis. The antigen was extracted in saline, and heterologous antisera was prepared. The antiserum was thoroughly absorbed with pooled normal human plasma and pooled lyophylized normal cervical tissue extract. Cervical carcinoma extracts showed the presence of tumor antigen while normal cervical tissue extracts failed to react with such antiserum. Extracts of other types of cancer did not show lines of identity with cervical carcinoma. Similar reports of other gynecologic tumor antigens have been published by others (Bhattacharya and Barlow 1975; Dorsett et al. 1975; Chen, Koffler, and Cohen 1975; Pattillo et al. 1979; Imamura et al. 1978; DiSaia et al. 1972; Levi, Parshley, and Mandl, 1968).

Ovarian cancer tumor associated antigens were demonstrated in the author's laboratory in 1979 (Pattillo et al. 1979) using cell mediated cytotoxicity tests in patients with ovarian epithelial malignancies. The Hellstrom type assay (1971), used in this instance for immunodiagnosis and for tumor monitoring, provided a well-documented rationale for identifying ovarian tumor antigens. The assay was quantitated by postlabeling with tritiated thymidine. The four epithelial ovarian cancers, constituting 90% of ovarian malignancies, were grown in tissue culture. Lymphocytes from ovarian cancer patients and normal controls were incubated for 24 hours with these target tumor cells in the presence and in the absence of the patient's serum. Because of prior sensitization of ovarian cancer patients' lymphocytes to a tumor of similar histologic type, their lymphocytes recognized antigens on tumor cell surfaces similar to their own. Because of a spectrum of cell types in many ovarian tumors—serous, mucinous, endometrid, and clear cell—some degree of cross-reactivity was seen in some of the target tumor systems. Seventy-one percent of serous and mucinous ovarian cancer patients showed recognition on an ovarian cancer cell line derived from a seromucinous ovarian cyst adenocarcinoma. Patients with progressive tumor growth showed blocking of cytotoxicity when autologous serum was added to the incubation, whereas active cytotoxicity was manifest in the absence of their own blocking serum factor. Further laboratory work produced the same pattern of blocking when antigens shed from the surface of the ovarian cancer cells in culture were added to the assay system. This suggested that blocking factor may be free tumor associated antigen or an antigen specific suppressor molecule.

Nonspecific Immunity

Although the host defense systems of immunity consist of two major components, the cellular and the humoral immune process, an important component of nonspecific immunity is also essential in maintaining internal homeostasis. When the organism is confronted by "nonself-antigens," the nonspecific system is the first line of defense. This system is phylogenetically derived and consists primarily of immediate reaction to offending pathogens or foreign antigens. Chemotaxis and energy requiring processes are the means by which neutrophils, basophils, eosinophils, and monocytes (circulating phagocytes) are specifically directed to migrate to the site of inflammation. Phagocytosis and ingestion of microbes or foreign substances follow and cytoplasmic lysosomes fuse within vacuoles, completing the ingestion process. Foreign antigens are also processed by the macrophages for activation of the specific immune system through antigen processing. This is the beginning of cell mediated and antibody mediated immunity to foreign antigens (Unamue 1972). Although nonspecific immunity forms the core of the major host defense mechanism, "specific immunity," which is specific to the inciting antigen and involves primarily T and B lymphocytes, is the host's major defense beyond inflammation.

T and B Cells Origin and Function

T cells derive originally from epithelial cells in the third and fourth pharyngeal pouches and are concentrated in the fetal thymus, where they synthesize the thymic hormone thymosin. Lymphocytes developing in the thymus are dependent upon thymosin for the development of characteristic T cell functions. Included in these functions are (1) immunosurveillance, a major aspect of cancer immunity; (2) delayed hypersensitivity reactivity; (3) transplantation immunity, as in graft rejection; and (4) cell mediated host defenses against certain viruses, fungi, and intracellular facultative bacteria. In addition, the activity of these T cells is stimulated by persistent antigens, or indirectly by antigen processed by macrophages (Feldman et al. 1975).

Three major subsets of T lymphocyte expansion may occur. (1) After being stimulated by their antigenic determinant "effector" T cells are generated, which upon encountering their antigenic determinant on cell surfaces produce a cytotoxic response. This cell mediated lymphocyte toxicity (CML) produces the typical delayed hypersensitivity skin reaction, as is seen in the PPD reaction. (2) Helper T cells develop with the ability to cooperate with B lymphocytes in promoting antibody synthesis. (3) Suppressor T cell proliferation is also generated, which suppresses or impedes synthesis of immunoglobulin by B cells.

"B lymphocytes" derive directly from the bone marrow, and in birds their maturation is dependent upon the bursa of Fabricius, a rudimentary blind pouch in the gut. The precise location of the B cell maturing factors is not clearly understood in the human, and accordingly B cells are said to be under the control of bursal equivalents in the mammalian species. B cell encounter with antigen, for which it has a receptor, stimulates proliferation similar to the previously described T cell proliferative response; however, the end product is the production of immunoglobulin from cells which have been stimulated to undergo proliferation and morphologic change to become plasma cells with characteristic marginal chromatin in the nucleus and highly basophilic cytoplasm. Five classes of immunoglobulins are secreted by these cells, including IgG, IgM, IgA, IgD, and IgE. These antibodies all combine with the antigenic determinant and constitute the major portion of the antibody mediated immunity (AMI) system, which requires complement for activation. B cells make up 15% to 30% of circulating lymphocytes, have abundant surface immunoglobulin, and bind both complement and the Fc fragment of gammaglobulin. By contrast, T cells, which make up the remaining 70% to 85% of circulating lymphocytes, have little surface immunoglobulin, but form rosettes when incubated with sheep red blood cells and proliferate when stimulated with PHA and con-A.

Lymphokines

After stimulation by specific antigens, T lymphocytes release a series of substances involved in the amplification of the antigen-specific immune process. These soluble antigens affect surrounding cells. They are released from activated lymphocytes and include (1) blastogenic factor; (2) migration inhibition factor; and (3) macrophage aggravation factor.

Complement

Antibody mediated cytolysis requires the activation by complement. This involves a series of cascading enzymes, ultimately to permit antibody combination with antigen on the target cell surface. This process produces defects in the cell membranes and ultimate lysis.

Immunocompetence and Prognosis in Gynecologic Cancer Patients

Immunocompetence and prognosis have been found to be related at each stage of human cancer. The first major correlation is the finding that immunoincompetent patients have a worse prognosis than immunocompetent patients (Eilber and Morton 1970). Although a deficiency of tumor specific immunity appears to exist in these cases, the deficiency is believed to be based on multiple factors; including genetic, nutritional, stress infection, and others. Immunosuppressive factors, including blocking factors thought to represent tumor antigen, are found in the ascitic fluid and in the serum of patients bearing progressive tumors. These factors produce immunosuppression detected in typical immunologic evaluation schemes.

T and B Lymphocytes in the Immune Response

Lymphocytes comprise the major cell type of the immune reaction. The lymphocyte is characterized by its unique surface receptors or recognition sites which allows it to pick out particular three-dimensional molecular configurations known as "antigenic determinants." A single lymphocyte is believed to be programmed for only one or two antigenic determinants. The contact of a quiescent lymphocyte with its corresponding antigenic determinant activates its cell membrane. This event triggers metabolic activation, which is followed by blast transformation and DNA synthesis. The cell enlarges and divides, giving rise to daughter cells with the same recognition site as the parent cell. This expansion continues until a whole colony of lymphocytes with the same recognition sites is produced.

T lymphocytes are thymic dependent. They mature under the influence of the thymus through the action of single peptide hormones of thymic origin. These cells are programmed to recognize particular antigenic determinants.

Immunological Work-Up

The routine laboratory is capable of performing a portion of indicated tests of immune function. Special immunological laboratories are being established

Table 17.2
T Cell Monitoring

In Vivo:

1) D.H. skin tests (Candida, mumps, PPD, SK/SD, DNCB)
2) Absolute lymphocyte count (% Lymphs × WBC)

In Vitro:

1) PHA
2) CON-A
3) MLC
4) T-B Rosettes-SRBC agglut c̄ T-B cell in Rosette
5) MIF - G.P. Mig. inhibit. by MIF from Ag. Stim. Lymph.

to handle the remainder. The immunologic work-up can be divided into two major categories, T and B cell tests performed to evaluate in vitro or in vivo function.

The absolute lymphocyte count is determined by calculating the absolute number of lymphocytes by multiplying the percentage of lymphocytes by the total white count.

T cell function can be evaluated in vivo by determining delayed hypersensitivity or recall antigen status. Over 85% of the population will have been exposed to one of a battery of skin test antigens, including common fungal antigen (candida and tricophytin) a viral antigen (mumps), an encapsulated bacteria (PPD), and a common skin organism (SK/SD—streptokinase-streptodornase). By the addition of a primary skin test antigen, Dinitrochlorobenzene (DNCB) nearly 100% of the population would be expected to react to at least one of these antigens.

In vitro assessment of T cell function (table 17.2) can be evaluated by the mitogens PHA and con-A, mixed lymphocyte cultures (MLC's), T cell ro-

Table 17.3
B Cell Monitoring

In Vivo:

1) Ig Levels, Quant. Ig.,
2) Typhoid H & O Response.

In Vitro:

1) B Cell Rosettes-Sens. SRBC Coated c̄ Antibody.
2) Rim Fluorescence

settes, and the production of lymphokines such as Migration Inhibition Factor (MIF) (David et al. 1964).

B cells or humoral immunity can be evaluated in vivo (table 17.3) by testing primary antibody responses to antigens, such as flagellin (Hersh et al. 1971). Secondary antibody responses can be evaluated to antigens, such as diphtheria and tetanus. Quantitative immunoglobulins, isoantibody titers, and complement levels can also be measured. In vitro assessment of B cell function includes the evaluation of B cell mitogen responses, such as pokeweed mitogen (PWM), detection of cell surface immunoglobulin by immunofluorescence, and rosette formation (Stjernsword et al. 1972).

Cytotoxicity can be evaluated by determining specific lymphocyte target cell recognition and cytolysis (fig. 17.8). The Hellstrom type assay is the major model for this evaluation, and the killing or the growth inhibition of target cells is the end point (Hellstrom et al. 1968).

Programs in immunotherapy are rapidly developing to address the problem of immunodeficiency found in the above evaluations. Extreme complexity still exists in the "sorting out" of immunotherapy induced changes, but the increasing refinement of immunologic techniques is making this more and more feasible.

Figure 17.8

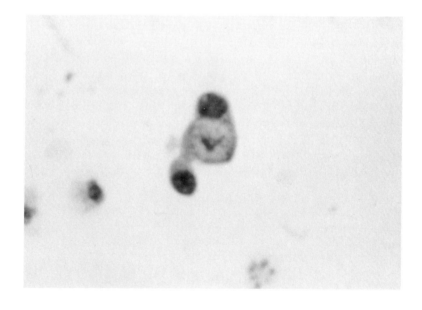

Lymphocyte recognizes antigen on surface of cervical cancer cell. (Pattillo 1976. Reprinted with permission.)

References

Bhattacharya, M., and Barlow, J. Tumor associated antigen for cystadeno-carcinoma of the ovary. *Natl. Cancer Inst. Monogr.* 42:25–32, 1975.

Chen, S.Y.; Koffler, D.; and Cohen, C.J. Cellular hypersensitivity in patients with squamous cell carcinoma of the cervix. *Am. J. Obstet. Gynecol.* 121:91–95, 1975.

David, J.R. et al. Delayed hypersensitivity in vitro: the specificity of inhibition of migration by antigens. *J. Immunol.* 93:567–576, 1964.

DiSaia, P.J. et al. Cell mediated immunity to human malignant cells, *Am. J. Obstet. Gynecol.* 114:979–989, 1972.

Dorsett, B.H. et al. Isolation of tumor specific antibodies from effusion of ovarian carcinoma cells. *Int. J. Cancer* 16:779–786, 1975.

Eilber, F.R., and Morton, D.L. Impaired immunologic reactivity and recurrence following cancer surgery. *Cancer* 25:362–367, 1970.

Feldman, M. et al. Cell collaboration between T and B lymphocytes and macrophages in antibody production in vivo. In *Lymphocytes and their interactions: recent observations.* ed. R.C. Williams, Jr. New York: Raven Press. 1975.

Foley, E.J. Autogeneic properties of methylcholanthrene-induced tumors in mice of the strain of origin. *Cancer Res.* 13:835–837, 1953.

Gall, S.A.; Walling, J.; and Pearl, J. Demonstration of tumor associated antigens in human gynecologic malignancies. *Am. J. Obstet. Gynecol.* 115:387–393, 1973.

Hellstrom, I. et al. Cellular and humoral immunity to different types of human neoplasms. *Nature* 220:1352–1354, 1968.

Hellstrom, I. et al. Demonstration of cell mediated immunity to human neoplasma of various histologic types. *Int. J. Cancer* 7:1–16, 1971.

Hersh, F.M. et al. Host defense mechanisms in lymphoma and leukemia. In *Oncology 1970: diagnosis and management of cancer, general considerations,* vol. 3. Chicago: Year Book Medical Publishers, 1971.

Hess, A.D.; Gall, S.A.; and Dawson, J.R. Inhibition of in vitro lymphocyte function by cystic and ascitic fluids from ovarian cancer patients. *Cancer Res.* 39:2381–2389, 1979.

Imamura, N. et al. Analysis of human ovarian tumor antigens using heterologous antisera: detection of new antigenic systems. *Int. J. Cancer* 12:570–577, 1978.

Klein, G. et al. Demonstration of resistance against methylcholanthrene-induced sarcomas in the primary autochthonous host. *Cancer Res.* 20:1561–1572, 1960.

Levi, M.M.; Parshley, M.S.; and Mandl, I. Antigenecity of papillary serous cystadenocarcinoma tissue culture cells. *Am. J. Obstet. Gynecol.* 102:433–439, 1968.

Pattillo, R.A. Immunotherapy and chemotherapy of gynecologic cancers, *Am. J. Obstet. Gynecol.* 124:808–817, 1976.

Pattillo, R.A. et al. Immunodiagnosis in ovarian cancer: blocking factor activity. *Am. J. Obstet. Gynecol.* 133:791–802, 1979.

Pattillo, R.A.; Story, M.T.; and Ruckert, A.C.F. Expression of cell-mediated immunity and blocking factor using a new line of ovarian cancer cells in vitro. *Cancer Res.* 39:1185–1191, 1979.

Pietsch, J.B.; Meakins, T.; and McLean, L.D. The delayed hypersensitivity response. Application in clinical surgery. *Surgery* 82:349–355, 1977.

Prehn, R.T., and Main, J.M. Immunity to methychlanthrene-induced sarcomas. *J. Nat. Cancer Inst.* 18:769–778, 1957.

Seltzer, M.H. Parenteral nutrition. *J. Parent. Enter. Nutr.* May–June 1979.

Stjernsword, J. et al. Lymphopenia and change in distribution of human B and T lymphocytes in peripheral blood induced by irradiation for mammary carcinoma. *Lancet* 1:1352–1356, 1972.

Ueda, K. et al. The prognostic value of serum immunosuppressive effect in patients with ovarian cancer. *Obstet. Gynecol.* 53:480–483, 1979.

Unamue, E.R. Regulatory role macrophages in antigenic stimulation. In *Advances in immunology,* ed. F.J. Dixon and H.G. Kunkel. New York: Academic Press, 1972.

PERSPECTIVE:

The Importance of an Immunologic Assessment of the Gynecologic Cancer Patient

W. Gary Smith

Investigation of cellular and humoral immunity in patients with gynecologic cancer has taken two directions. On the one hand, there has been a great deal of interest in the quantitation and isolation of tumor specific antigens, while on the other, investigators have attempted to measure the repudiated immune response of the host to these antigens. Collectively, most of the data suggest that host immunity may have a dual role in its response to cancer and its metastases. The immune system is an incredibly complex network of interacting cells and their molecular products which counterbalance one another and are influenced in their relative effectiveness by contact with antigenic molecules of the internal environment. Neoantigens, both tumor associated and tumor specific, stimulate the production of immune reactive cells that may be capable of inhibiting tumor spread (DiSaia et al. 1972). Unfortunately stimulation of immunologic reactivity in a tumor bearing host might also enhance metastatic spread of the disease as various inhibitors of cell mediated tumoricidal effector mechanisms are activated by exposure to these antigens.

Immune Surveillance

The role of the immune system as a primary control mechanism for the elimination of malignant cells is still very controversial. Burnet, in 1970, incorporated varied observations within his concept of "immune surveillance" to suggest that the major role of the immune system is to recognize and reject neoplastic cells developing de novo in a host. Somatic mutation from whatever cause is characterized by the development of new surface antigens on the cell membrane. These neoantigens can be recognized by the host as non-self and can result in the production of specific antibodies and specialized effector lymphocytes directed against them. Malfunction of the recognition and effector function of the immune system may lead to uncontrolled tumor growth. Burnet did not take into account that the function of the immune system may, at times, be harmful and lead to enhancement of tumor growth. It is quite possible that one population of tumor reactive lymphocytes might be tumoricidal while a second may have no detrimental effect, or even a growth promoting effect, on the tumor. The postulated suppressor activity of the immune system may serve as an immunologic escape mechanism for malignant cells and lead to micrometastases and primary tumor growth (Prehn 1972).

It has been relatively easy to demonstrate cancer restraining properties of tumor sensitized lymphocytes in laboratory animals, but translation of these data to the human situation is difficult. In the laboratory rat, initial sensitization of the immune system is accomplished by injection of a tumor bolus, providing a large but singular exposure of the host to tumor antigens; in man, abrogation of immune responsiveness is gradual and related to a prolonged and constant shedding of antigen and antigen-antibody complexes into the lymphoid system. Although the mechanisms of sensitization are quite different, there is circumstantial evidence that the human host-tumor immunologic interplay is beneficial to control of the oncologic process. For instance, many of the hereditary immune deficiency diseases result in a marked increase in subsequent malignancies (Kersey, Spector, and Good 1973). Patients who receive iatrogenic immune depression to prevent transplanted organ rejection have an incidence of malignancy 100 times greater than individuals in the general population (Penn 1974). Twenty-one percent of these cancers occur in the uterine cervix and include both in situ and invasive malignancies. Prolonged and quiescent periods of cancer growth not attributable to any therapeutic or pathological event strongly suggest that host defense mechanisms can operate in recognizing and destroying neoplastic cells.

If immune surveillance is a separate mechanism for tumor control, then the post-factum immune response of the tumor bearing host aimed against its own growing tumor may be an identifiable immune function (Mitchell 1975). In many tumor systems, documented immunologic responsiveness of the host directed at its growing tumor has encouraged the view that cancer cells might be eradicated by nonspecific stimulation of the immune system (Richman, Gutterman, and Hersh 1979). Immunotherapy fails, however, to take into account the potential activity of the suppressor network of immune reactive cells; thus, until immune testing can adequately define the intricate and sometimes contradictory immune reactivity between the host and its primary neoplasm, immunotherapy must only be used as a controlled and investigational treatment.

414

Delayed Hypersensitivity Skin Test Reactivity

Although studies of the immune response in patients with gynecologic cancer have been random and inundated by poor experimental technique, variegated patient populations, and a dichotomy of results, there does appear to be a relationship between the immunologic competence of the host and the prognosis of the disease. As early as 1926 it was noted that cancer patients have a significantly reduced delayed hypersensitivity reaction to tuberculin (Renaud 1926). Further interest in skin test experiments remained dormant until Graham, in 1962, demonstrated that patients with gynecologic malignancy have deficient hypersensitivity responses when tested intradermally with a group of nonspecific antigens. Cutaneous delayed hypersensitivity reactions test three separate components of the immune response necessary for elimination of antigenically foreign material. For a positive reaction to occur, the antigen must be initially processed by circulating macrophages and then presented to effector cells in the regional draining lymph node. The resultant antigen induced immunological reactivity of the host is then translated into circulating immunoreactive cells capable of attacking the foreign invader (Billingham and Silvers 1971). Any defect in the initial processing of the antigen, central lymph node reactivity, or the efferent active limb of this immunologic reaction will cause an impaired skin test response. Defects in any arm of the response infer that the host has impaired recognition and effector components of the immune system.

There are several skin test antigens in use today. A response to a fungal, viral, or bacterial agent is dependent upon previous exposure to these antigens. Although greater than 90% of the general population will show skin reactivity to at least one of the panel of antigens (Nalick et al. 1974), there are other chemical agents such as Dinitrochlorobenzene (DNCB) (Catalona et al. 1972) and 1-nitro and 2, 4-difluorobenzene (DNFB) (Kligman and Epstein 1959) that do not require previous exposure to elicit immune responsiveness in the normal host. Theoretically, testing patients for response to a panel of these nonspecific antigens might provide valuable information concerning the tumor host immunologic relationship. Although skin test reactivity is not specific, testing is easy to perform, reproducible, and usually not injurious to the patient. In 1970, Eilber studied delayed hypersensitivity reactivity in a group of patients with various malignancies. Fourteen patients with squamous carcinoma of the cervix were included in this study and the cervical cancer group showed a markedly reduced skin test reactivity to a battery of viral, bacterial, and fungal antigens. Nalick, in 1974, studied an additional 36 patients with invasive squamous cancer of the cervix and later expanded his study to include 81 patients with cervical cancer, 24 patients with epithelial ovarian cancer, and 20 patients with adenocarcinoma of the endometrium. All patients were skin tested prior to definitive treatment. The incidence of reactivity to one or more skin test antigens in patients with carcinoma of the cervix was significantly less than that of the control group of patients. Skin test anergy was more marked in patients with large volumes of tumor. In addition, patients with ovarian cancer had depressed immune responsiveness, often in the presence of only small volumes of tumor. There was no statistical difference in skin test reactivity between patients with endometrial cancer and their controls. The immune system as measured by delayed hypersensitivity reactivity does not appear to be influenced by adenocarcinoma of the endometrium (Chen, Cohen, and Koffler 1976), but squamous carcinoma of the cervix (Levy et al. 1978) and squamous cancers in several other sites are characterized by an overwhelming anergy to the various skin test reagins (Catalona, Sample, and Chretien 1973).

It appears that the histology of the tumor may be a major determining factor in the presence or absence of measurable immune reactivity. A second, yet important, variable that influences immunologic reactivity is the volume of tumor present at the time of testing. Morton (1970) has shown that anergy appears to reflect increasing tumor burden in patients with melanoma, and that after operative tumor reduction the anergic state may be reversed. Unfortunately, many studies of tumor induced anergy fail to take into account different anatomical sites and the volume of active tumor present. These variables must be considered in assessing results of immune testing.

Nutritional and debilitating effects of the tumor burden itself may depress immunologic reactivity. The proposed tumor induced immunologic depression as measured by skin test anergy may only be the result of debility induced by the growing tumor rather than an initiating cause of uncontrolled metastases. Unfortunately, Nalick's studies used nondebilitated patients as controls, and the observed immunologic differences between the cancer patients and the control group may not be attributable to the disease but rather a result of the tumor induced debilitation. If immunologic skin testing is to be of predictive value, then control subjects must be matched for age, chronicity of illness, and severity of disease. Recent weight loss alone can lead to depressed, delayed hypersensitivity reactivity to skin test antigens (Law, Dudrick, and Abdou 1973). Protein depletion can cause malfunction of both the afferent and efferent limbs of the cell mediated immune response (Edelman et al. 1973) and nutritional repletion can restore skin test reactivity (Law 1974).

Peripheral Lymphocyte Reactivity

These vagaries of delayed hypersensitivity skin test reactivity in patients with gynecologic cancer make it imperative to define more specifically immunologic reactivity in the tumor bearing host. Without isolation and purification of tumor-specific antigens, however, most studies measure nonspecific parameters of disease induced immunologic depression. For instance, measurement of the total number of circulating lymphocytes in the peripheral blood of patients with cervical (DiSaia et al. 1978) and ovarian cancer

(Wolff and DeOliveira 1975) correlated with the duration of survival. When lymphocyte counts are below 1000 prior to treatment, the prognosis is significantly worse than for patients with total peripheral lymphocyte counts over 2000. Riesco, in 1970, found that five-year cure rates for 589 patients with assorted malignancies (35 female genital tract) were significantly better in patients with high peripheral lymphocyte counts. Unfortunately these studies also fail to differentiate histologic tumor types and the inanition and debility associated with large tumor masses.

To further define the lymphocyte composition of the peripheral blood, Ueda, in 1977, measured both T and B cell populations in patients with ovarian cancer. There was a significantly reduced number of T cells when tumor volumes were large but there was no discernible reduction in the T cell population when the tumor volume was small and the stage of disease was early. Lack of early suppression of T lymphocytes negates the value of this test for early detection and screening of occult disease. It is interesting to note that in spite of a lowered T cell population in patients with advanced disease, curability of the tumor is reduced when the number of peripheral neutrophils is elevated (Riesco 1970). This unexpected negative correlation between neutrophil number and survival further emphasizes our present inadequacies in assessing the activity of the immunologic system in man.

When lymphocytes are removed from a cancer bearing host and tested in vitro, they show various measurable activities directed against autochthonous and allogeneic tumor cell preparations. DiSaia (1972) has demonstrated that peripheral lymphocytes from patients with ovarian and cervical cancer show cytotoxicity to allogeneic tumor cell lines. Although he observed a trend to increased cytotoxicity with increasing tumor burden, DiSaia was unable to correlate cytotoxic reactivity with stage and tumor grade. Cytotoxicity tests are difficult to perform and suffer from extreme variability in laboratory technique and subsequent results. Inability to define the effector cell population and the occurrence of spontaneous cytotoxicity in lymphocytes from normal individuals greatly hampers the usefulness of this assay for monitoring disease related factors in cancer patients (Heberman and Oldham 1975). It is also not uncommon for patients to obtain marked clinical remission of their disease in the presence of reduced in vitro lymphoid cell cytotoxicity.

In addition to in vitro cytotoxicity, lymphocyte responsiveness to the plant lectins shows various activity in accordance with the disease status. Patients with carcinoma of the cervix have decreased lymphocyte blastogenesis when the cells are mixed in vitro with phytohemagglutinin and concanavalin-A (Jenkins et al. 1975). Since, however, the number of T lymphocytes in the peripheral blood varies with each patient, it is difficult to determine whether this lack of responsiveness is due to fewer numbers of competent lymphocytes or to normal numbers of poorly responding lymphocytes or both. Daunter, in 1979, found both decreased lymphocyte responsiveness to PHA, and normal responsiveness to con-A in a patient group with carcinoma of the cervix. Response to these agents measures T cell activity, and opposing test results found in the same patient further challenge the credibility of immune testing in the cancer patient. Decreased mitogen responsiveness is also related to nutritional depletion, and it is impossible to separate inactivity related to cancer from inactivity related to the debility of the disease (Halili et al. 1976).

To define further the specificity of measured immune deficiency, lymphocyte function has been assessed by a variety of tests designed to measure lymphocyte antigen interaction. Unfortunately, mediator release by lymphocytes after exposure to tumor cell lines is difficult to measure, and results vary from laboratory to laboratory. Chen, in 1976, could show no increase in lymphocyte hypersensitivity as measured by leukocyte migration inhibition tests in patients with endometrial cancer; yet Menzer, in 1978, found that lymphocytes from patients with large volumes of endometrial tumor had an increased capacity to inhibit macrophage migration. Following tumor removal, lymphocyte reactivity was markedly decreased. If this assay could be standardized and reproduced, then it could be used for follow-up and screening of patients with endometrial cancer.

Regional Lymphocyte Reactivity

The present data suggest that there is both in vitro and in vivo sensitization of the immune system by neoplasms. The magnitude of cancer-related immunologic responsiveness is controversial, however, and at times may only reflect nonspecific immune mechanisms. As early as 1953 it was recognized that the presence of lymphocyte invasion into the primary tumor correlates with increased patient survival (Black, Kerpe, and Speer 1953). When the cells are separated from the tumor and immunologically typed, the majority of cells are found to be thymus dependent, but paradoxically they lack cytotoxic activity in vitro (Husby et al. 1976). Van Nagell, in 1977, showed that sinus histocytosis (macrophage activity) and paracortical hyperplasia (T cell activity) present in the regional lymph nodes of patients with gynecologic cancer are indicative of antitumor reactivity and correlate with an improved survival. The histologic appearance of an unstimulated and lymphocyte depleted lymph node implies a less favorable prognosis. In addition to these morphologic studies, lymphoid cells have also been isolated from regional draining lymph nodes (DiSaia 1975). It was originally hypothesized that these nodes contain large numbers of presensitized lymphocytes that might induce a marked cytotoxic effect on target tumor cells, but lymphocyte suspensions made from pelvic lymph nodes excised at laparotomy from patients with cervical cancer had very little cytotoxic effect on allogeneic tumor cells. In fact, lymphoid cells present in the regional draining lymph nodes may enhance tumor growth. Recently lymphocytes have been isolated from regional lymph nodes of patients with bladder tumors, and instead of cytotoxic activity the lymphocytes suppressed antibody dependent cell mediated target cell lysis. Lymphocytes separated from lymph nodes of control patients failed to

418

show suppressor activity (Catalona et al. 1978). Activation of lymphocytes within the draining lymph node may stimulate the production of suppressor cells, which may in turn provide an immunologic escape mechanism for metastatic tumor cells.

Immunoglobulins

Evaluation of immunoglobulin levels and isoantibody titers in patients with malignancy are relatively simple and easy to perform. However, except in chronic lymphocytic leukemia and multiple myeloma, they are of limited value in assessing tumor prognosis. In most patients with either solid or lymphoreticular neoplasms, the ability to form humoral antibodies to a variety of antigenic substances, even in the presence of advanced disease, is not impaired. There have been few data from gynecologic tumor patients, but there appears to be no evidence of antibody suppressive activity in the serum of patients with carcinoma of the cervix (Levy et al. 1978). Lymphocyte reactivity to PHA in the presence of autochthonous plasma is normal. The relatively obscure area of antigen, antigen-antibody complexes, and blocking factors needs to be defined further in an in vivo situation, for there is suggestive in vitro evidence that these complexes exist and may in fact abrogate cellular immunologic reactivity (Good and Fisher 1973).

Conclusion

Measurement and quantitation of immunologic reactivity in gynecologic oncology patients are often contradictory and confusing. It does appear that many patients with gynecologic cancer can mount an effective immunologic response directed toward their neoplasm. Whether this response is sufficient for the clinical control of the neoplastic process is the subject of considerable debate. In some tumors, immunocompetence may correlate with prolonged survival and stage of disease. The data from one tumor system, however, cannot be easily extrapolated to other types of tumors. Different histologic subtypes of tumor may give varying degrees of delayed hypersensitivity responses (Hersh et al. 1976). In studies showing a statistical correlation between immunocompetence and prolonged survival, there are several exceptions, that is, clinical response of the tumor to therapy in spite of impaired immunologic responsiveness. It may be that the functional capacity of the peripheral and circulating lymphocytes are quite distinct from that of lymphocytes in and around the lymph nodes draining the regional tumor bed. (Mavligit et al. 1974).

There is a need for more specific means of assessing immunocompetence in vivo. Skin testing with nonspecific antigens and various in vitro test systems fail to measure the patient's response to her own tumor. Depressed immunologic reactivity may be attributed to a variety of nonspecific factors related to genetic background, nutrition, age, and stress. It is imperative to consider the role of other important cells—the macrophage, for example—in attempting to dissect the responsiveness of the immune system to cancer. For the future, tumor specific antigens must be identified and isolated so that they may be used to define specific immunologic reactivity directed against them. Selection of the optimum immunologic test on a clinical basis will require further research and multifactoral correlations between existing data so that an immunologic index might be established for each patient to predict responsiveness to therapy.

Explanations for the anergy seen with malignancy are unknown but seem closely associated with the volume and extent of the primary disease. It is possible that anergy precedes the development of metastatic disease and facilitates the early occurrence of metastases, but critical analysis of the present data seems to indicate that immunologic suppression is the result rather than the cause of the tumor growth.

The current interest in immunotherapy demands further definition of the immune status of patients with cancer. The immune system is a vast array of interrelated cell activity, and stimulation of the wrong cell could lead to enhancement of tumor growth. The relationship of the immune system and tumorigenesis is just being defined. Coordination of research and standardization of investigative techniques over the next decade will help clear the murky water surrounding the status of immunologic competence of patients with malignancy. Immune testing of patients with cancer should continue, but in an organized, institutionally shared fashion in hopes of defining a more specific and therefore more sensitive indicator of the responsiveness of the host to the various cancer therapies.

References

Billingham, R.E., and Silvers, W.K. In *The immunobiology of transplantation* eds. A. Osler and L. Weiss. Englewood Cliffs, N.J.: Prentice-Hall, 1971.

Black, M.M.; Kerpe, S.; and Speer, F. Lymph node structure in patients with cancer of the breast. *Am. J. Pathol.* 29:505–521, 1953.

Burnet, F.M. *Immunological surveillance.* Oxford: Pergamon Press, 1970.

Catalona, W.J. et al. A method for dinitrochlorobenzene contact sensitization. *N. Engl. J. Med.* 286:339, 1972.

Catalona, W.J. et al. Suppressive effects of regional lymph node cells and extracts on antibody-dependent cellular cytotoxicity. *J. Urol.* 119:396–402, 1978.

Catalona, W.J.; Sample, W.F.; and Chretien, P.B. Lymphocyte reactivity in cancer patients. Correlation with tumor histology and clinical stage. *Cancer* 31:65–71, 1973.

Chen, S.Y.; Cohen, C.J.; and Koffler, D. Cellular hypersensitivity in patients with adenomatous hyperplasia and adenocarcinoma of the endometrium. *Am. J. Obstet. Gynecol.* 126:370–373, 1976.

Daunter, B.; Khoo, S.K.; and Mackay, E.V. Lymphocyte response to plant mitogens. II. The response of lymphocytes from women with carcinoma of the cervix to phytohemagglutinin-P, concanavalin A, and poke weed. *Gynecol. Oncol.* 7:314–317, 1979.

DiSaia, P.J. Immunological aspects of gynecological malignancies. *J. Reprod. Med.* 14:17–20, 1975.

DiSaia, P.J. et al. Cell-mediated immunity to human malignant cells. *Am. J. Obstet. Gynecol.* 114:979–989, 1972.

DiSaia, P.J. et al. Immune competence and survival in patients with advanced cervical cancer: Peripheral lymphocyte counts. *Int. J. Radiat. Oncol. Biol. Phys.* 4:449–451, 1978.

Edelman, R. et al. Mechanisms of defective delayed cutaneous hypersensitivity in children with protein-calorie malnutrition. *Lancet* 1:506–508, 1973.

Eilber, F.R., and Morton, D.L. Impaired immunologic reactivity and recurrence following cancer surgery. *Cancer* 25:362–367, 1970.

Good, R.A., and Fisher, D.W. Immunologic defenses against cancer. In *Immunobiology,* eds. R.A. Good and D.W. Fisher. Stamford, Connecticut: Sinauer Associates, 1973.

Graham, J.B., and Graham, R.M. Autogenous vaccine in cancer patients. *Surg. Gynecol. Obstet.* 114:1–4, 1962.

Halili, M. et al. The long-term effect of radiotherapy on the immune status of patients cured of a gynecologic malignancy. *Cancer* 37:2875–2878, 1976.

Heberman, R.B., and Oldham, R.K. Problems associated with study of cell-mediated immunity to human tumors by microcytotoxicity assays. *J. Natl. Cancer Inst.* 55:749–753, 1975.

Hersh, E.M. et al Immunocompetence, immunodeficiency and prognosis in cancer. *Ann. N.Y. Acad. Sci.* 276:386–406, 1976.

Husby, G. et al. Tissue T and B cell infiltration of primary and metastatic cancer. *J. Clin. Invest.* 57:1471–1482, 1976.

Jenkins, V.K. et al. In vitro lymphocyte response of patients with uterine cancer as related to clinical stage and radiotherapy. *Gynecol. Oncol.* 3:191–200, 1975.

Kersey, J.H.; Spector, B.D.; and Good R.A. Immunodeficiency and cancer. *Adv. Cancer Res.* 18:211–230, 1973.

Kligman, A.M., and Epstein, W.L. Some factors affecting contact sensitization in man. In *Mechanisms of hypersensitivity,* ed. J.H. Shoffer, G.A. Lo-Grippo, and M.W. Chase. Boston: Little, Brown, 1959.

Law, D.K.; Dudrick, S.J.; and Abdou, N.I. Immunocompetence of patients with protein-calorie malnutrition: *Ann. Intern. Med.* 79:545–550, 1973.

Law, D.K.; Dudrick, S.J.; and Abdou, N.I. The effect of dietary protein depletion on immunocompetence. *Ann. Surg.* 179:168–173, 1974.

Levy, S. et al. Cellular immunity in squamous cell carcinoma of the uterine cervix. *Am. J. Obstet. Gynecol.* 130:160–164, 1978.

Mavligit, G.M. et al. Immune reactivity of lymphoid tissues adjacent to carcinoma of the ascending colon. *Surg. Gynecol. Obstet.* 139:409–412, 1974.

Menzer, J. et al. Cell-mediated immunity in patients with endometrial adenocarcinoma. *Gynecol. Oncol.* 6:223–228, 1978.

Mitchell, M.S. Role of suppressor T lymphocytes in antibody induced inhibition of cytophilic antibody receptors. Presented in International Conference on Immunobiology of Cancer, New York Academy of Sciences, New York, November 1975.

Morton, D.L. Cancer immunology and the surgeon. *Surgery* 67:396–398, 1970.

Nalick, R.H. et al. Immunologic response in gynecologic malignancy as demonstrated by the delayed hypersensitivity reaction: clinical correlation. *Am. J. Obstet. Gynecol.* 118:393–405, 1974a.

Nalick, R.H. et al. Immunocompetence and prognosis in patients with gynecologic cancer. *Gynecol. Oncol.* 2:81–92, 1974b.

Penn, I. Occurrence of cancer in immune deficiencies. *Cancer* 34:858, 1974.

Prehn, R.T. The immune reaction as a stimulator of tumor growth. *Science* 176:170–171, 1972.

Renaud, M. La cutiréaction à la tuberculine chez les cancéreaux. *Bull. Soc. Med. Paris* 50:1441, 1926.

Richman, S.P.; Gutterman, J.U.; and Hersh, E.M. Cancer immunotherapy. *J. Cancer Med. Assoc.* 120:322–329, 1979.

Riesco, A. Five-year cancer cure: relation to total amount of peripheral lymphocytes and neutrophils. *Cancer* 25:135–140, 1970.

Ueda, K. et al. Immunosuppressive effect of serum in patients with ovarian carcinoma. *Obstet. Gynecol.* 51:225–228, 1977.

Van Nagell, J.R. et al. The prognostic significance of pelvic lymph node morphology in carcinoma of the uterine cervix. *Cancer* 39:2624–2632, 1977.

Wolff, J.P., and DeOliveira, C.F. Lymphocytes in patients with ovarian cancer. *Obstet. Gynecol.* 45:656–658, 1975.

PART VIII

TECHNIQUES OF OVARIAN CONSERVATION

As we achieve increasing rates of control in certain human tumors, quality as well as length of life becomes an important consideration. The ability of radiation therapy and chemotherapy to cure many young women afflicted with Hodgkin's disease has led to concerns regarding their ability to preserve menstrual and childbearing capabilities. Drs. Nahhas and Donaldson review their respective techniques for ovarian conservation in women undergoing treatment for Hodgkin's disease. Dr. Nahhas also comments on the preservation of hormonal function in women undergoing treatment of reproductive tract tumors, while Dr. Donaldson emphasizes the successful childbearing capabilities of many of her patients with Hodgkin's disease.

The issue of potential damage to the fetus through disruption of the genetic apparatus by gonadal radiation and/or chemotherapy is alluded to. Clinical evidence suggests, however, that with sophisticated techniques of radiation dosimetry the outcome for the fetus should be favorable. This chapter serves to emphasize the role of gynecologic oncologists in the treatment of patients rather than their diseases.

Chapter 18

The Preservation of Ovarian Function in Patients Undergoing Pelvic Irradiation: Indications and Technique

PERSPECTIVE:

William A. Nahhas

In July 1969, a program of planned diagnostic laparotomy, splenectomy, and liver and lymph node biopsies was instituted at the Memorial Hospital for Cancer and Allied Diseases in New York as a method of accurately staging patients with Hodgkin's disease prior to radiation therapy. The opportunity became available to examine a new method of reducing ovarian exposure by surgically relocating the ovaries outside of the radiation field in young women subjected to staging laparotomy. The technique of "lateral ovarian transposition" was thus developed by the Memorial Hospital Gynecology Service under the direction of Dr. John L. Lewis, Jr., in an effort to avoid ovarian sterilization in young women who may later need pelvic radiation therapy as treatment for Hodgkin's disease. A preliminary report describing this technique and its success was published by us in 1971 (Nahhas et al.), and more recently by Lewis (1976).

Recently, patients with carcinoma of the uterine cervix have been undergoing laparotomy for surgical staging or for radical therapy of their cervical tumors (Nelson et al. 1974; Piver and Barlow 1977; Van Nagell, Roddick, and Lowin 1971; Wharton et al. 1977; Nelson et al. 1977). Because early cervical carcinoma rarely metastasizes to the ovaries, it became logical to consider the use of lateral ovarian transposition as an integral part of the operative procedure in young women in order to prevent castration should subsequent radiation therapy be planned or become necessary. In this group of patients continued ovarian function is essential in preventing the early onset of osteoporosis, relieving vasomotor symptoms, and promoting psychological and general well-being.

Since July 1977 lateral ovarian transposition has been used by the Division of Gynecologic Oncology of the Milton S. Hershey Medical Center in patients below the age of 36 with epidermoid carcinoma of the cervix in conjunction with surgical therapy or operative staging prior to radiation therapy. The purpose of this chapter is to discuss the present indications and to describe the technique of lateral ovarian transposition in this group of patients and in other young women with malignancies necessitating pelvic radiation therapy.

Background and Rationale

Premenopausal women receiving therapeutic doses of pelvic irradiation will invariably become sterile and amenorrheic if the ovaries are not protected in some way. The radiation dose necessary to sterilize the ovaries has been estimated to vary from 325 to 625 tissue roentgens (Glücksmann 1947; Peck et al. 1940). Peck reported a 90% sterilization rate when a dose of 500 tissue roentgens was delivered to the pelvis. In the past, loss of ovarian function in young females receiving radiation therapy to the pelvis was thought to be inevitable. During the past 30 years, however, clinicians and their patients have become increasingly aware of the value of continued hormonal function following radiotherapy in young women with curable malignancies of the pelvis (McCall, Keaty, and Thompson 1958; Krebs, Blixenkrone-Moller, and Mosekilde 1963; Kovacev 1968; Trueblood et al. 1970).

Ovarian conservation is one of the most compelling reasons for choosing surgical instead of radiation therapy as primary treatment for early carcinoma of the uterine cervix in young women (Rutledge 1969). Several procedures have been devised to protect ovarian function in patients undergoing operation or radiation therapy for cervical tumors or other malignancies affecting organs in the female pelvis (Nahhas et al. 1971; Krebs, Blixenkrone-Moller, and Mosekilde 1963; Kovacev 1968; Bieler, Schnabel, and Knobel 1976; Ray et al. 1970). In 1958 McCall, Keaty, and Thompson championed the cause of ovarian conservation in patients having radical surgery for carcinoma of the cervix. Webb, in 1975, confirmed these observations. In his series, early invasive carcinoma of the cervix did not metastasize to the ovaries. Kovacev preserved ovarian function during the Wertheim-Meigs operation for carcinoma of the cervix by exteriorizing the ovaries under the skin. Ovarian function was preserved, but the exteriorized ovaries developed cystic changes causing moderate pain and necessitating repeated needle aspiration.

Technically the ovaries and their blood supply can be adequately preserved at the time of radical operation, or at the time of operative staging. Although these ovaries will function normally, a small number of patients may require further therapy for benign conditions directly related to the retained ovaries. Unlike recurrent or advanced cervical cancer, most studies indicate that early cervical carcinoma does not metastasize to the ovaries, thus making ovarian conservation in most patients both safe and worthwhile (Brunschwig and Pierce 1948; Henriksen 1949; Nahhas, Abt, and Mortel 1977).

In 1970 Ray and associates described the procedure of oophoropexy as a means of preserving ovarian function following pelvic radiotherapy in patients with Hodgkin's disease. The procedure consists of suturing the ovaries and their attached vascular pedicles to the midline of the pelvis and marking them with metal clips so that they may be effectively shielded during radiation therapy. In this procedure each ovary is sutured to the serosal surface of either the anterior or the posterior wall of the uterus. The authors noted that oophoropexy itself did not cause amenorrhea or dysmenorrhea and that patients who did not undergo pelvic radiation therapy continued to menstruate normally. In their discussion, however, they mentioned that if great care is not taken in positioning the ovarian block, a potential complication of this procedure would be the accidental shielding of involved pelvic lymph nodes. This problem is of course obviated by the use of the technique of lateral ovarian transposition.

Trueblood and associates, in 1970, described 23 young women who had oophoropexy prior to pelvic radiation therapy for Hodgkin's disease. Twelve patients continued to have normal periods following radiation, giving a 52% rate of continued menstrual function. At the time of that report one of the patients was in her fifth month of a normal pregnancy. One explanation given for the low ovarian preservation rate was that the repositioned ovaries received as much as 9% of the radiation dose by scatter and by penetration of the shield. Additionally, the ovaries did move from the midline position in some cases, as detected by the change in position of the metallic marker. Other technical difficulties were also mentioned.

In 1976, Bieler and associates described 10 premenopausal women with stage I_b to II_b cervical cancer whose ovaries were repositioned away from the irradiated field and he compared them to 8 similarly aged patients whose ovaries were not transposed. Using pituitary gonadotrophin levels, it was demonstrated that ovarian transposition preceding radiotherapy was an effective means of preserving ovarian function in these young women, whose malignancies of the pelvic region demanded radiation. The technique used was quite similar to the one previously described by us. One slight modification was the retroperitoneal placement of the transposed ovary.

Indications for Lateral Ovarian Transposition

In the 1971 report from the Memorial Hospital for Cancer and Allied Diseases a procedure for ovarian relocation was devised for, and utilized in, young females with Hodgkin's disease undergoing staging laparotomy. One ovary was relocated out of the pelvis, leaving the uterus, other ovary, and both tubes in their original position. The purpose of lateral ovarian transposition (LOT) was to preserve ovarian function should pelvic radiation therapy become necessary because of the presence of Hodgkin's disease within pelvic lymph nodes. The uterus, tubes, and other ovary were preserved in their normal anatomic location in order to maintain future reproductive function if pelvic radiation therapy was found to be unnecessary. In this group of young patients with Hodgkin's disease, normal cyclic menstrual function was maintained and term pregnancies and deliveries were achieved (Nahhas 1971; Lewis 1976; Ray et al. 1970).

Young women with invasive carcinoma of the cervix will invariably lose their ability to bear children following adequate surgical or radiation therapy. Childbearing, therefore, ceases to be an important indication for ovarian relocation, and the procedure is modified and simplified to preserve only hormonal ovarian function. Lateral ovarian transposition in patients below the age of 36 with invasive carcinoma of the uterine cervix is therefore indicated in the following situations:

1. Patients with stage I_b or II_a disease undergoing radical hysterectomy and pelvic lymphadenectomy with ovarian conservation. One or both ovaries and tubes are located out of the pelvis in case postoperative radiation therapy becomes necessary because of depth of tumor penetration into the cervical stroma, with inadequate surgical margins, or due to the presence of metastatic carcinoma in lymph nodes.

2. Patients with stage I_b and II_a disease explored for the purpose of doing radical hysterectomy and lymphadenectomy who are found to have unresectable disease due to local extension or due to metastases to the pelvic and/or paraaortic lymph nodes. The radical procedure is abandoned and right lateral ovarian transposition is performed.

3. Patients with stage II_b or greater disease who undergo abdominal laparotomy for staging and paraaortic lymph node sampling. Patients who have only retroperitoneal paraaortic lymph node sampling in an effort to reduce the surgical and radiation therapy complications of the transperitoneal approach cannot benefit from the technique of lateral ovarian transposition (Berman et al. 1977).

Technique of Lateral Ovarian Transposition

The technique of lateral ovarian transposition uses to advantage the dual blood supply of the ovary from the ovarian vessels contained within the infundibulopelvic ligament and from branches of the uterine vessels (fig. 18.1). The procedure is indicated for young women with invasive carcinoma of the cervix, Hodgkin's disease, or any other pelvic malignancy necessitating pelvic radiation therapy where ovarian conservation is both desirable and safe.

In Invasive Carcinoma of the Cervix

Future reproductive function is not a consideration in young women with invasive carcinoma of the cervix. The technique of lateral ovarian transposition is therefore considerably simplified. In those patients whose disease is thought to be unresectable, the utero-ovarian ligament and tube are divided

Figure 18.1

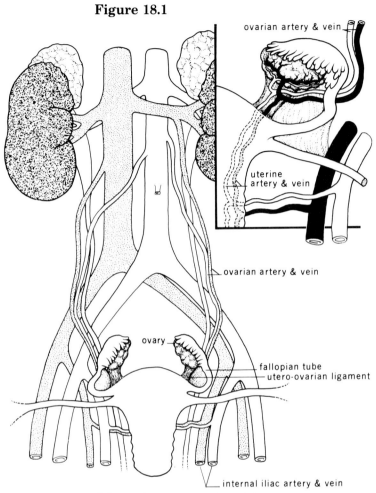

ovarian artery & vein

ovarian artery & vein

uterine
artery & vein

ovarian artery & vein

ovary

fallopian tube
utero-ovarian ligament

internal iliac artery & vein

*Schematic representation of the pelvic organs and
their vascular relations. Inset demonstrates the
dual blood supply of the ovary from the uterine and
ovarian vessels.*

at the uterine cornu, and the parietal peritoneum on each side of the infundibulopelvic ligament is slit cephalad until an adequate length of ligament is
freed. The ovary is then swung laterally and sutured to the parietal peritoneum overlying the lower pole of the kidney (fig. 18.2A).

Following radical hysterectomy and pelvic lymphadenectomy, the procedure can be performed on one or both sides by swinging the ovary and tube
as one unit laterally on the long infundibulopelvic ligament (fig. 18.2B). To
prevent ovarian infarction, care should be taken not to twist the ligament
and not to angulate it acutely. It is important to move the ovary as laterally
and as superiorly as possible in order to minimize scatter radiation. Lateral

transposition alone without a significant superior motion will cause the ovary to rest more medially because of the curvature of the parietal peritoneum. In all cases the borders of the ovary are marked with metal clips for identification by the radiotherapist.

In Hodgkin's Disease

In young women with Hodgkin's disease the procedure of lateral ovarian transposition is complicated by concern over the maintenance of future reproductive capacity. It is important, therefore, to preserve the integrity of the fallopian tube on the side of the transposed ovary. After dividing and securing the utero-ovarian ligament, the meso-ovarium is cut and all fine bleeding points are clamped and tied. Ligatures should be placed so as not to distort the normal contour of the fallopian tube. The insertion of the infundibulopelvic ligament beneath the fimbriated end of the fallopian tube is divided between clamps and secured with fine chromic sutures, leaving the ovary attached to its major blood supply provided by the ovarian vessels contained within the infundibulopelvic ligament. This ligament is then lifted off its ret-

Figure 18.2

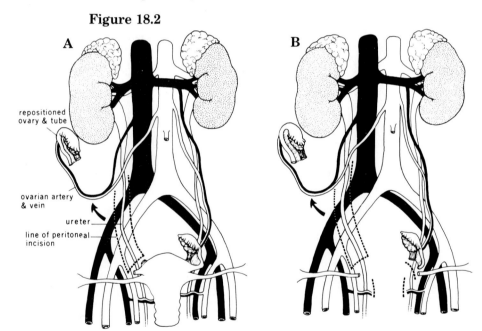

A, *schematic representation showing the line of peritoneal incision and the final location of the repositioned right ovary and fallopian tube. The uterus and left ovary and tube remain in place.*

B, *the uterus is removed. The right ovary and tube are repositioned. The left ovary and tube may be removed, repositioned, or left in place.*

432

roperitoneal bed by sharp and blunt dissection, thus providing the ovary with a long pedicle which can be swung laterally over the ureter and common iliac vessels. Silk sutures are used to secure the ovary to the parietal peritoneum lateral to the psoas muscle and just beneath the pole of the kidney. The lateral and medial borders of the ovary are marked with metal clips, and the ovarian vascular pedicle is sutured to the posterior peritoneum to obliterate the space beneath it, thus preventing potential bowel herniation and strangulation. Closure of the defect created in the posterior parietal peritoneum by lifting the infundibulopelvic ligament is then effected (fig. 18.3).

Technique of Radiotherapy

For invasive carcinoma of the cervix, external radiation therapy is delivered, using a 10 Mev linear accelerator. For stages I and II_a, 4250 rad are given over five weeks, using 170 rad per day. For stage II_b and over, or for patients with metastases to the pelvic and/or paraaortic lymph nodes, 5100 rad are given over six weeks, using 170 rad per day. Anterior and posterior opposing fields are used, except in obese patients where the therapy is delivered by a four field "box technique." Pelvic ports usually measure 17 to 18 cm in each dimension. The superior margin is at the level of the fifth lumbar vertebral body and the inferior margin is usually at the midportion of the obturator foramen or at the lowest extension of disease with an adequate margin. The field extends to at least 1 cm beyond the lateral margin of the bony pelvis as

Figure 18.3

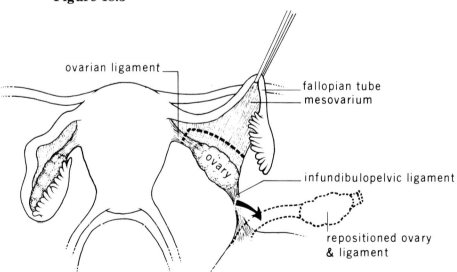

Line of meso-ovarial incision and final location of the repositioned ovary in patients with Hodgkin's disease.

Figure 18.4

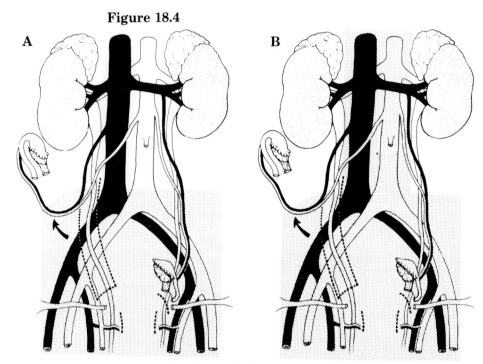

A, *the pelvic radiation field in relation to the transposed right ovary and tube.*

B, *the pelvic and paraaortic radiation field in relation to the transposed right ovary and tube.*

measured at the widest plane. The paraaortic field is 8 cm in width and extends to the superior border of the twelfth thoracic vertebral body. The transposed ovary is shielded by a Cerrobend block with a 7.5-cm thickness allowing 5% transmission of any scatter radiation to the area (fig. 18.4).

Two intracavitary applications of cesium[137] are given at the end of the external radiation therapy, each lasting 48 hours and separated by an interval of two weeks. A maximum of 6500 mg hours are given if the external therapy dose is 4250 rad and 5500 mg hours are delivered if external therapy totals 5100 rad.

Conclusions

Lateral ovarian transposition should be seriously considered in young women with pelvic malignancies necessitating pelvic radiation therapy. The procedure is simple and safe, and ovarian function can be maintained in nearly all patients.

By using the technique of lateral ovarian transposition, the ovary can be lifted a distance of more than 15 cm from its normal position in a lateral and superior direction. This reduces the ovarian dose to about 1% to 3% of the total dose to the pelvis (Bieler, Schnabel, and Knobel 1976). Shielding allows only 5% of this scatter dose to reach the ovary. The transposed ovary of a patient treated by paraarotic radiation therapy in addition to a pelvic field will receive a higher dose. In fact, one out of a recent group of eight Hershey Medical Center patients with carcinoma of the cervix having lateral ovarian transposition followed by radiation therapy lost ovarian hormonal function, as evidenced by vasomotor symptoms and elevated gonadotrophin levels. A few patients treated only through a pelvic field lost ovarian hormonal function. This was due to moving the ovary only in a lateral direction without a significant cephalad component, causing the ovary to rest close to the edge of the radiation field.

The procedure of lateral ovarian transposition, therefore, can be regarded as an important part of surgical staging in patients with Hodgkin's disease and in young patients with invasive carcinoma of the cervix subjected to radical operation or to operative staging.

References

Berman, M.L. et al. The operative evaluation of patients with cervical carcinoma by an extraperitoneal approach. *Obstet. Gynecol.* 50:658–664, 1977.

Bieler, E.U.; Schnabel, T.; and Knobel, J. Persisting cyclic ovarian activity in cervical cancer after surgical transposition of the ovaries and pelvic irradiation. *Br. J. Radiol.* 49:875–879, 1976.

Brunschwig, A. and Pierce, V. Necropsy findings in patients with carcinoma of the cervix. *Am. J. Obstet, Gynecol.* 56:1134–1137, 1948.

Glücksmann, A. The effects of radiation in germ cells with special reference to man. In: Certain aspects of the action of radiation on living cells, ed. F.G. Spear. *Br. J. Radiol. (Suppl.)* 1:101–109, 1947.

Henriksen, E. The lymphatic spread of carcinoma of the cervix and of the body of the uterus. *Am. J. Obstet. Gynecol.* 58:924–942, 1949.

Kovacev, M. Exteriorization of ovaries under the skin of young women operated upon for cancer of the cervix. *Am. J. Obstet. Gynecol.* 101:756–759, 1968.

Krebs, C.; Blixenkrone-Moller, N.; and Mosekilde, V. Preservation of ovarian function in early cervical cancer after surgical uplifting of the ovaries and radiation therapy. *Acta Radiol. (Ther.)* 1:176–182, 1963.

Lewis, J.L., Jr. Surgical transposition of the ovaries as part of staging laparotomy for Hodgkin's disease. In *Hodgkin's disease,* ed. M.J. Lacher. New York: John Wiley, 1976.

McCall, M.L.; Keaty, E.C.; and Thompson, J.D. Conservation of ovarian tissue in the treatment of carcinoma of the cervix with radical surgery. *Am. J. Obstet. Gynecol.* 75:590–605, 1958.

Nahhas, W.A. et al. Lateral ovarian transposition: ovarian relocation in patients with Hodgkin's disease. *Obstet. Gynecol.* 38:785–788, 1971.

Nahhas, W.A.; Abt, A.B.; and Mortel, R. Stage I$_b$ glassy cell carcinoma of the cervix with ovarian metastases. *Gynecol. Oncol.* 5:87–91, 1977.

Nelson, J.H., Jr. et al. The incidence and significance of para-aortic lymph node metastases in late invasive carcinoma of the cervix. *Am. J. Obstet. Gynecol.* 118:749–756, 1974.

Nelson, J.H., Jr. et al. Incidence, significance, and follow-up of para-aortic lymph node metastases in late invasive carcinoma of the cervix. *Am. J. Obstet. Gynecol.* 128:336–340, 1977.

Peck, W.S. et al. Castration of the female by irradiation: the results in 334 patients. *Radiology* 34:176–186, 1940.

Piver M.S., and Barlow, J.J. High dose irradiation to biopsy confirmed aortic node metastases from carcinoma of the uterine cervix. *Cancer* 39:1243–1246, 1977.

Ray, G.R. et al. Oophoropexy: a means of preserving ovarian function following pelvic megavoltage radiotherapy for Hodgkin's disease. *Radiology* 96:175–180, 1970.

Rutledge, F.N. Surgery versus x-ray for treatment in cancer of the cervix. In *Controversy in obstetrics and gynecology,* ed. D.E. Reid and T.C. Barton. Philadelphia: W.B. Saunders, 1969.

Trueblood, H.W., et al. Preservation of ovarian function in pelvic radiation for Hodgkin's disease. *Arch. Surg.* 100:236–237, 1970.

Van Nagell, J.R., Jr.; Roddick, J.W., Jr.; and Lowin, D.M. The staging of cervical cancer: inevitable discrepancies between clinical staging and pathologic findings. *Am. J. Obstet. Gynecol.* 110:973–978, 1971.

Webb, G.A. The role of ovarian conservation in the treatment of carcinoma of the cervix with radical surgery. *Am. J. Obstet. Gynecol.* 122:476–484, 1975.

Wharton, J.T. et al. Preirradiation celiotomy and extended field irradiation for invasive carcinoma of the cervix. *Obstet. Gynecol.* 49:333–338, 1977.

PERSPECTIVE:

The Preservation of Ovarian Function in Patients Undergoing Pelvic Irradiation: Indications and Technique

Sarah S. Donaldson

Introduction

A major therapeutic challenge to an oncologist today is cure of tumor with minimal sequelae from the treatment administered. When dealing with women who have abdominal or pelvic neoplasms, the issue of preservation of ovarian function invariably appears when one considers therapeutic options which may, in some way, impact upon the ovaries. When treatment options include therapeutic radiation directed to the abdomen or pelvis, oncologists must consider ways of minimizing ovarian dysfunction secondary to radiation as they plan treatment with curative intent. Such therapeutic strategies require the close interplay and collaboration of surgical oncologists, medical oncologists, and radiation oncologists. It is because of the close team effort of individuals from these three modalities that we now can discuss the subject of preservation of ovarian function in women undergoing pelvic irradiation.

The advent of operative staging by laparotomy with splenectomy for Hodgkin's disease has provided an opportunity to perform elective abdominal-pelvic surgery on young women who have excellent opportunities for cure. It was this procedure, pioneered by Kaplan (1972) and investigators at Stanford University Medical School, which prompted the use of oophoropexy as a means of shielding the ovaries with subsequent preservation of ovarian function in female patients who require radiation to the pelvic lymph nodes.

This chapter will outline the indications for and technique of oophoropexy with midline transposition of the ovaries, as developed by the Stanford investigators for the management of women with Hodgkin's disease. The dosimetry of pelvic radiation with midline shielding will be described, along

Supported in part by U. S. Public Health Service grant CA-05838 from the National Institutes of Health.

with a review of the results of this surgical technique, which has allowed the preservation of ovarian function with pregnancy in a population of young women with projected long-term survival.

Indications

The advance of elective surgical staging for Hodgkin's disease created the opportunity to consider an operative means of identifying, localizing, and manipulating the ovaries so as to optimize their position to allow therapeutic doses of radiation to the areas at risk for Hodgkin's disease, while the surrounding normal tissues including the ovaries could be effectively shielded from the radiation. Surgical staging for Hodgkin's disease is now an established part of the total therapeutic plan in all patients with the exception of those with bone marrow involvement at presentation. Approximately 30% of all patients will have their clinical stage altered by findings at surgical staging, which includes splenectomy, liver, and selected lymph node biopsies and an open bone marrow biopsy (Hellman 1974; Kaplan 1972). Thus, if treatment decisions are based upon accurate staging, surgical staging should be performed.

Operative morbidity from surgical staging in experienced hands has been minimal, and in large series mortality has been zero (Cannon and Nelson 1976). This is undoubtedly due to the fact that surgical staging for years was not considered routine, and was undertaken in centers where large numbers of patients were referred for diagnosis, evaluation, and treatment. The operative technique was developed by surgeons who performed large numbers of these procedures and who had particular expertise in identifying the location and extent of disease, as well as the normal anatomic structures. As a result, accurate and precise radiotherapy could be planned.

When the major therapeutic modality used for Hodgkin's disease is radiation, extended field treatment is now the established therapy for essentially all patients. Subsets of asymptomatic patients with localized disease, that is, pathologic stages I_a and II_a supradiaphragmatic disease, can be safely treated with subtotal lymphoid irradiation of a mantle and spade fields (splenic hilar and paraaortic lymph node treatment down to the level of the pelvic brim). However, patients with systemic "B" symptoms and those with advanced disease, above and below the diaphragm, require total lymphoid irradiation (Kaplan 1972). Thus pelvic irradiation must be considered as a therapeutic possibility for all patients with Hodgkin's disease. Subtotal lymphoid and total lymphoid radiation have now contributed to prolonged survival and disease-free survival rates for patients with Hodgkin's disease. In fact, 80% to 90% of all patients will be cured, provided that they have optimal staging and therapy for their disease (Donaldson 1980; Rosenberg et al. 1978). Thus, when considering the management of patients with Hodgkin's disease, it is clear that surgical staging has made a large contribution and is considered routine; that total lymphoid irradiation is the established treat-

438

ment of choice for large numbers of patients with Hodgkin's disease; and that with these techniques close to 9 out of 10 patients will be long-term survivors.

In addition, it is known that in female patients ovarian function is essentially permanently abolished if doses in excess of 500 to 800 rad are delivered to both ovaries (Kaplan 1972). Thus, considering the extreme gonadal radiosensitivity of the ovaries, the value of abdominal-pelvic surgical staging, the necessity of pelvic irradiation, and the likelihood of prolonged survival and cure of these young women, there is little need to justify the value of oophoropexy as a means of preserving ovarian function in premenopausal women requiring radiotherapy.

Technique

Surgical Technique

Oophoropexy, the operative procedure describing the midline transposition of the ovaries, was pioneered at Stanford University Medical Center (Ray et al. 1970; Trueblood et al. 1970). The procedure, initially developed as an adjunct to the staging laparotomy, is performed at the termination of the surgical staging procedure. It consists of the movement of one or both ovaries and their attached vascular pedicles to the midline of the true pelvis. The ovaries normally lie in close proximity to the iliac vessels, as shown in figure 18.5A. There is sufficient mobility to the ovaries and sufficient length in the broad ligament so that one or both of the ovaries with attached tube and blood vessels can be lifted without difficulty from their normal lateral position to a position close to the midsagittal plane. The uterus is held anteriorly with a tenaculum; a 2-0 braided stainless steel wire suture is placed through the right ovary, through the lowest portion of the uterus or cervix, and then through the left ovary during bilateral oophoropexy (fig. 18.5B). By tying the wire suture, the ovaries are pulled into a position posterior to the uterus in the midline (fig. 18.5C). Alternatively, the ovaries may be attached to the anterior surface of the uterus, or with one ovary attached anteriorly and one posteriorly (fig. 18.5D). The entire procedure adds approximately five minutes to the total operative time of surgical staging laparotomy. Ovarian placement low on the uterus, on or near the cervix, allows a more generous pelvic shield to be used. When the ovaries are inadvertently placed higher on the uterus, they receive an additional contributing dose of radiation from therapy to the iliac lymph node chain.

A midline vertical incision is most appropriate when oophoropexy is performed as an adjunct to the staging laparotomy; however, a horizontal Pfannenstiel incision can also be used for the procedure if one is not doing an exploration of the upper abdomen including splenectomy. In rare instances, there may not be enough length in the broad ligament to allow for movement to the midline, in which oophoropexy is technically more difficult, and the

Figure 18.5

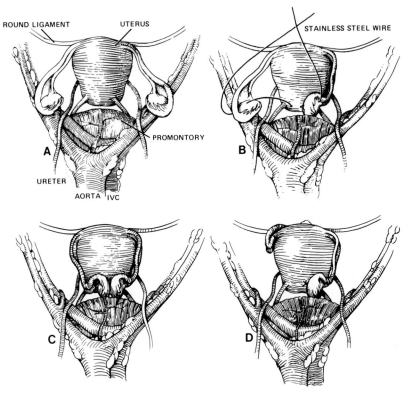

Surgical Stages in Oophoropexy: A, *normal anatomic structures;* B, *wire suture being placed through the right and left ovaries during bilateral oophoropexy;* C, *the right and left ovaries sutured to the posterior aspect of the uterus;* D, *one ovary attached anterior to the uterus and one posterior to the uterus.*

ovaries may not be sutured quite to the midline. In such instances the broad ligament can be divided to provide further mobility. Other technical difficulties have occurred in women with prior pelvic inflammatory disease in which extensive scarring of the tubes or broad ligament shortens the tubes and thus makes transposition impossible. On rare occasions, oophoropexy has not been possible in women with uterine pathology, such as uterine fibroids.

Lateral transposition of the ovaries has been recommended by some as an alternative technique, as is discussed elsewhere in this text (Nahhas et al. 1971). The lateral transposition technique does not suffice, however, for women with the diagnosis of lymphoma, in whom the mesenteric lymph nodes are at risk and require treatment by whole abdominal radiation portals (Goffinet et al. 1976).

Routinely, a bilateral oophoropexy is performed. Initially, however, before the technique had proved itself successful, only a unilateral oophoropexy was recommended in an attempt not to alter normal anatomy needlessly. Some patients have had ovarian pathology, such as cystic disease, in one ovary and thus only unilateral oophoropexy was performed. But since bilateral oophoropexy had been demonstrated to be safe in terms of subsequent reproductive function, routinely bilateral oophoropexies are recommended in all premenopausal women who undergo surgical staging for Hodgkin's disease.

Radiographic Technique and Dosimetry

By transposition of the ovaries to the midline and localization with radiopaque wire markers, one can construct an individually designed central block to shield the ovaries while simultaneously allowing treatment to the iliac, inguinal and femoral lymph nodes opacified and visualized by the ethiodol

Figure 18.6

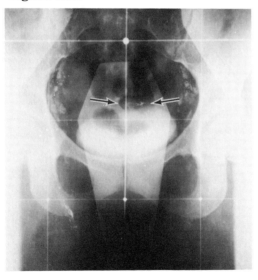

A simulator film demonstrating the pelvic irradiation field. Note the placement of the midline pelvic block effectively shielding the central structures while the iliac, inguinal, and femoral lymph nodes are treated. Arrows point to the radiopaque wire placed on the right and left ovaries at the time of oophoropexy.

441

Figure 18.7

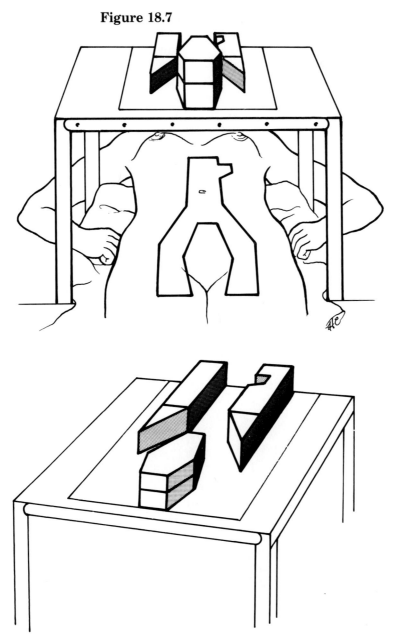

Diagram of a patient in the treatment position during the inverted-Y field of irradiation. The lead blocks are placed on the overlying coffee table. The ovaries are shielded with two 5 cm (10 cm) thick blocks. (LeFloch et al. 1976. Reprinted with permission.)

dye in the lymph nodes from a previously performed lymphogram. Figure 18.6 demonstrates the pelvic field localization procedure showing the shielding of the soft tissues in the midline of the true pelvis, from the pelvic brim down to the symphysis pubis. The technique at Stanford incorporates two 5-cm thicknesses of lead shield of appropriate width which are placed on an overlying coffee table (fig. 18.7). Figure 18.8 shows examples of three typical pelvic blocks that are precut and frequently used. It is possible, however, to cut different blocks, specifically adapted to an individual patient's anatomy to accommodate the positioning of the ovaries. The dose to the ovaries has been measured by reconstructing the anteroposterior and posteroanterior inverted-Y x-ray treatment fields and exposing Kodak RP/V (rapid processing therapy verification) film at midline depth in a flat Presdwood phantom. The inverted-Y x-ray fields can be easily reconstructed by drawing templates from the simulator and port films taken at the time of treatment. Since the ovaries are identified with wire sutures at oophoropexy, these areas can be identified in the phantom film exposures and quantitatively evaluated by photodensitometry. Radiographs demonstrate that there is no shift in the location of the ovaries from the supine to the prone position.

Figure 18.8

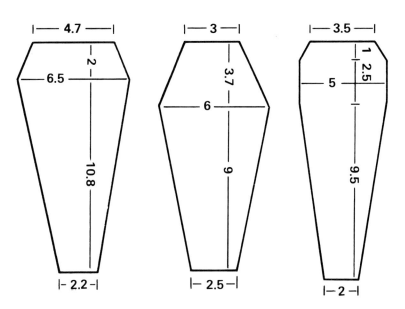

Examples of three precut lead blocks that are frequently used for ovarian shielding. The dimensions indicated are in centimeters. (LeFloch et al. 1976. Reprinted with permission.)

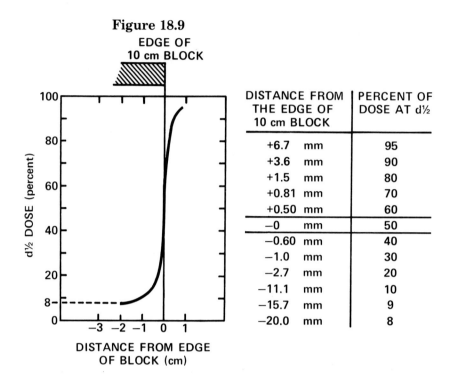

Figure 18.9

EDGE OF
10 cm BLOCK

DISTANCE FROM THE EDGE OF 10 cm BLOCK		PERCENT OF DOSE AT d½
+6.7	mm	95
+3.6	mm	90
+1.5	mm	80
+0.81	mm	70
+0.50	mm	60
−0	mm	50
−0.60	mm	40
−1.0	mm	30
−2.7	mm	20
−11.1	mm	10
−15.7	mm	9
−20.0	mm	8

The rapid decrease of the radiation dose from the edge of the block to midline. D1/2 indicates the midline dose. Beneath the center of the block, the radiation dose is 8% of the primary dose. (LeFloch et al. 1976. Reprinted with permission.)

Figure 18.9 shows the rapid decrease in the radiation dose from the edge of the block to the midline. When a 10-cm lead pelvic block is used, the x-ray dose at the extreme lateral edge of the block is 50% of the primary dose; 11 mm within the edge it is 10% of the primary dose; and at 20 mm from the edge to the middle of the block, the dose is 8% of the primary dose. The dose to the ovaries calculated as a minimum dose and a maximum dose for that part of the ovary located closest to the edge of the block can be calculated. Table 18.1 shows the minimum and maximum ovarian radiation dose and pelvic lymph node dose for nine women in whom calculations were made, and who later became pregnant. The dose under the center of the 10-cm lead ovarian shield using this technique is 8% of the unshielded dose, of which 0.5% is due to primary transmission and the remainder to scatter radiation. If, however, standard 5-cm thick lead blocks were used, the dose under the center block would be 14% to 15% of the unshielded dose, with 6% due to primary transmission through the shield and the remainder from scatter radiation. Thus the dose to the ovaries using the technique with a 10-cm thick midline shield is due mostly to scattered radiation and depends on the area shielded relative to the total field size and the energy of the photons. Further increase in the thickness of the ovarian shield would not significantly change the dose to the ovaries. There have been no cases of pelvic relapse of Hodgkin's disease among 177 women who have had oophoropexy and pelvic radiotherapy at Stanford using the specifically designed double thickness pelvic midline block.

Results

Oophoropexy

The operative procedure is technically not difficult to perform in young women who have normal anatomy and no prior history of gynecologic pathology. Since July 1968, oophoropexy has become a routine procedure at Stanford University Medical School as an adjunct to the surgical staging for premenopausal women with Hodgkin's disease. To date more than 300 women have undergone oophoropexy at Stanford University Medical Center with no complications directly related to the operative procedure. The radiopaque wire sutures used to outline the ovaries provide for an easy assessment of ovarian placement. On occasion in the postoperative period movement of the wires has been observed and on rare occasion a second surgical procedure has been performed to resuture the ovaries in place prior to pelvic radiotherapy. The second procedure has been technically successful and has not inter-

Table 18.1
Minimum and Maximum Ovarian
Radiation Dose

Patient	Dose to Ovaries in Rad		Dose to Pelvis in Rad*	Duration of Pelvic Treatment in Days
	Minimum	Maximum		
1	396	485	4400	39
2	374	660	4400	46
3	352	462	4400	43
4	393	656	4375	36
5	396	660	4425	43
6	396	550	4375	43
7	352	440	4410	39
8	352	440	4425	35
9	352	—	4400	41

*At D 1/2 (midplane dose).

fered with subsequent pelvic radiotherapy. Similarly, oophoropexy is not a contraindication to later pelvic surgery. Women who, following oophoropexy, pelvic radiotherapy, and successful pregnancy, have desired permanent contraception have successfully undergone pelvic surgery with tubal ligation without difficulty.

Hormonal Function

Approximately two-thirds to three-fourths of women will maintain ovarian function following oophoropexy and pelvic radiotherapy (Donaldson, Glatstein, and Kaplan 1976; Kaplan 1972; Ray et al. 1970). Some women will maintain normal menses throughout treatment; others not uncommonly will experience a temporary amenorrhea from 2 to 12 months following completion of radiotherapy (LeFloch, Donaldson, and Kaplan 1976). Still others have been observed following pelvic radiotherapy to experience irregular menses, which have become regular again following cycling by oral contraceptive agents. In series where gonadotrophin concentrations have been investigated as an indication of intact ovarian function, normal basal gonadotrophin concentrations have been observed following oophoropexy itself as well as among patients receiving paraaortic irradiation and among some patients receiving inverted-Y irradiation (Thomas et al. 1976). Further interference with ovarian function can be anticipated in those women who receive combination chemotherapy. Sherins and colleagues (1975) have shown that 8 of 14 (57%) of women become amenorrheic as a consequence of functional castration secondary to nitrogen mustard, oncovin, prednisone, and procarbazine (MOPP) chemotherapy. Furthermore, Chapman and associates (1979) have demonstrated that only 7 of 41 (17%) of women have functioning ovarian activity following MOPP, the remaining 34 (83%) being categorized as having failed or failing ovarian activity, with absent or irregular menses, elevated follicle stimulating hormone and luteinizing hormone levels, and low estradiol levels. These alterations in ovarian activity are clearly age related and require effective hormonal replacement and patient counseling.

Pregnancy

To date, 50 women with Hodgkin's disease have become pregnant following oophoropexy with or without pelvic radiotherapy. Of these, three women who have had oophoropexy followed by subtotal nodal radiation (no pelvic irradiation) have had ectopic pregnancies. One 24-year-old woman with a history of pelvic inflammatory disease had an incidental ectopic pregnancy discovered at the time of staging laparotomy and subsequently has had two additional ectopic pregnancies. One woman, following oophoropexy and subtotal nodal radiation, has had three pregnancies, two normal, full-term pregnancies and one ectopic pregnancy; one young woman, following oophoropexy and subtotal nodal radiation, had a tubal pregnancy thought to be related to an intrauterine device. It is possible that ectopic pregnancy may be related to the

446

Figure 18.10

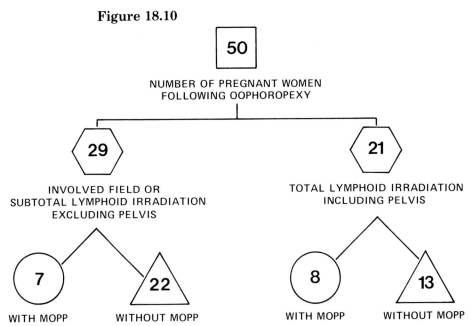

The treatments administered are diagramed for 50 women with Hodgkin's disease who have become pregnant following oophoropexy.

surgical procedure with transposition of the ovaries in the woman who has no prior history of abnormal pregnancies or prior illnesses which might complicate a normal pregnancy.

Of the 50 women in the Stanford series who have become pregnant, 29 had involved field or subtotal nodal radiation only, thus omitting pelvic radiation (fig. 18.10). Seven of these 29 had six cycles of adjuvant MOPP chemotherapy in addition to their radiotherapy; the remaining 22 were treated with radiotherapy only. As there is no significant radiation to the ovaries in women who receive subtotal nodal radiation in which the inferior border of the field is at the pelvic brim and does not include the true pelvis, one would not anticipate a fertility problem related to radiation in this group of women.

Of significance is the observation that 21 women have had oophoropexy followed by total lymphoid radiation, including radiation to the pelvis, and have become pregnant (fig. 18.11). The pelvic lymph node dose in these women has ranged between 3000 to 5500 rad. Of these 21 women, 8 received, in addition, six cycles of MOPP chemotherapy; the remaining 13 were treated with radiation alone. The patients became pregnant at follow-up periods of 12 to 60 months after completion of pelvic radiotherapy. Fifteen of the 21 pregnant patients had uncomplicated term pregnancies and gave birth to 20 healthy children. Six women had abortions, two of which were spontaneous abortions occurring four to eight weeks following conception. Five women elected to have therapeutic abortions, one patient on two occasions.

It is not possible to know the incidence of pregnancy inasmuch as we do not have a reliable denominator for the number of patients who were sexually active, trying to become pregnant, or those not using birth control measures. Although treatment may decrease fertility or possibly result in early undiagnosed abortion, the number of recognized cases of spontaneous abortion (two) does not seem greater than that observed in a normal population. All children born of women who have previously had oophoropexy and pelvic radiation with or without chemotherapy are normal. One of the babies had a cytogenetic study by amniocentesis revealing a normal female karyotype. In addition, the products of conception were observed to be cytogenetically normal in one of the cases ending in abortion. Thus whereas a risk of malformation of the offspring of these patients certainly does exist, the incidence appears too low to be detected in this small series. Holmes (1978) compared pregnancy outcomes for treated Hodgkin's disease patients with matched sibling controls and was unable to detect differences in numbers of spontaneous abortions or abnormal offspring among radiated patients as compared to controls; however, he did observe an increased risk of these

Figure 18.11
HODGKIN'S DISEASE
OOPHOROPEXY – PELVIC IRRADIATION – PREGNANCY

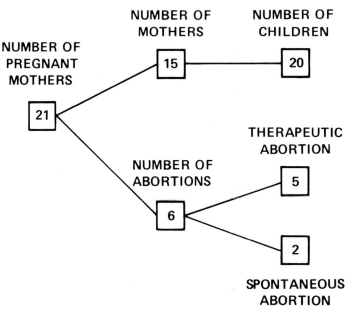

Pregnancy has occurred in 21 women who have had oophoropexy followed by high-dose pelvic radiation.

events among a group of 13 patients treated with chemotherapy and radiotherapy. Fetal abnormalities have been reported when conception occurred during treatment with chemotherapy (Mennuti et al. 1975; Nicholson 1968; Shepard 1974; Sokal and Lessman 1960); however, to date no significant increase in abnormalities has been detected in children born of mothers with previously treated Hodgkin's disease who were not under active treatment prior to conception.

Summary

Twenty-one women have become pregnant following midline transposition of the ovaries and high-dose pelvic irradiation, and have given birth to 20 healthy offspring. The dosimetry as calculated to the ovaries is precise, with little variation from patient to patient. The technique is simple, and in experienced hands has proved to be accurate. Thus we conclude that oophoropexy by midline transposition of the ovaries, followed by pelvic radiotherapy using an individually designed midline block, is safe, effective, and practical. The Stanford experience demonstrates that it is indeed possible to preserve ovarian function in women undergoing pelvic radiotherapy by midline transposition of the ovaries. We recommend oophoropexy be performed in all women with Hodgkin's disease of reproductive age as a means of preserving hormonal function and fertility.

References

Cannon, W.B., and Nelsen, T.S. Staging of Hodgkin's disease: a surgical prospective. *Am. J. Surg.* 132:224–230, 1976.

Chapman, R.M.; Sutcliffe, S.B.; and Malpas, J.S. Cytotoxic-induced ovarian failure in women with Hodgkin's disease. I. Hormone function. *JAMA* 242:1877–1881, 1979.

Donaldson, S.S. Pediatric Hodgkin's disease—focus on the future. In *Status of the curability of childhood cancers,* ed. J. vanEys and M.P. Sullivan. New York: Raven Press, 1980.

Donaldson, S.S.; Glatstein, E.; and Kaplan, H.S. Radiotherapy of childhood lymphoma. *Trends in childhood cancer,* ed. M.H. Donaldson and H.G. Seydel. New York: John Wiley, 1976.

Goffinet, D.R. et al. Abdominal irradiation in non-Hodgkin's lymphomas. *Cancer* 37:2797–2806, 1976.

Hellman, S. Current studies in Hodgkin's disease. Laparotomy has wrought. *N. Engl. J. Med.* 290:894–898, 1974.

Holmes, G.E., and Holmes, F.F. Pregnancy outcome of patients treated for Hodgkin's disease. *Cancer* 41:1317–1322, 1978.

Kaplan, H.S. *Hodgkin's disease.* Cambridge: Harvard University Press, 1972.

LeFloch, O.; Donaldson, S.S.; and Kaplan, H.S. Pregnancy following oophoropexy and total nodal irradiation in women with Hodgkin's disease. *Cancer* 38:2263–2268, 1976.

Mennuti, M.T.; Shephard, T.H.; and Mellman, W.J. Fetal renal malformation following treatment of Hodgkin's disease during pregnancy. *Obstet. Gynecol.* 46:194–196, 1975.

Nahhas, W.A. et al. Lateral ovarian transposition. Ovarian relocation in patients with Hodgkin's disease. *Obstet, Gynecol.* 38:785–788, 1971.

Nicholson, H.W. Cytotoxic drugs in pregnancy. *J. Obstet. Gynaecol. Br. Comm.* 75:307–312, 1968.

Ray, G.R. et al. Oophoropexy: a means of preserving ovarian function following pelvic megavoltage radiotherapy. *Radiology* 96:175–180, 1970.

Rosenberg, S.A. et al. Combined modality therapy of Hodgkin's disease. A report on the Stanford trials. *Cancer* 42:991–1000, 1978.

Shepard, T.H. Teratogenicity from drugs an increasing problem. *DM* June 1974, pp. 3–33.

Sherins, R. et al. Surprisingly high risk of functional castration in women receiving chemotherapy for lymphoma (abstr.). *Clin. Res.* 23:343A, 1975.

Sokal, J.E., and Lessmann, E.M. Effects of cancer chemotherapy agents on the human fetus. *JAMA* 173:1765–1771, 1960.

Thomas, P.R.M. et al. Reproductive and endocrine function in patients with Hodgkin's disease: effects of oophoropexy and irradiation. *Br. J. Cancer* 33:226–231, 1976.

Trueblood, H.W. et al. Preservation of ovarian function in pelvic radiation for Hodgkin's disease. *Arch. Surg.* 100:236–237, 1970.

PART IX

THE GYNECOLOGIC ONCOLOGY NURSE

In 1979, I had the privilege of serving on a committee to evaluate a thesis entitled "Role Functions of a Nurse Clinician in Joint Practice with Gynecologic Oncologists," which was submitted in partial fulfillment of the requirements for the degree of Master of Nursing. Thirty-three nurses were identified as being involved in the practice of gynecologic oncology nursing and were asked to respond to a variety of questions regarding the scope of their professional conduct. Although data from this thesis clearly indicate that a role model for the gynecologic nurse oncologist is still lacking, the identification of a group of nurses in joint practice with gynecologists has, in itself, given clarity to this area of specialization in the nursing profession.

It seems quite natural that a group of physician specialists dedicated to the comprehensive care of women with cancer should require the assistance of nurses with similar goals. The areas of interest and expertise of the gynecologic oncology nurse parallel those of the gynecologic oncologist and include pre- and postoperative assessment, the administration and monitoring of cytotoxic chemotherapy, and serving as a mediator between the patient, her family, and her physician. Although only one chapter has been dedicated to the training of the gynecologic nurse oncologist, one can foresee the appearance in the nursing literature of an entire volume on the subject and the gradual emergence of specialized registered nurses who will function together with gynecologic oncologists in the care of women with cancer of the reproductive system.

Chapter 19

Specialized Training of Nurses in the Care of Gynecologic Cancer Patients

PERSPECTIVE:

Dorothy C. Donahue and
June A. O'Hea

This chapter will focus on the evolution of gynecologic oncology nurses and their specialized training at Memorial Sloan-Kettering Cancer Center (MSKCC). The advantages and disadvantages of preparing all gynecologic oncology nurses in this manner will be discussed together with recommendations for methods of standardized preparation.

Evolution of the Role of the Gynecologic Oncology Nurse

The advent of radical pelvic surgery as treatment for gynecologic cancers brought about the need for a more specialized base of both medical and nursing knowledge. Physicians acquired this knowledge through completion of formal training programs in the specialty of gynecologic oncology. These programs have progressed to a point of national standardization and board certification. In contrast, nurses acquired knowledge in the specialty through on-the-job training, which varied according to institution and patient population. Nursing titles and responsibilities grew at a rapid pace without standardization. Today, among major cancer treatment centers, the role of the gynecologic oncology nurse currently varies significantly because it evolves from the increasing complexity of patient care and changing treatment modalities. For example, the role of the staff nurse at MSKCC, on a unit comprised solely of gynecologic oncology patients, may be comparable to that of a gynecologic nurse oncologist in an alternate care setting. At Memorial, the staff nurse is responsible for coordination of aspects of patient care which include physical, psychosocial, and discharge planning needs. Staff

pists, and all other health team members. Through the information contributed by all disciplines, a patient profile is compiled which includes a review of her nursing and medical histories, treatment, socioeconomic status, and family environment. A written nursing care plan is developed for all new patients, and existing nursing care plans are updated. Long- and short-term goals are reevaluated and revised as indicated. Goals and the plan of care are discussed with the patient and family to insure compliance and eliminate fears and anxiety generated by lack of knowledge.

Patient teaching is accomplished primarily by the staff nurse. Teaching skills are utilized to ascertain the patient's level of understanding of her disease and treatment and to develop an individualized teaching plan. The ultimate goal of the teaching plan is to rehabilitate the patient so that she is able to resume her former life-style or adapt to limitations imposed by her illness. The examples of the teaching cards in figures 19.1, 19.2, and 19.3 are representative of the standardization of patient teaching and care performed by the nurse. Through ongoing review of treatment protocols, teaching guides and nursing management of these patients are updated. The staff nurse also is involved in evaluating the nursing care delivered. In keeping with the philosophy and objectives of the Department of Nursing, standards of care and specific audit criteria are established. Through this process of evaluation, the staff nurse is able to revise the plan of care so that it is specific to a patient's needs.

The training program also promotes collegial relationships between nurses and physicians, through which optimum patient care is delivered. Schaffrath states that collaboration by physicians and nurses "strongly implies something other than a master-servant relationship. It implies a relationship into which both parties are entering freely and voluntarily with mutual respect (Appelbaum 1978). By adhering to this concept, nurse-physician collaboration is facilitated in decisions effecting patient care.

Training Program Deficiencies
and Recommendations

The design of the MSKCC program, as is true of any specialized training, is less than optimal. The deficiency most obvious to us is fragmentation of nursing responsibilities, which does not afford total involvement of the professional nurse in all phases of patient care. For example, the outpatient nursing staff, practicing exclusively in the office-clinic setting, has no involvement in inpatient care. Conversely, the inpatient nursing staff, with the exception of observation in the outpatient department and postdischarge telephone inquiries, has limited contact with the patient before admission and after discharge. Ideally, provision should be made for scheduled rotation of professional nursing personnel to office and clinic settings to provide optimal coordination of patient care. With this rotation, patient-nurse rapport is initiated at a time when patient counseling is crucial. During this period of anxiety and uncertainty, a patient often does not fully understand the information imparted to her by the physician at the time of the office visit. The nurse can assess the level of the patient's understanding, clarify information, provide emotional support, and begin preoperative instruction. Continuity of care is facilitated as the patient identifies with this nurse, who, in turn, communicates information and potential problems to other health team members.

A second deficiency of the program involves the lack of preparation of nurses in physical assessment skills. This preparation would allow selected nurses to monitor physical parameters, which in turn would lead to early identification of problems. The extent to which the nurse would become involved in physical assessment would be determined by guidelines mutually agreed upon by nurses and physicians. A primary consideration in establishing the guidelines would be to define clearly the responsibilities of these nurses so that patients are not subjected to repetitive physical examinations.

A third deficiency of the program concerns the limited opportunity it affords the professional nursing staff to participate in conferences and meetings outside the institution. This problem must not be underemphasized, for it promotes job satisfaction and provides opportunity for communication and expansion of the staff nurse's knowledge pertaining to the specialty. Provision of opportunities to attend conferences and meetings should be included as an integral part of any specialized training program.

The system of staff development and training employed at MSKCC may not be feasible in all oncology settings, as patient populations and institutional limitations may not be conducive to its implementation. The goals could be met, however, through alternate methods designed to fit the needs of a particular institution. The following are additional recommendations made for the purpose of developing standardized programs for the specialized training of gynecologic oncology nurses.

It is necessary for nurses currently working in the specialty to convene under the auspices of an association for gynecologic oncology nurses. It is suggested that the association be established through an existing nursing group and be closely aligned with physician gynecologic oncology groups. By organizing within an existing nursing group, such as the Oncology Nursing Society or the American Nurses' Association, a new specialty group would be able to benefit from the parent organization's already formulated bylaws. A specialty group for gynecologic oncology nurses would unite this segment of the nursing community for the purpose of identifying the educational needs of this nursing population, standardizing training to meet these needs, and identifying methodology for standardization. In addition, the specialty group could provide a tool for ongoing review of patient care and initiate nursing research to evaluate the progress made in specialized training programs. In-

Figure 19.1

<u>MEMORIAL SLOAN-KETTERING CANCER CENTER</u>

<u>DIVISION OF NURSING</u>

<u>DEPARTMENT OF NURSING EDUCATION</u>

<u>PREOPERATIVE TEACHING CHECKLIST</u>

Patient's Name_____

	Date Taught	R.N. Initials
1) Coughing and deep breathing:		
A) Rationale		
B) Demonstration		
C) Return demonstration		
D) Splinting incision		
2) Exercises: Lower Extremity		
A) 1) Ankle circles		
2) Knee bends		
3) Flexion & extension of feet		
B) Purpose of T.E.D.'s or Ace bandages		
3) Activity:		
A) Positioning		
B) Ambulation		
4) Equipment:		
A) Nasogastric Tube		
B) Foley Catheter		
C) I.V. Therapy		
D) Specific Drainage Tubes		
5) Night before surgery:		
A) Send home or lock valuables		
B) Operative area shaved		
C) Betadine shower & scrub		
D) Wear hospital gown		
E) Sleeping medication		

(over)

460

Figure 19.1 (cont.)

	Date Taught	R.N. Initials
6) Morning of Surgery:		
A) Remove all jewelry, make-up, nail polish		
B) Remove dentures, prosthesis and lock		
C) Void - on call to O.R.		
D) Vital signs before surgery		
E) Purpose of pre-operative medication & need to remain in bed		
F) Two family members may visit		
G) Holding area		
7) Recovery Room:		
A) Use of O_2 mask		
B) Vital signs		
C) Pain medication		
D) ↓ temperature		
E) Throat irritation		
F) Length of stay		
8) Return to Floor:		
A) Family visit		
B) NPO		
C) Pain medication:		
1) Purpose		
2) How to obtain it		
3) Frequency		
D) Reinforce - coughing, deep breathing, turning, leg exercises, early ambulation		

DOCUMENT AREAS TAUGHT AND UNDERSTOOD IN NURSE'S NOTES.

Figure 19.2

MEMORIAL SLOAN–KETTERING CANCER CENTER

OSTOMY TEACHING GUIDE

Topic Discussed	Date	By Whom	Notes regarding Progress
Pre-operative Preparation:			
1) Explanation of procedure to patient and/or family			
2) Review post-operative expectations, fears, concerns			
3) Mark stoma site			
Post-operative Care:			
1) Skin care:			
a) patient able to look at stoma			
b) care of suture line			
c) observation of stoma			
1) color			
2) moisture			
3) protrusion			
4) output			
d) technique of care of stoma			
1) agents used:			
2) Ostomy appliances:			
a) patient observed appliance			
b) patient applied bag with assistance			
c) patient applies bag independently			
d) family observed application			
e) family applied independently			
f) measuring of bag observed			
g) patient measured bag with assistance			
h) odor problems discussed			
i) type of temporary bag used:			
size			
kind			

Figure 19.2   (cont.)

Topic Discussed	Date	By Whom	Notes Regarding Progress
Post-operative Care: (cont'd)			
3) Colostomy irrigation:			
a) time of day performed			
b) frequency_____			
c) equipment used_____			
d) solution used_____			
e) amt. of solution___cc			
f) irrigation technique			
1) patient observed			
2) patient assisted with irrigation			
3) patient performed with assistance			
4) patient performed independently			
5) family observed			
6) family person performed			
4) Diet			
a) type of diet ordered			
b) explanation of foods affecting output			
c) diet reviewed with patient family			

Topic Discussed	Date	By Whom	Notes Regarding Progress
Post operative Care: (cont'd)			
5) Discharge information:			
a) equipment ordered for home			
b) where equipment can be obtained & list of suppliers			
c) permanent appliance to be used			
d) how often appliance is to be changed			
e) how to make up an emergency kit			
f) what to do about traveling			
g) activities permitted			
h) marital relations			
i) bathing, swimming			
j) clothing			
k) review of skin care, leakage, & odor problems			
l) written booklet(s) given			
m) visiting nurse referral			

Summary:

Figure 19.3

MEMORIAL SLOAN-KETTERING CANCER CENTER
DEPARTMENT OF NURSING

(KEEP IN NURSING CARE KARDEX)
USE IN CONJUCTION WITH STANDARD CARE PLAN FOR RADICAL VULVECTOMY AND
GROIN DISSECTION

NAME: _____

POINTS IN TEACHING & CHARTING	TAUGHT	DATE CHARTED	R.N.
1. PERSONAL HYGIENE			
2. ACTIVITY SCHEDULE			
3. DIET TEACHING			
4. SEXUAL INFORMATION			
5. WOUND OBSERVATION			

asmuch as we believe that nurses are best qualified to evaluate nursing, a specialty group would provide the means for sharing experiences and knowledge with nursing colleagues and for establishing a basis for peer review and certification.

By establishing a specialty group in close alignment with physician gynecologic oncology groups, the nursing community would be more aware of current medical trends and advances in gynecologic oncology treatment. Delivery of optimal patient care requires a collegial relationship between nurse and physician. This collaborative mechanism will enhance the nurse's ability to inform physicians of constructive changes in nursing practice for the purpose of improving the quality of patient care.

Summary

The information we have presented encompasses the program for specialized training of the gynecologic nurse oncologist at Memorial Sloan-Kettering Cancer Center. Development of a training program in alternate settings should take into consideration the patient population, the professional interests of the nursing staff as they pertain to gynecologic oncology, and the limitations of the institution. With consideration of these points, it is possible to structure a program that will meet the needs of patients with gynecologic cancers.

References

Appelbaum, A.L. Commission leads way to joint practice for nurses and physicians in hospitals. *J. Am. Heart Assoc.* 52:78–81, 1978.

Craytor, J.K.; Brown, J.K.; and Morrow, G.R. Assessing learning needs of nurses who care for persons with cancer. *Cancer Nurs.* 1:211–220, 1978.

Van Scoy-Mosher, C. The oncology nurse in independent practice. *Cancer Nurs.* 1:21–28, 1978.

INDEX

emergence of, 20–24
within obstetrics and gynecology, 2
Suit, H., 216
Surgery, *See also specific procedures*
combined with radiation therapy, xxii
in gynecologic oncology, 6
in training programs for gynecologic
oncology, 3
tumor reductive, 321–324
Survival curves, plotting, 240–241. *See
also* Statistical evaluation
Symmonds, R. E., 185, 190, 313, 357

T

Taft, P. D., 95
Taft, R. A., 298
Takasugi, N., 118
Talerman, A., 357
Tamimi, H. K., 36, 39, 40
Tamoxifen, 201
Taussig, F. J., 59, 62, 69, 72
Taylor, H. B., 355, 357
T:B lymphocyte ratio, and tumor
growth, 67
T boost technique, of radiation therapy,
305
T cells
in immune response, 408
monitoring, 409
origin and function of, 406–407
Teaching, gynecologic oncologists, 9–10
Teilum, J., 86
Tepper, E., 338, 339, 341
Teratologic changes
of intrauterine DES exposure, 119
management of, 99–100
Testicular carcinoma, associated with
DES exposure, 101
Thigpen, T., 250, 272, 275
Thiotepa, in chemotherapy for ovarian
cancer, 353, 256, 275
Thoeny, R. H., 357
Thomas, P. R. M., 446
Thompson, B. H., 147
Tobias, J. S., 273, 313
Total parenteral nutrition, and ovarian
cancer, 314, 317
Towler, C. M., 387

Townsend, D. E., 133, 138, 148, 152
Trabin, J. R., 29, 30
Training programs, 2
contents of, 3
development of, 4
growth of, 30
for gynecologic oncology nurses,
458–464
length of, 17
qualifications for, 18
in university hospitals, 11
Transformation zone (t-zone), 140
defined, 131
effect of cryotherapy on, 144
Tredway, D. R., 138
"Triad of trouble," 182
Trophoblastic neoplasms, 369–370
Trout, 127
Trueblood, H. W., 428, 429, 439
Truskett, I. D., 219, 224
Tsakraklides, V., 68
Tsuruhara, T., 377, 378
Tuboendometrial cells, 90
incidence of, 89–90
in vaginal adenosis, 100
Tumor immunology, development of,
403–405
Tumor marker
free alpha subunit as, 384–386
free beta subunit as, 386–387
HCG as, 369–370, 391
potential, 391
pregnancy specific B_1-glycoproteins as,
387–390
Tumor, nodes, metastases (TNM)
system, 158. *See also* Staging
systems
Tumor reductive surgery,
321–324
t-zone. *See* Transformation zone

U

Ueda, K., 402, 403, 417
Unamue, E. R., 406
Underwood, P. B., 138, 214, 226
University hospitals
core residency programs in, 16